A **NEW WAY** *to* **FOOD**

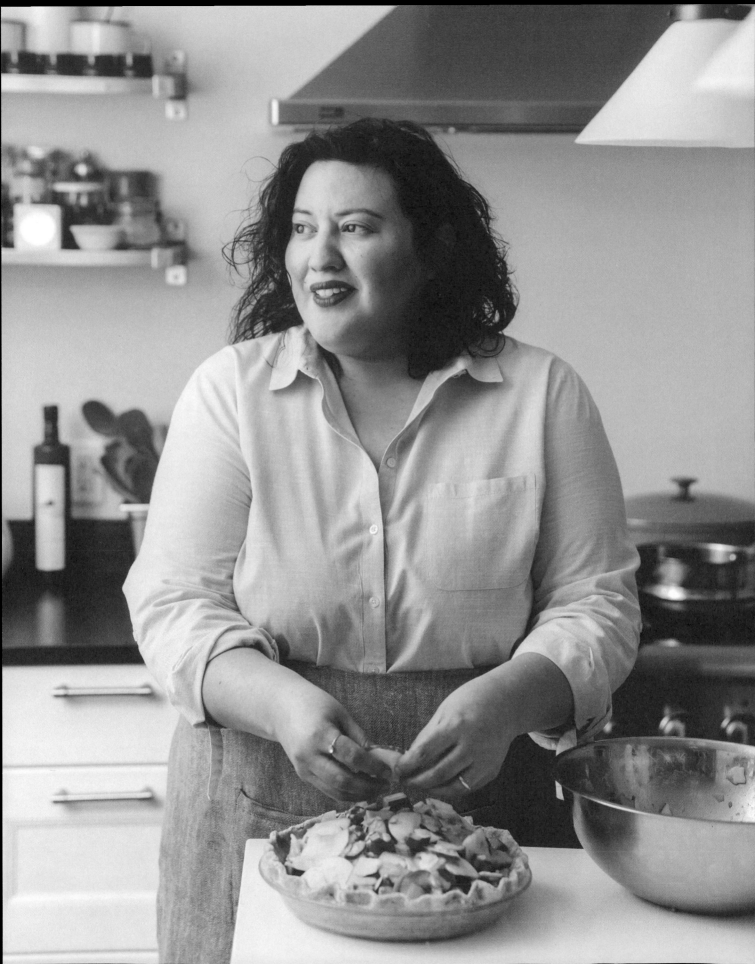

A NEW WAY *to* FOOD

100 Recipes to Encourage a Healthy Relationship
with Food, Nourish Your Beautiful Body,
and Celebrate Real Wellness for Life

························

MAGGIE BATTISTA

Photographs by KRISTIN TEIG

ROOST BOOKS

BOULDER

2019

ROOST BOOKS
An imprint of Shambhala Publications, Inc.
4720 Walnut Street
Boulder, Colorado 80301
roostbooks.com

©2019 by **MAGGIE BATTISTA**
Photographs ©2019 by **KRISTIN TEIG**
Photographs on pages 2, 6, and 296 ©2019 by **GABI VALLADARES**
Food styling by **HEIDI ROBB**

9 8 7 6 5 4 3 2 1

First Edition
Printed in the United States of America

♾This edition is printed on acid-free paper that meets the American National Standards Institute Z39.48 Standard.
♻Shambhala Publications makes every effort to print on recycled paper. For more information please visit www.shambhala.com.

Roost Books is distributed worldwide by Penguin Random House, Inc., and its subsidiaries.

Designed by **CAT GRISHAVER**

Library of Congress Cataloging-in-Publication Data
Names: Battista, Maggie, author.
Title: A new way to food: 100 recipes to encourage a healthy relationship with food, nourish your beautiful body, and celebrate real wellness for life /
Maggie Battista; photographs by Kristin Teig.
Description: Boulder: Roost Books, 2019. | Includes index.
Identifiers: LCCN 2018013407 | ISBN 9781611806175
(hardcover: alk. paper)
Subjects: LCSH: Self-care, Health. | Nutrition. | LCGFT: Cookbooks.
Classification: LCC RA776.95 .B37 2019 | DDC 613—dc23
LC record available at https://lccn.loc.gov/2018013407

To every girl,
I see all your beautiful potential.

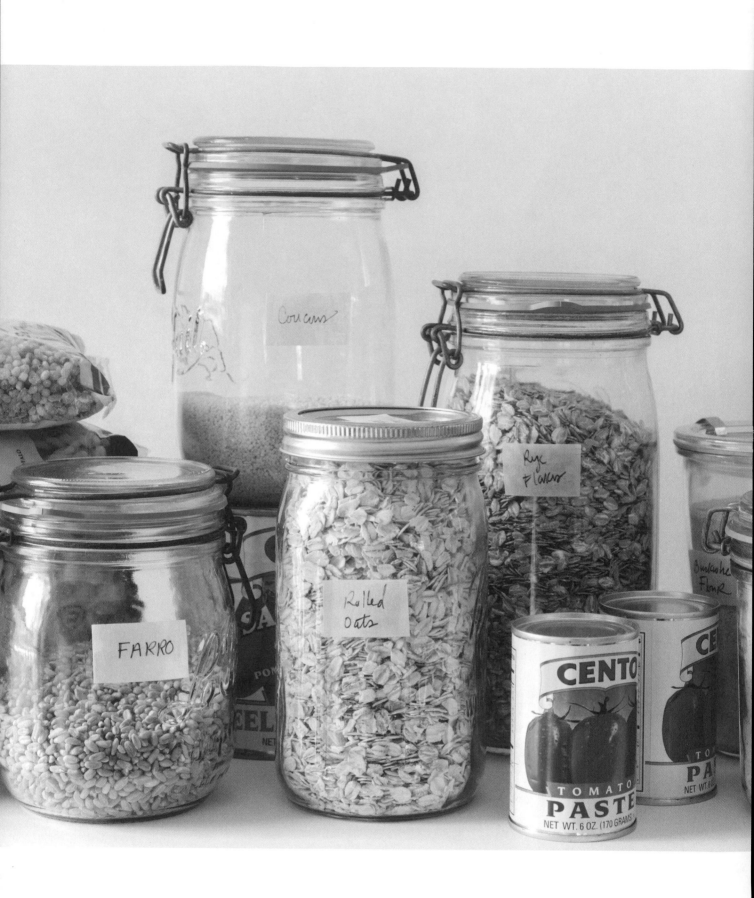

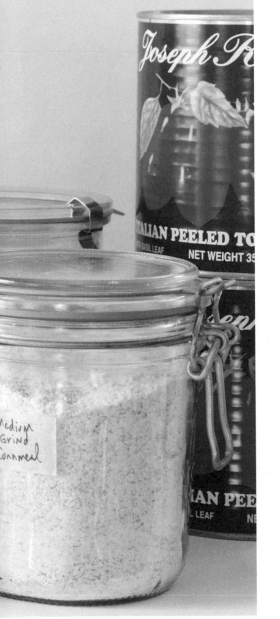

CONTENTS

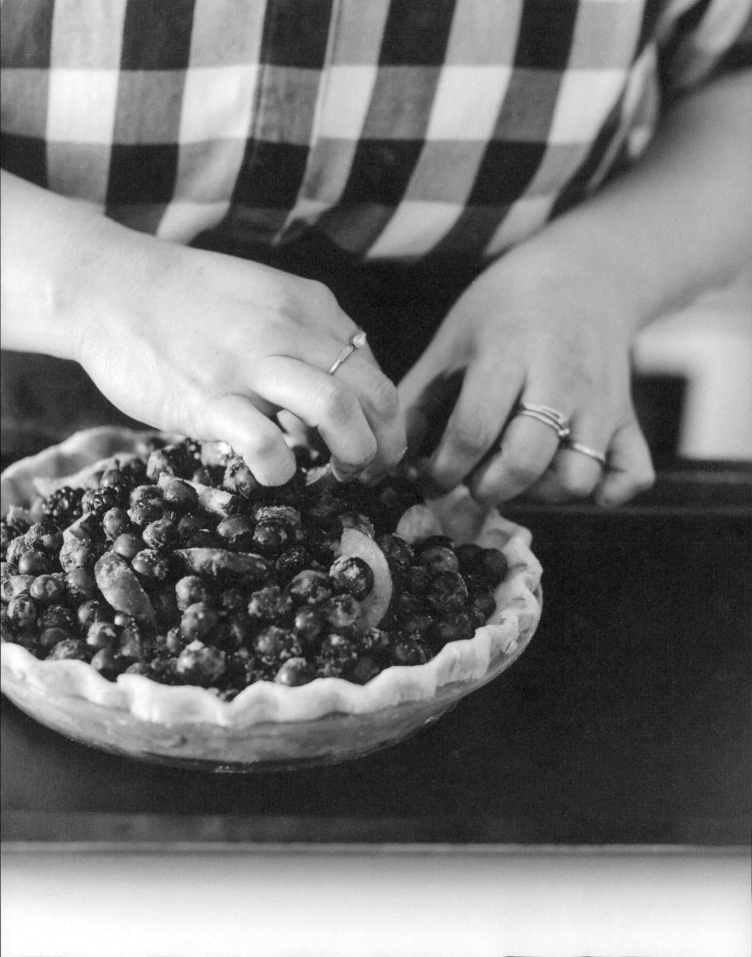

A NEW WAY to FOOD

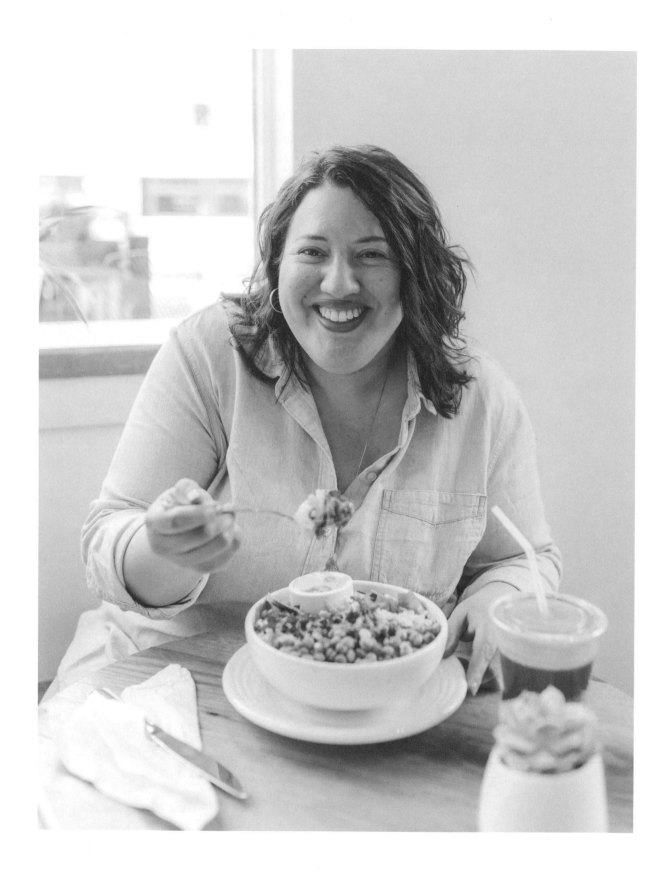

How I Finally Realized My Beautiful Potential

Raise your hand if you've struggled with your health, and perhaps your weight, for some or all of your life. I'm waving both arms in the air because it feels like fixing my body has been the unequivocal purpose of every one of my days on planet earth.

You see, I've been big most of my life, the kind of big that's definitely fat but slightly adorable, in an I'm-not-so-threatening, sidekick sort of way. When I was way younger, I wasn't even given a sideways glance by . . . anybody. In fact, most people would look past me, the fat girl, to the thin girl at my side, whether she was an exotically beautiful member of my family or a pretty, preppy school friend.

I suppose being ignored would have been okay for a wallflower type who wanted to fade into the background, maybe partially covered by a jacket or a whole human being. But as I got older, I never really stomached being the snubbed sidekick.

I'm just not shy. I'm vocal and opinionated, doling out what's on my mind like all the pepperoni on an extra-large pie—the more, the better. I'm enthusiastic and chatty, and usually enter a room with a big smile on my face, ready to make new friends and, you know, make life happen.

In my teens, when I realized that people weren't going to notice me for my figure, as was the case for most of the women in my life (my mother had been a model, after all), I boosted my personality, quite inadvertently, to get noticed. Eventually, my all-too-friendly disposition stuck and became the way I got folks to like me and, I'd like to think, got them to appreciate the content of my character over the imperfection of my frame. Honestly, I didn't want people to look at my body or notice that I was 100+ pounds larger than I really wanted to be.

I've spent decades trying to get a handle on my weight. I have been on every diet or lifestyle plan ever invented, or so it seemed, some of which I had no business trying. I went low fat, low carb, mostly grapefruit, and high protein. I even did Jenny Craig and Weight Watchers (multiple times). On occasion, I stopped eating entire food groups, fasted, and even hid food away—a trick I picked up from my parents who hid all the delicious, indulgent food groups like sandwich cookies and potato chips from their big-little kid (yes, insert sad face here).

I don't blame anyone for my lifelong body issues. I accept full responsibility for the state of my body. But listen, it's hard to lose weight. It's difficult to be on a diet at age nine, at age twelve, at age nineteen, or in adulthood— whatever the age, it's hard. And if it were as easy as eating a common sense selection of foods and exercising regularly, I promise you that I'd be looking svelte in a swimsuit 365 days a year, and so would all of you.

In my personal experience, being fat wasn't just the state of my body; it was who I was—it became a state of mind. After being bullied by kids for being bigger; after being ignored by boys at all the school dances; after being picked last for every sporting activity; after being told, "You're pretty for a big girl," for the thousandth time; I convinced myself that everyone was right.

Being in that state of mind, and after so many years of trying to be smaller, healthier, prettier, and stronger, I finally hit my bottom. At the time, my main feeling wasn't frustration or shame, though both were in the mix. Only now, after years of thoughtful review, journaling, therapy, and just plain time, do I recognize that one feeling overshadowed and trumped every other feeling: I felt desperate, desperately desperate. My lowest of low points looked something like this:

1. *I was in pain every day.* I couldn't walk a block, let alone a mile, because my heels were consistently sore, my calves were tight and strained, my knee joints were angry at me, and my back and thighs experienced the sort of daily agony that made it hard to get up out of bed, step into the shower (or out), or bend down to tie my shoes. I wish no disease on anyone, ever, but especially chronic pain. Chronic pain will make you hate your body for all the trouble it causes you and all the life it holds you back from living.

2. *I experienced tingling in all my limbs,* but especially in my fingertips and toes. I could never find the cause, and neither could my doctors. Tingling in your limbs is scary; it makes you feel like you're prime for a heart attack at any moment.

3. *I was so lonely.* There were so many people around me, but I was so tired of being excluded from all the fun lady-type activities in life. I couldn't shop for clothes in the same places as my friends. I wouldn't even think to buy nice lingerie—nor ever walk into one of those types of boutiques. Shoe shopping was even a drag—my feet were wide and impossible to fit. I was reluctant to get manicures, pedicures, and especially massages, worried that someone would see my big body. And I never saw girls like me in fashion magazines; they just weren't made for big girls.

4. *I wanted to prove everyone wrong.* If you're a fat girl, you get used to everyone chiding you about your size. Every year, someone had a new diet for me to try. Every month, a new food to gulp down or eliminate. And every day, people would tell me how pretty I'd be if I'd only lose weight. I was so used to hearing everyone say something about my weight that I didn't even notice when it all stopped. I don't know if it was when I moved out on my own or met my love and got married. I think I used to ignore the comments but eventually, as I got older, I'd hold my own, telling whomever to mind their own business, get out of my face, worry about their own body, and so on. Regardless, at some point the comments stopped, and I'm sure I felt a sense of relief at first. Soon after, I realized, they had given up on me—all of them. They didn't want to fight and left me to figure it out on my own. I wanted to show them that I could do it, on my own. In fact, I could only *really* do it on my own.

5. *After so many years trying to figure out what I wanted to do* professionally, I finally had the formulas and business plan to open a food retail space to provide a new way to shop for food. But I was frightened I wouldn't have the health to bring it to life. Launching a boutique requires a lot of physical energy, the ability to walk without pain, the strength to lift boxes that weighed more than ten pounds, at least a few days a week without lower back pain, and the critical thinking and mindfulness to lead a team to bring this vision to life. I wanted to be healthy enough—full of passion, spark, and vigor—to make it all happen.

6. *I was unhappy being so large.* I don't want to dis anyone who's happy in their skin—we should all be so lucky to be happy and healthy at any size. I, however, was not happy. I hated my thighs rubbing together, I hated how difficult it was to shop for clothes, and I hated how people judged me. Hell, I hated how *I* judged me for taking an extra scoop or three of ice cream. I needed, so desperately, to find a way to stop that hate.

. . . .

And I did. Now, many years into the story of my life, something has changed. Now I see myself skinny. That doesn't mean I am skinny by popular definition, because I'm far from a size 4. That means I see myself skinny in the way that I see the potential in me to be healthy, to be deserving of a fit physique, to be proud and beautiful in the sort of clothes I want to wear. I stopped being disgusted by my skin, stopped thinking the worst of my body, and started really loving my skin for what it was and what it could be. Instead of the negative image of being too big or not small enough, I saw myself as I truly was: a body with so much beautiful potential. The change didn't come in an instant but through an intentional process, combined with eating all the good foods, which I will share in this very personal cookbook.

Once I saw myself as something more than a fat girl—like as a girl who could finally tackle all her proverbial demons; as a lady with something to say; as a businesswoman with a vision to bring to life; as a food professional with a real purpose; as a person worth loving and giving love; and, as a human with a physical body that deserved care and attention—I finally began to seriously tackle my weight issues, to understand the reasons why I put food in my mouth, and to ultimately lose some of the weight that I've carried all of my life. I saw my full potential, my beautiful potential. I learned to love me, at last. And if I can love me, at last, I know you can love you, too.

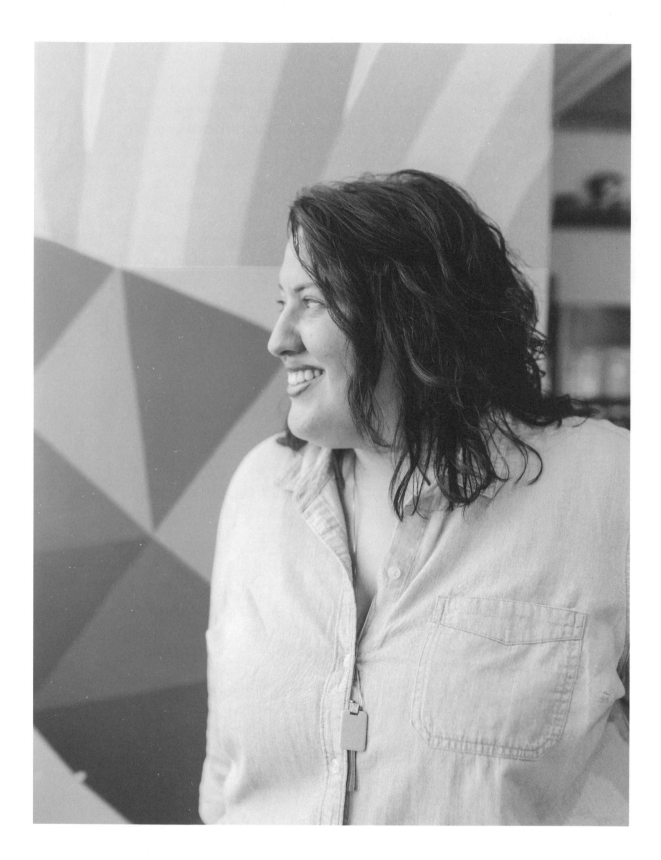

Finding a New Way to Food

My relationship with food and my understanding of my body is tragic and triumphant. This journey has been filled with great highs and too many lows to count. And when I say low, I mean hiding candy bars in my childhood dresser to sneak sweet bites before bed, I mean eating three burgers from the drive-through in my car after a bad date or because I had no date, and I mean feeling so sick from overeating that the only way I knew to feel better was to eat even more because a full belly was the only way I knew how to care for myself.

If you picked up this cookbook, I bet you've been on a journey, too. Maybe you've found some way to reckon how you see yourself and what foods you put in your mouth. Or perhaps you're holding this cookbook because you're still searching for a way to know and love yourself. Perhaps you haven't stumbled upon your right way to nourish yourself—and all the ways that you've tried haven't worked long-term. Perhaps you're on a traditional diet right now and the scale is flat or going up rather than down. Perhaps you think processed food is the cheapest or fastest option for you at this time. Perhaps you're in so much pain every single day that just walking outside to your car or to the bus stop on the corner feels like the world is going to end. Or maybe you're at your lowest of low points and you think you have no options anymore.

I am tearing up for you, for us, while I type this. I want to hug you. I want to share a cup of tea and cry it out with you. I want to bake you a cookie from this cookbook and show you how good food makes you feel strong and powerful. And I want to whisper in your ear right now: "That was me."

This cookbook is a bit like my diary. It shares my life-changing journey from fat girl to mostly well and happy-to-be-just-me lady. It's full of a bunch of tiny victories, a few aha moments, and perhaps some all-too-raw thoughts that, played out in my own personal sequence, got me to my other side, the side where I finally see a me who is worthy of good food and good health.

Now, this is not a diet book. In fact, as someone who's been on and off every kind of diet possible, I wholeheartedly believe that diets do not work. After decades of restrictions, of endless yo-yo dieting, of putting a gigantic pause on all the good things in life until I was smaller, faster, and healthier, I'm so done with diets.

Because this is not a diet book, please don't look for a strict food plan or an exercise regime. Instead, you'll find something far less confining. I'll walk you through the steps and the recipes that freed me from a life of restriction and empowered me to find a new way to food and, ultimately, real wellness. What ultimately worked for me was a two-part approach to wellness: healthier eating *and* a shift in mindset.

HEALTHIER EATING

Instead of dieting, I see life through two modes. During *active wellness mode*, I try to be a bit more balanced—that could mean a bit lighter, a bit stronger, a bit more in tune with my body. In this phase, I'm on a quest to take better care of myself—through eating differently or maybe moving more. I could be in this mode at any time; I just like to actually say the words to myself—"I am in active wellness mode"—before I begin, as a gentle but clear intention.

Once I've learned to add more balance into my life and relish a pause, I go into *everyday wellness mode*. This means I'm just living my daily life in a wholesome way, not hugely restrictive but not damaging all the progress I've made. I'm just trying to stay lighter, stronger, connected to my body, healthier, and ultimately, balanced. It's during this mode that I aim to turn any new eating or movement habits into a permanent part of my healthy life. During everyday wellness mode, I eat all the good-for-you foods in excess and enjoy the other stuff in moderation. I won't deny myself some of the foods I love, but I will think before I put any ingredient into my mouth because my good health matters more than the fleeting flavor of . . . anything.

Today, I eat dairy-free all of the time—the reduced inflammation in my joints and reduced lethargy was too grand to make eating dairy again a priority—and I eat a plant-based diet most of the week. When I lost all the weight originally, I started an elimination diet, only putting plants in my mouth and avoiding sugar, caffeine, animal protein, dairy, gluten, alcohol, and processed foods. Over time (meaning months), I added eggs, fish, and gluten back in—though I still keep gluten-free pasta in my pantry because I like the texture in certain dishes. I also added in

a weekend glass or two of wine, but steered clear of cocktails because of the added, sometimes unnatural, sugars.

All that said, my meal plan is mine and not yours. I am not a nutritionist and don't know your unique health concerns. For me, I feel my lightest, my most mindful, pain-free, and extremely energetic when I eat mostly plants—and most of my friends and family say the same. I do eat animal protein—eggs often; fish and beef once or twice per month; and duck or turkey on special occasions—but I keep it in check to ensure I don't overindulge. I make sure I get ample protein each day (45 to 60 grams for an adult woman who doesn't exercise daily) but I do it in various ways via beans, nuts, and certain vegetables. I remember the day my cousin-chef Vanessa told me, "greens have protein." At first, I didn't believe her. But as I researched their nutritional value and ate big steaming bowls of chard greens drizzled with sea salt and lemon or a swig of sesame oil, I realized, "I've got energy and, wow, she was right."

The recipes in this cookbook are mostly plant-based and many of them are dairy-free. Some recipes work better with a little animal dairy, so a few recipes using ghee (clarified butter) appear in this cookbook, too. Since I eat animal protein on occasion and serve it to family and friends regularly, I've included a smattering of my favorite recipes using eggs, seafood, chicken, and beef.

Because I now eat a plant-based diet, I also don't worry about portion control. I generally eat all the vegetables I want, whenever I want them. Sometimes I want two bowls of my Instant Faux Pho (page 248) and I never feel guilty about it. If I want a big salad with two eggs instead of one, then I'll have it. If I want another homemade scone, then leave me to it. I remain mindful about all the food

I take in during a given day. If I have had a slice of thick grainy bread with lunch, I may avoid eating any bread for dinner. If I do munch down on two scones, then I'll probably cut out any extra flour for the rest of the day.

I see my eating as a continuous ocean wave—sometimes I'm eating more than enough (high tide) and sometimes I'm eating less (low tide), and it's up to me to feed my beautiful body in a balanced, nutritional way and keep that wave flowing. Since I've generally limited or eliminated many of the foods that could make me less healthy (pork, sugar, animal dairy, etc.), I feel okay eating all the vegetables all the time.

A SHIFT IN MINDSET

I started to see a real difference in my health when I paired a change in the food I ate with a change in my thinking. Instead of seeing a wobbly gross body that required all sorts of food restrictions in order to be healthy fast, I found my way to see a wobbly beautiful body that required all the best foods in order to be well for life. I started to love myself enough to see my positives instead of my negatives.

That mindset shift occurred only because I did the work to acknowledge all my issues around food and throughout my life in general, and sort them out bit by bit. I claimed every one of my issues, stared at them straight on, and stared at *me* straight on.

I began the work to love my body many months before I realized what all my issues were, and I began to love myself when I confronted each issue and started to do the hard work required to just exist through it all. The very moment I made it through week one of a hardcore elimination diet successfully was the moment I started to see all my beautiful potential. When you see yourself tackle the biggest issue of your life with some success, you learn to like yourself. And, in the ideal situation, if all the (potato) chips fall where they are destined to (and you also work on the hard issues simultaneously), you learn to love yourself.

Learning to love yourself is no easy task, especially if you've been raised in an environment that fights that potential love daily. There are so many forces in this universe telling us that we're not enough, that we're not worthy of love. To really make a full-on health change, you need to shut the universe out, quiet the voices in your head, and go through the steps in this book to find a full and real love for yourself.

As you move through the chapters in this cookbook, you'll discover what I learned and ways in which I think you can make some or all of my approach work for you. However, you have to be ready for real change, and just saying the words won't always do the trick. You have to believe it deep down in places you didn't even know existed.

It took me years to believe I was ready and a full year to begin my transformation. Eventually, I came to a place of understanding with each issue that had me so desperately desperate. In turn, I was finally able to maintain a significant weight loss and, most importantly, a more wholesome outlook on wellness. I don't know if this approach will work for you because I don't understand all the burdens you carry, but I hope the stories in this cookbook provide solid insight that helps you get from where you are to something way better.

SIX WAYS TO GET READY FOR A NEW WAY TO FOOD

If you're ready to make this approach work for you, consider taking some of these initial steps, which will pave the way for all the explicit advice and suggestions in the upcoming chapters.

1. *Remove obstacles to wellness.* If you are consistently making excuses for why you can't revamp the way you eat or just the way you see yourself, then start eliminating those excuses one by one.

For example, I loved to drink water but had taste issues with tap water, so I set up a monthly filtered water delivery to my home. I also wanted to take long walks but felt that my personal walking goals sometimes conflicted with my dog's walking goals; she wanted to stroll and do her business, I wanted to walk quickly to exercise or very slowly to browse shop windows. I opted to bring on a dog walker to ensure my dog got her perfect daily walk, which freed me up mentally to just walk for me.

My biggest obstacle involved parting with all the not-so-amazing foods in my kitchen; I hated the idea of tossing or wasting sugar or flour or chocolate chips—after all, who knows when a baking itch would kick in and wasting food is so, well, criminal. I did give myself permission to just toss some of the less-than-stellar fats and oils, but I focused on giving the good stuff away to friends and family quickly. Knowing that my chocolate collection and various sugars went to good homes removed that as an obstacle to wellness. Find your obstacles and make them go away.

2. *Make your health a top priority.* I know your job is intense and may require every bit of your brain. I also know that society has convinced you and me that family comes first, and maybe work comes second. However, if you are not well and whole and healthy, you won't be able to properly care for your family nor maintain your commitment to your work.

It's really as simple as this: if you make your health a top priority, you'll be strong enough to support the folks around you and certainly alert enough to excel at your job. Schedule health-related activities just as you would a work meeting or weekend date. I simply used the same calendar as my work calendar to make sure I took a break here and there, walked around the block two or three times per week, and made the time to both cook and eat regularly.

3. *Revamp your mind for the life you want.* If there is something big that you want to accomplish in order to love yourself more and it's been tough to make it so, it may be that your mind is holding you back. For example, some of us are fat or stay fat because we've got non-food issues to work on. Figure out what your issues are and face them. Take a quiet moment to write them all down and really dwell on them. Are these issues within your control to fix or change? Can you work on them on your own, or do you need help from a coach, therapist, or family friend? I am a big fan of pulling in a total stranger—hiring them if you must—to get the perspective and help you need to trudge through the issues that may be standing between you and good health.

4. *Eat regularly.* Whether you're a five-star chef or a home cook struggling to get dinner on the table each evening, you cannot forget to eat. Real self-love is derived from doing good things for yourself, and eating is at the top of the list.

Skipping breakfast or lunch or both deprives you of the nutrients and energy you need to do excellent work or get through a long day. Food is filled with vitamins and nutrients to feed your organs, including your brain. When you're fed, you'll be equipped to make good choices throughout the day as well as better choices on self-care.

I typically eat four smaller meals per day, with one of those meals being a sweet or savory smoothie. I eat regularly so I don't come upon any time of day when I'm *hangry*; it's in those moments that I may make bad choices just to get the quickest thing into my belly. Because I eat often I rarely feel any hunger pangs.

I also prefer to eat before grocery shopping. An empty stomach is like a call from the wild that seems to attract every sort of food into my market basket; I may not buy the best stuff and I may spend more than my budget. If I happen to arrive at the market hungry, I shop for something to eat first. Once I have my smoothie or sushi or hard-boiled egg in my stomach, I carry on with my shopping, pangs in check.

5. *Toss out all thoughts that promote self-degradation.* This is an especially difficult tip for all of us to fully commit to. I battle harsh words in my head every day and sometimes they slip into my writing and out of my mouth. A little of this is okay and perhaps a touch funny—remember, no beating ourselves up—but since there are enough forces in the world telling us what's wrong with us on the regular, our jobs is to be friendly and sweet to ourselves. If you sense a negative thought in your head or negative word about to slip from your lips, pause and reframe it in a positive way. This tiny edit will clean up your self-degradation program promptly.

6. *Don't put yourself in unsupportive situations.* This may sound obvious, but it isn't to everyone. If you have food issues <raising hand>, don't put yourself in places where you'll be tempted. If you have booze issues or body issues, avoid situations that won't help you stay well. Just say no, seriously.

I used to taste food products daily and judge food competitions regularly. Once I made a commitment to taking good care of myself, I had to avoid situations that would tempt me or totally undermine my progress. I turned down invites that made it impossible for me to stick to my plan. If a cocktail or dessert event was imperative, I'd eat at home first; having a good base in my belly meant I was less interested in all the booze or dairy presented to me.

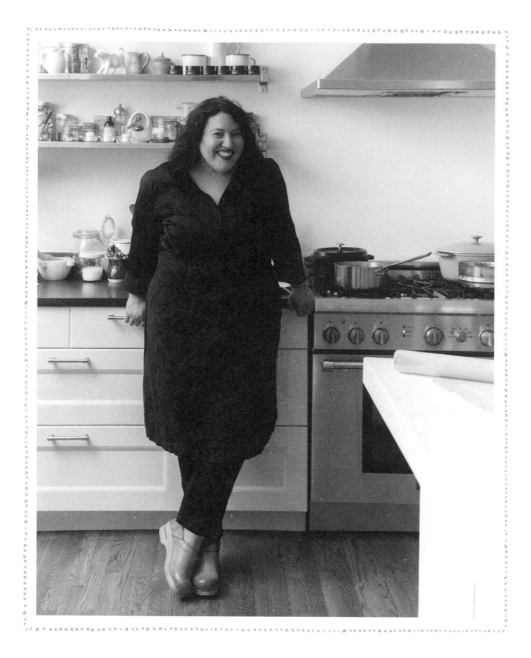

About the Recipes

This cookbook is an amalgamation of all my years on diets, off diets, and the in-between times. The recipes included are pertinent to my evolution of learning to love my body and myself, and are precious reminders of the important food moments in my life. Some of these recipes are effortless and require little explanation—i.e., toss everything into a blender—and some require more detailed steps.

Over the years of eating the wholesome food my body deserves, I developed most of these recipes on my own—with inspiration from the travelers, supporters, or cheerleaders in my life who perhaps made something similar for me or advised me to eat a particular food frequently. If a recipe was developed by other cooks, friends, or family, I mention the original adaptation in the headnote and point out how I've manipulated the recipe to suit my food preferences. Every recipe has gone through extensive recipe testing with a wide group of testers at varying skill levels.

HOW OFTEN I MAKE EACH RECIPE

While I cringe at the thought of telling you precisely what to eat and when, this is indeed a cookbook about my health journey; I believe some loose direction is required, especially since I'm fairly aware of what I eat when I'm in active wellness mode. Some of you may opt to follow this way of eating very directly, while others may just want to add certain recipes to how you already eat today. I've assembled some guidance in the form of a legend that calls out the frequency at which I make each recipe. Look for one of these on every recipe throughout the recipe chapters of this cookbook:

ALMOST EVERY DAY: *I eat this more wholesome dish whenever I want*

ONCE PER WEEK: *I make and eat this meal weekly*

A COUPLE TIMES PER MONTH: *This comfort food is on rotation in my kitchen*

ONCE A SEASON: *I enjoy this seasonal recipe at just the right moment*

ONLY ON A SPECIAL OCCASION: *I usually enjoy this dish on a birthday or holiday*

ONCE PER YEAR, REALLY: *I didn't give this up forever so I indulge in a serving annually*

FOOD PREFERENCE CATEGORIES

Each recipe is also labeled with the appropriate food preference category:

DAIRY-FREE *(DF)*

GLUTEN-FREE *(GF)*

NUT-FREE *(NF)*

REFINED-SUGAR FREE *(RSF)*

VEGAN *(V)*

VEGETARIAN *(Veg)*

Many of these recipes allow for lots of flexibility, as I believe that half the fun of cooking is improvising. Feel free to swap ingredients in and out to meet your food preferences or whatever you have in the fridge at the moment. Cooking is an exploration of tastes and texture, and finding your new way to food is definitely part of that journey.

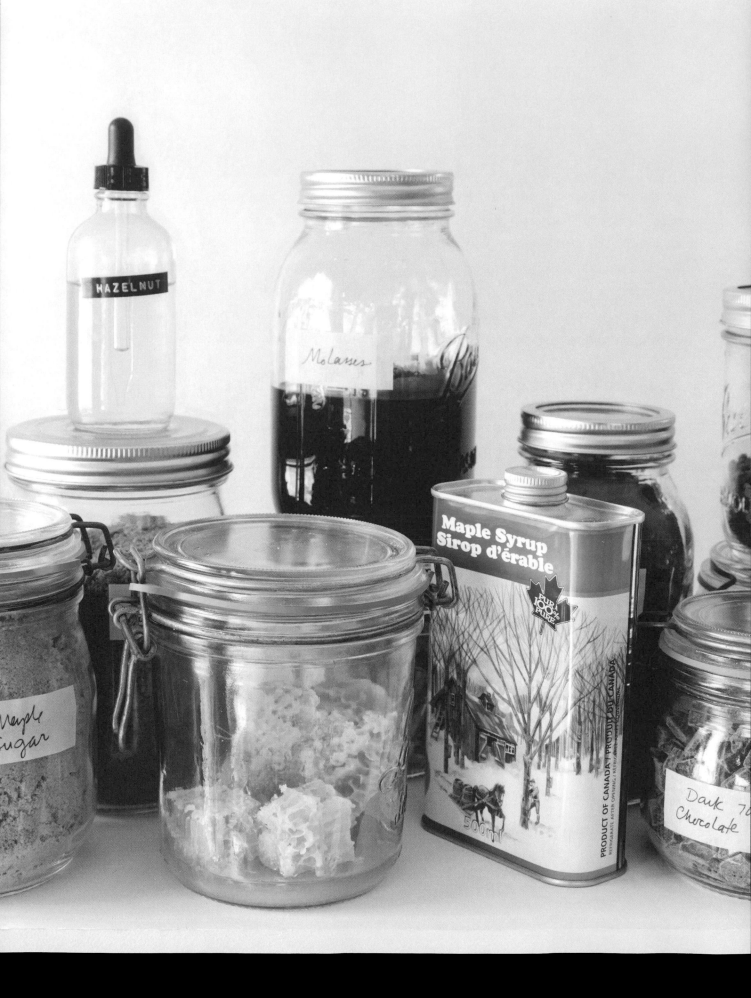

PART ONE

A New Kind of Pantry

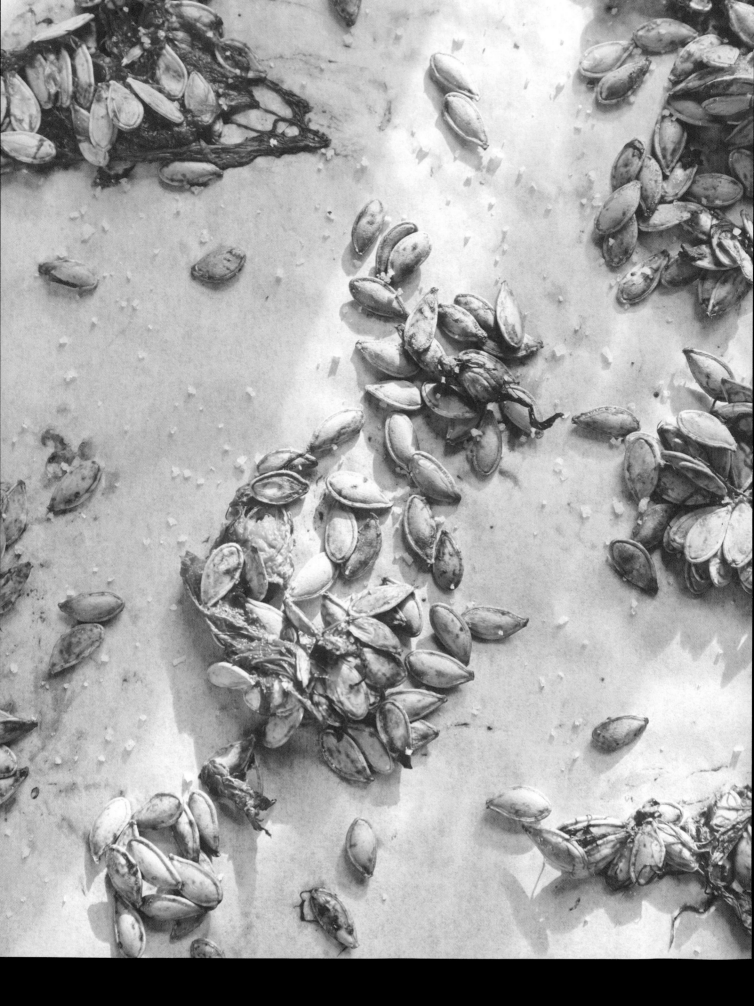

1

REVAMP YOUR PANTRY

As a cookbook author and food professional, my kitchen was traditionally filled with flour, sugar, and chocolate; animal proteins including bacon, pork, and beef; butter, milk, cream, yogurt, and every kind of cheese imaginable; and plenty of cloying cocktail ingredients and booze for my evening drink(s). During my transformational journey from fat girl to happy-to-just-be-me lady, the entire contents of my pantry, fridge, and freezer morphed considerably.

The most radical change was in the dairy and sweetener categories. I switched from animal milks to plant milks and from regular sugar to no sugar at all or small doses of specific sugars that didn't throw my glycemic levels so out of whack. As you transform the way you eat, I encourage you to explore my suggestions for getting the creamy texture and the sweet flavor that we all crave naturally in a more wholesome way.

This book isn't about deprivation—it's about making smarter choices that support your beautiful body and long-term wellness. You'll see that my pantry is as abundant as ever, just a lot more wholesome. Here are the building blocks for all the meals I make in my kitchen and the keys to making more wholesome versions to fit any creamy, sweet, and savory cravings.

SWITCH UP YOUR SWEETENERS

The glycemic index measures how rapidly digestible a food is or the extent to which it raises blood sugar levels after eating it. Diabetics watch this measure very closely, and while I've never been a diabetic, I find it super helpful to be mindful of this. The more stable and lower my glycemic levels, the longer I feel full and the less I want to eat. A food that registers high on the glycemic index (like a piece of milk chocolate cake sweetened with white sugar) may give me a sugar high and then crash, and may send me looking for more food sooner. Since I wanted to stuff myself with good foods that kept me fuller longer, I changed the sugars in my pantry to natural sweeteners, which are lower on the glycemic index. I also take care to avoid purchasing any foods with added sugar (for example, most prepared foods have even just a little sugar, including many types of bread, tortillas, and wraps).

Although a little organic cane sugar certainly remains in my pantry (because I work in food and need access to everyday ingredients), I prefer to stock and only consume these lower glycemic sweeteners:

APPLES *(whole, fresh; and shredded, frozen)*

BANANAS *(whole, fresh; and peeled/chopped, frozen)*

BROWN RICE SYRUP

COCONUT SUGAR

DATES

DATE NECTAR

DATE SUGAR

DATE SYRUP

HONEY *(light, wildflower, chestnut, hazelnut, raw, simple syrup)*

MAPLE SUGAR

MAPLE SYRUP

MOLASSES

All of these sweeteners are still forms of sugar so use as little as possible in your everyday cooking. And, to be clear, during active wellness mode, it's best to consume only natural sugars via fruit and wholesome carbohydrates.

DITCH DAIRY FOR PLANT-BASED MILKS AND CHEESES

Now that I only eat plant-centric dairy, my body feels so much better—the inflammation in my joints is non-existent and I rarely get sinus infections. And since most store-bought desserts are made with animal dairy, I am compelled to steer clear of desserts generally. The switch was a huge win for me.

Plain, unsweetened plant milk, typically the home-made variety, forms the base of all of my smoothies and is always in my fridge. I use it in baked goods, scrambled eggs, and to make creamy dishes even creamier. I also add a splash to coffee or tea. Of the many varieties I've tried, cashew and almond milk are my top choices.

I usually make nut milks from scratch in my kitchen. I also stock boxed plant milk from the grocery store for using in a pinch—read the label to ensure it has no added sugar. I make other plant milks, as needed, for specific dishes.

These are the milks I use regularly:

ALMOND MILK

CASHEW MILK

COCONUT MILK

HAZELNUT MILK

OAT MILK

PISTACHIO MILK

In lieu of dairy-based cheeses and condiments, I now use plant-based cheeses in my cooking. They really are delicious and add enough creaminess to support my craving. I typically make Almond Ricotta (page 39) and Crème Fraîche (page 43) from scratch, and purchase plant-based cheese shreds at the store to use sparingly on a pizza.

GET YOUR FAT
FROM HEALTHY SOURCES

Healthy oils and fats have been proven to be essential to weight loss, brain function, and strong muscles. While I don't use gallons of oil in my home cooking, I do use as much as I need—just healthier, mostly unrefined oils.

I prefer using extra-virgin olive oil to sauté at lower heats. I use grape seed or coconut oil to sauté over high heat, as well as in my baking. (For those who don't love the taste of coconut, know that refined coconut oil tastes less like actual coconut.) I use light sesame oil at higher heats; toasted sesame oil is better to just flavor dishes, as the seeds have already been cooked and the oil turns rancid quickly over heat.

I love to use ghee when butter is useful in a certain recipe. Ghee is essentially clarified butter—the milk solids have been removed through a heating process and the golden fat has been toasted up beautifully. It tastes a little like browned butter, aromatic and nutty. It is neither vegan nor dairy-free because some milk solids inevitably remain in the golden liquid. You can buy ghee in most markets or make your own (see page 44).

These are all the oils I use regularly:

    AVOCADO OIL
    COCONUT OIL *(refined and unrefined)*
    GHEE
    GRAPE SEED OIL
    OLIVE OIL *(extra-virgin, cold-pressed)*
    SAFFLOWER OIL
    SESAME OIL *(light and toasted)*

Pay close attention to the temperature guides on the bottles of each oil you use and do not use oil outside of those suggested temperatures. If oil ripples in a hot pan or smokes, it's turned toxic and should be tossed.

As for other healthy fats, I stock the sort that I crave daily like avocados, shredded and flaked coconut, all types of olives, and nut butters. I also eat sustainably sourced wild salmon about once a month.

MAKE PRODUCE THE STAR
OF EVERY DISH

Since the bulk of my dishes are filled with produce, my home is always filled with fruits and vegetables. While I will buy a beautiful tub of strawberries when they're in season or a pile of just-dug parsnips from the local farmers market, I stock a fairly standard roster of produce—like onions, carrots, celery, potatoes, greens, greens, and more greens, etc. Except for the greens, I store most of these ingredients in a cool pantry—a space in the kitchen that is dark and away from any heat. I am hyper concerned about food waste so I buy more perishable produce in very small quantities.

I also keep a lot of unsweetened dried fruit on hand to top smoothies, grain bowls, or salads—and to add to savory stews. Fruit is sweet enough naturally so search out the sort with no added sugar. I store dried fruit in the refrigerator but bring it to room temperature before using so it's soft and pliable in my dish.

EAT MEAT SPARINGLY

I eat animal protein only occasionally—a bit here or there—most likely when I am cooking for guests or family. I buy organic, pasture-raised, and grass-fed meat from a trustworthy farmer in bulk a few times per year; I freeze it and thaw as needed.

This is the animal protein most typically in my kitchen:

    BEEF *(organic feed, grass-fed):* consumed 1 to 2 times per month
    CHICKEN *(organic feed, pasture-raised):* consumed 1 to 2 times per year
    DUCK *(organic feed, pasture-raised):* consumed 1 to 2 times per year
    EGGS *(organic feed, cage-free):* consumed 1 to 2 times per week

SALMON *(wild caught):* consumed 1 to 2 times per month

TURKEY *(organic feed, pasture-raised):* consumed 1 to 2 times per year

I get plenty of protein from all the plant-based ingredients in my pantry, so I have no concerns with making meat a special-occasion ingredient.

FILL UP ON BEANS, LEGUMES, AND WHOLE GRAINS

The bulk of my plates are filled with scoops of beans and legumes, as they pack a nutritional punch that keeps me fuller longer.

I prefer to stock dried beans as they require no preservatives and, when simmered slowly, develop a beautiful creaminess. I also stock canned beans since they make a meal in minutes. Search out canned beans that have not been genetically modified and that come in cans lined without Bisphenol A (BPA). Drain and rinse canned beans before using.

I eat grains to help me feel fuller longer, too. I stock a variety of grains and prefer to cook with many types—like basmati rice, quinoa, rye flakes, and couscous—to make my dishes interesting and nutritionally varied.

You'll notice a few alternative flours throughout the recipes. I like to substitute buckwheat, spelt, and rye flours for some or most of the all-purpose flour in some of my recipes, to add just a little more nutritional value to a baked treat.

ADD A NUTRITIONAL CRUNCH WITH NUTS AND SEEDS

I use nuts for everything from adding a little crunch to a salad to pureeing for plant milk, using as egg substitutes in baking, or to make creamy sauces and salad dressings. I prefer to source raw, shelled, whole nuts and do any roasting or salting when I'm ready to use them. The only variant is almonds, which I tend to stock in multiple states: sliced, slivered, whole, ground, and flour.

I often source whole seeds—like flax seeds and chia seeds—as well, always organic, and grind or chop just before use. Whole seeds stay fresher longer, maintain their bite, and keep their unique flavor.

Nuts and seeds are sensitive and can become rancid after just a few months at room temperature. I store most of my nuts and seeds in labeled glass jars in the back of my fridge.

TRY SOMETHING TART AND TANGY IN YOUR DISHES

Vinegars contribute so much to my new way of cooking. I splash a little on vegetables at the end of a sauté and even drink well-diluted shots during allergy season. I tend to use apple cider vinegar and coconut vinegar most frequently and, often, interchangeably.

If I happen to have extra hulled strawberries, I'll slide them into a container of white wine vinegar for up to a week to impart their sweet flavor into the vinegar and, subsequently, into my dishes.

In addition to vinegars, I'm a big fan of adding pickles and ferments to my plates, often just before serving to offer a healthy probiotic punch or dynamic flavor contrast. For example, pickled onions perk up a bowl of plain rice and add a vibrant punch.

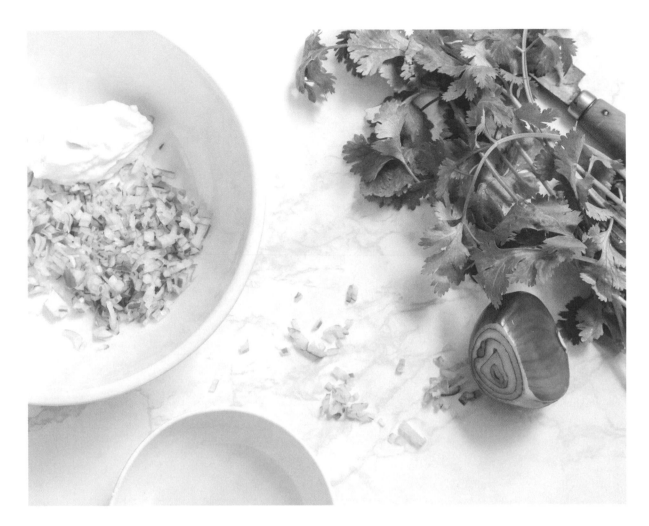

STOCK CONDIMENTS AND SPICES FOR FURTHER FLAVOR

I keep a variety of condiments on hand—too many to count—to make my bowls and plates feel powerful and taste delicious. Pureed garlic and ginger are essential, as most dishes dazzle with a little cooked in. I also prefer to use flavors from my childhood that are spicy and punchy like chipotle in adobo, chili oil, and all kinds of hot sauce—a little stirred into a fried rice dish or splashed on an egg can make a meal more exciting. As well, miso paste, nutritional yeast, and Mushroom Powder (page 54) add that hard-to-recognize umami that many dishes need to make them savory and appetizing. You'll see them used throughout my recipes.

You'll find a bunch of other ingredients in my pantry as well as some never-fail foods like dark chocolate for nibbling and teas to ease anxiety or perk me up. But it's with all of these major ingredient shifts that my recipes became way more wholesome and pleasurable, on the palate and on the plate.

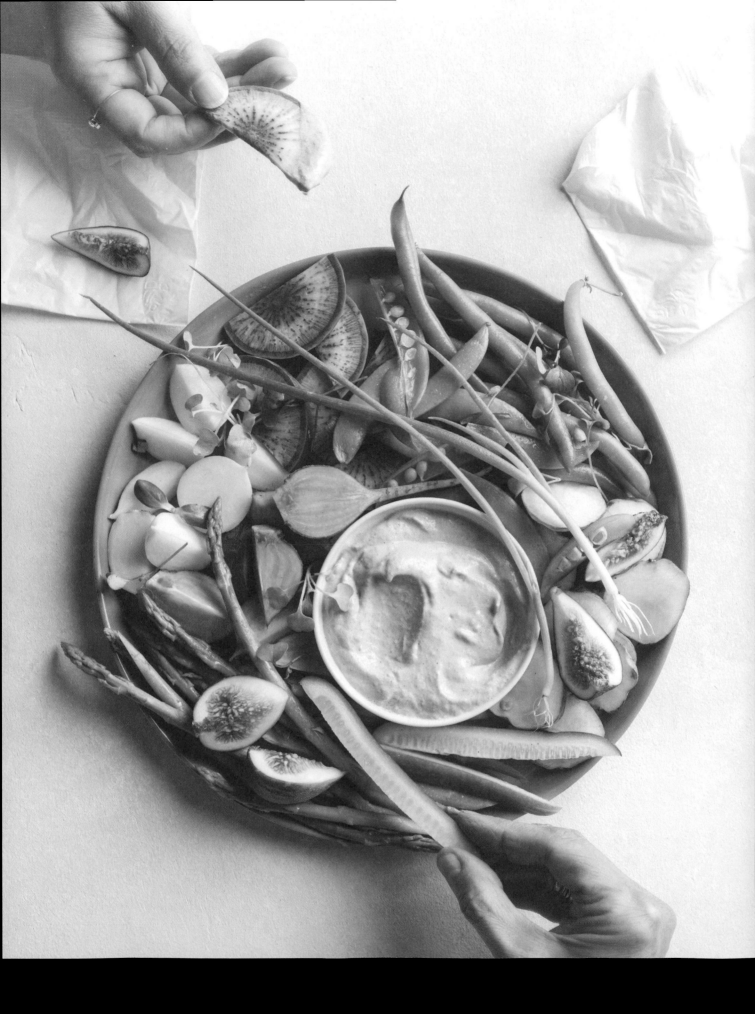

2

REVAMP YOUR MEAL PLANNING

With a revamped pantry, wholesome meals come to life far faster than all those nights when you stared into a half-empty fridge, shivering, wondering what to make for dinner yet again. Meal planning has become one of my favorite parts of the week—and not just because it feels like I'm crafting really easy nightly dinner parties.

I'm fond of meal planning for how effortless it is now and for how it brings my little tribe of two together to reconnect and plan for good food moments. And despite what you may witness on social media, planning meals for the week does not mean spending eight hours in the kitchen to create ten containers filled with enough food for a long road trip. Proper meal planning is simply about helping your future self out just a little bit more.

For most of my professional life, I was a workaholic. Between my full-time job in the tech world and starting Eat Boutique, I worked hard all week for someone else and typically spent the weekends taking care of my passion project—shipping food gift orders, making web site updates, sampling and selecting food, scheduling social marketing updates, and catching up on last-minute writing projects. I barely had time to eat, let alone cook.

All that changed when I learned to really love myself. To love yourself is to take care of yourself and be mindful of every single thing you put in your mouth. Yes, seriously. You have one body and if you fill it with greasy, processed fast food every day, your body will get big, lethargic, and perhaps give up on you sooner than you'd like. To love yourself is to feed yourself the very best food you can at every meal.

For me, part of my process was learning to slow down so that I can savor my meals. To start, instead of not-so-great food and brunch cocktails from my local diner for a leisurely weekend breakfast, I began cooking long Sunday breakfasts. My husband, Don, would hand-grind coffee beans for our slow pots of coffee—slow because I drink Bialetti-style coffee which cooks on the stove in about 10 minutes and he drinks pour-over coffee, which takes a while to drip-infuse; slow because we'd talk for a while over coffee and then decide what we felt like eating; slow because maybe instead of instant oatmeal, I'd steadily cook oats in plant milk and cinnamon to make a creamy porridge or maybe I'd decide to pull together some scones by hand (which takes 10 minutes) and then bake them off fresh (another 20 minutes). Those slow mornings were a treasure and a revelation—we can take the time to make and enjoy very good food at home, like wow.

When those Sunday mornings felt so good—not just delicious but a weekly sort of reconnection between us to remember what we loved (food and each other)—the good feelings drifted into the afternoon where we'd plan meals for the week, pick out recipes to try, decide who would make what, and cook in advance for the week. Sundays have really become my fun days.

Most Sunday afternoons, you'll find me cooking a big pile of brown rice for the week and Don foraging through our freezer for something to defrost. We may soak dried beans the day before to slow braise late Sunday afternoon, enough beans for that night's dinner and a couple meals later in the week. Sometimes I spend the afternoon chopping up onions, tomatoes, and cilantro for a big jar of Pico de Gallo, the Latin-style condiment that livens up basically everything, while he reads a book, tends to a roaring fire, or keeps the good tunes flowing in the background.

The only rules we abide by are to take it slow, make something delicious, and prepare at least one thing for the rest of the week's meals. While we do plan the entire week's worth of dinners, we don't try to make everything on Sunday—we just try to do something, one thing, that may ease the week. And our meal plans aren't complicated, as you'll see in a moment.

FIVE FOODS TO MAKE ON SUNDAY FOR MEALS ALL WEEK LONG

Since I want meal planning to be as easy as possible, I focus on prepping just one thing, not seven, on Sunday to help make dinner fast during the week. By making just one thing, you cut dinner prep to less than 30 minutes in most cases. These no-fuss meals are the sort of wholesome that makes you feel good, sleep better, and be energized for the next day. Here are five ingredient strategies to get started.

black beans

HOW TO MAKE: *Follow the Beans from Scratch recipe on page 33.*

HOW TO USE IN A MEAL:

1. Reheat some beans (without liquid) and spoon them into tortillas for quick tacos. Top with avocado, greens, or salsa.

2. Reheat some beans (with their liquid) and a few red pepper flakes to make soup. Top with extra-virgin olive oil, yogurt, and fresh chopped herbs.

3. Reheat some beans (with their liquid) and pile them on rice. Top with sliced avocado and lemon-and-oil-dressed greens.

cauliflower

HOW TO MAKE: *Follow the cauliflower preparation from the Cauliflower and Plantain Tacos recipe on page 91.*

HOW TO USE IN A MEAL:

1. Finely chop the cauliflower and use as a stand-in for rice in a bowl filled with roasted vegetables, sliced avocado, and salsa.

2. Finely chop the cauliflower and quickly sauté it with vegetables, pureed ginger, soy sauce, and sesame oil to make cauliflower-fried rice.

3. Reheat the cauliflower and add to a bowl. Top with a fried egg and hot sauce.

chickpeas

HOW TO MAKE: *Follow the Beans from Scratch recipe on page 33.*

HOW TO USE IN A MEAL:

1. Blend 2 cups of drained chickpeas with a little tahini, a little less lemon juice, a pinch of salt, and ¼ cup extra-virgin olive oil in a blender. Taste and add salt or lemon juice, to taste. Eat with pita wedges or sliced vegetables.

2. Sauté chickpeas with a little chopped white onion, garlic clove, and curry powder in olive oil. Add a can of tomato sauce, a can of coconut milk, and plenty of vegetable broth. Simmer until bubbly and hot to make an easy curry.

3. Add chopped lettuce leaves to a salad bowl. Add sliced cucumbers and tomatoes. Pile in some drained chickpeas. Toss with lemon juice, extra-virgin olive oil, salt, and pepper to make a hearty salad.

eggs

HOW TO MAKE: *Follow the egg preparation in the Avocado, Soft-Boiled Eggs, Thin Rice Cakes recipe on page 183.*

HOW TO USE IN A MEAL:

1. Eat them with sea salt and black pepper as a snack.

2. Slice them in half on top of toast as a more substantial meal.

3. Place an egg, sliced in half, on top of a bowl of noodles with broth to add extra protein to a dish.

tomato sauce

HOW TO MAKE: *Follow the Spicy Tomato Sauce recipe on page 35.*

HOW TO USE IN A MEAL:

1. Boil dried pasta according to package directions until al dente. Top with reheated tomato sauce.

2. Simmer tomato sauce with any leftover cooked veg. Break a couple eggs into the sauce and simmer until cooked. Serve from the pan with toast.

3. Sauté chopped garlic and seafood in olive oil. Add tomato sauce and simmer until warmed through. Serve on a deep platter with bread for dipping.

A WEEK'S WORTH OF MEALS

With simple strategies and a lot of determination, making meals that work with your new way to food doesn't need to be a chore. And once you've revamped your pantry and perhaps cooked some food ahead of time, meal planning will start to become a more seamless process.

To help you start visualizing how these meals can come together to form a week of menus, I created a chart to show some of the dishes I eat across six days in a given week; I always leave Sundays open for spontaneous cooking.

This style of chart may be just the thing you need to get you to cook, or it may seem way too daunting right now. Try just changing up one or two days per week, swapping in something you prepared at home, like an Instant Faux Pho Jar (page 248), for your normal deli takeaway sandwich. If that seems too hard, try to cook a few meals on the weekend, when you have the time and energy to bring it all to life, and play it by ear the rest of the week.

All the recipes listed appear in this cookbook. For the snacks, I point you to my guide on Simple Strategies for How to Snack (page 28).

	MONDAY	TUESDAY	WEDNESDAY	THURSDAY	FRIDAY	SATURDAY
FIRST MEAL	*Chocolate Zucchini Smoothie (page 82)—plus tea or coffee*	*My Special Oatmeal (page 119)—plus tea or coffee*	*Everything Green Smoothie (page 81)—plus tea or coffee*	*Avocado, Soft-Boiled Eggs, Thin Rice Cakes (page 183)—plus tea or coffee*	*Breakfast Toast Salad with a Fried Egg (page 87)—plus tea or coffee*	*Blueberry Buckwheat Pancakes (page 211)—plus tea or coffee*
FIRST SNACK	*Nuts*	*Banana*	*Nuts*	*Banana*	*Dried fruit*	*Avocado*
SECOND MEAL	*Italian-Style Leftover Rice Salad (page 219)—plus water*	*Instant Faux Pho Jars (page 248)—plus water*	*Beans in Olive Oil Broth with Tomatillo Salsa Verde (page 247)—plus water*	*Mega Kale Tartine with Smoky Mayonnaise (page 245)—plus water*	*Tuna Salad Lettuce Wraps (page 191)—plus water*	*Carpaccio-Style Vegetable Feast (page 101)—plus water*
SECOND SNACK	*Avocado—plus tea*	*Dark chocolate—plus tea*	*Olives—plus tea*	*Dark chocolate—plus tea*	*Blueberries*	*Dark chocolate—plus tea*
THIRD MEAL	*Spring Vegetable Stir Fry, Tortillas, Hot Sauce (page 195)—plus water*	*Eggs in Tomato Sauce (page 215)—plus water*	*Cauliflower and Plantain Tacos with Lemony Pesto Dressing (page 91)—plus water*	*Pasta with Cauliflower and Capers (page 160)—plus water*	*Veggie Fried Rice (page 156)—plus water*	*Smoky Paella with Fennel (page 262)—plus water or wine*
THIRD SNACK	*Dates—plus tea*	*Dark chocolate—plus tea*	*Olives—plus tea*	*Dates—plus tea*	*Dark chocolate—plus tea*	*Grapefruit Soda and Bitters (page 103)*

When I'm paying super close attention to all the food I eat during active wellness mode, I typically eat three meals per day with just one or two snacks tucked in between those larger meals. You can certainly create your own chart with as many meals as you need to get through your days. Focus on staying fuller longer and never letting yourself get too hungry.

SIMPLE STRATEGIES FOR
HOW TO SNACK

Lest you think my new way of eating is all thinly cut raw vegetables all of the time, take a look at my simple snacking strategies. I eat all sorts of good-for-you fats and I generally consume these snacks whenever I wish. You see, snacks, those tiny in-between meals, are way important to me. They provide satisfying energy and keep me going throughout the day. As well, snacks have always offered a little bit of comfort during stressful times; they often satiate whatever in me needs a good hit of textural foods now and again.

As a perennial snacker, I had to find ways to replace the treats from my old way of eating with new, rich, satisfying plant-based nibbles. Below, I present the fare I seek when a craving comes on and I offer a few no-recipe recipes (the sort with no measurements required) to make snacks way easy.

dark chocolate

An antioxidant powerhouse, dark chocolate is packed with minerals like potassium, zinc, and selenium. Recent studies have found that chocolate restores flexibility in the arteries, helping boost your heart and circulation. Chocolate also makes you feel better—it contains a chemical that your brain already creates when you feel like you're falling in love. I choose chocolate that's at least 67 percent or darker and that is made by people who care about their craft. Handmade chocolate is not mass-produced and it's not cheap, but I love knowing I've supported a small business that is hyper-aware of where the beans are sourced, how they're grown and harvested, and whether farmers have been properly rewarded for their work.

FAVORITE WAY TO EAT: *Dipped in no-sugar almond butter.*

olives

Most of the calories in olives come from fat, but it's the good kind of fat that helps to lower harmful cholesterol, raise beneficial cholesterol, and prevent heart disease. Some research shows that the phytochemicals in olives can help reduce inflammation (which contributes to arthritis). And they taste so darn good.

FAVORITE WAY TO EAT: *I'll pop olives, pitted or not, just as they are. Sauté them with a little orange zest, fresh rosemary leaves, and dried fennel seeds to get a little fancy or serve to guests during wine time.*

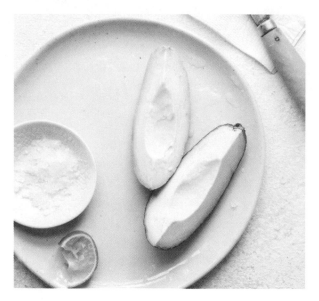

avocado

These lime-green orbs are a great source of vitamins, riboflavin, niacin, folate, magnesium, and potassium (they have more potassium than a banana). Avocados are good for your heart, great for your vision, and may help protect against certain cancers. They have a lot of fiber and even contain a chemical that signals the brain when you're full, which makes avocados a very useful snack.

FAVORITE WAY TO EAT: *I keep avocados on hand at all times to add into smoothies, whiz into dips and sauces, or just eat raw. Besides spreading avocado flesh on toast, I love to squeeze lime and sprinkle sea salt on a half or quarter wedge, eating it just like that with a spoon.*

nuts

Nuts are packed with protein and most of them contain heart-healthy unsaturated fats. Nuts contain the same chemicals that lower harmful cholesterol and raise beneficial cholesterol, and eating nuts may be linked with lowering levels of inflammation that can contribute to heart disease. Nuts are also packed with omega-3 fatty acids, fiber (which helps to make you feel full), and vitamin E. Most nuts are high in calories—so if you're watching calories then keep portions small—but they're way better for you than most other possible snacks.

FAVORITE WAY TO EAT: *I like to snack on raw whole almonds, pecans, pistachios, and walnuts. Sometimes, I'll keep a jar of nuts mixed with unsweetened dried fruit by my desk during long writing sessions.*

dried fruit

As with any fruit, dried fruit has both great and less optimal qualities. Dried apricots, dates, and figs can boost your fiber intake and supply your body with antioxidants. They are, however, high in sugar and calories. Make sure you choose unsweetened dried fruit exclusively and fruit without added preservatives that are used to maintain color. To keep them fresher longer, store dried fruit in the fridge.

FAVORITE WAY TO EAT: *I eat dried fruit just as it is but pay close attention to the quantities I consume. I'm less concerned with calories than with adding too much sugar to my way of eating. Treat dried fruit just like you would a piece of cake; enjoy it in friendly doses. For an appetizer, slice pitted dates in half, stuff them with a whole almond, and roast them in the oven for a few minutes.*

bananas

Bananas are a super fruit, loaded with essential vitamins and minerals like potassium, calcium, manganese, magnesium, iron, fiber, folate, niacin, riboflavin, and B6. They don't have much protein and contain no fat; they're mostly just water and carbohydrates. Bananas rank low on the glycemic index and don't spike your sugar levels quickly. Generally, bananas help me feel full and I consider them a wholesome part of my way of eating.

FAVORITE WAY TO EAT: *I'll certainly eat bananas just as they are, peeled, and always carry one around with me during the day. However, my favorite way to eat a banana is on a slice of toast with almond butter. This snack is more like a meal and keeps me full for hours.*

blueberries

These little blue gems are super fruits and are believed to have the highest antioxidant capacity of all produce. They may also help fight aging and certain cancers. They're low in calories and very high in nutrients like fiber, vitamins C and K, and manganese. Since they're mostly water, I eat them on the regular.

FAVORITE WAY TO EAT: *I prefer to freeze my blueberries, as they can degrade after a few days in the fridge. Once frozen, I pop a few in my morning oatmeal or bake them into something comforting. And there's nothing like a frozen blueberry on a warm summer day; when I mention frozen blueberries to kids, they tend to rid me of my harvest rather quickly.*

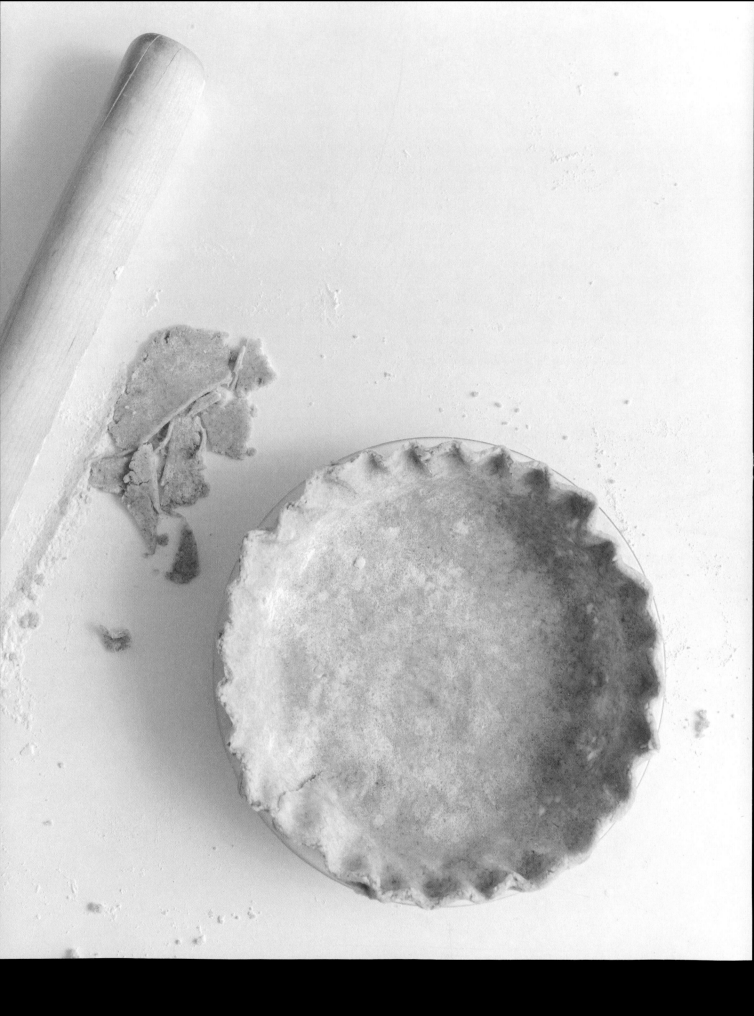

3

RECIPES FOR BETTER BASICS

As part of my new way to food shift, I decided that I no longer had time for diets, for counting calories, and for guilt around what I ate. What I do have time for is to cook better. I have time to make sure I eat a lot of produce every day. I have time to shop for food. And when I say I have time to do these things, I mean, I choose to make the time in my busy life because no one else will.

When I shop, I make sure to buy wholesome organic ingredients that are not processed in any way. I spend most of my available funds on produce, nuts, beans, seeds, good fats and oils, and grains, and far less on animal-based proteins. I keep my condiment door and spice drawers stocked so I can add lots of flavor to the food I cook.

Cooking many of my basics from scratch is one way I ensure that there are no unknowns in my dishes—instead of store-bought basics that may be filled with preservatives or hidden sugars, these homemade ones feel so good to eat and use in all my wholesome recipes. Many of them come together in a snap or are the sort of cooking you can do during the in-between time like when pausing a long movie or before switching the laundry to the dryer or when you're just passing through the kitchen for a few moments.

Easy Essentials

These are the hard-working, dependable ingredients in my pantry that I use daily. You'll find them in numerous recipes throughout this cookbook.

BASIC STOCK

I tend to only use homemade stocks since making them in between other cooking has become second nature to me. I store all homemade stock in 1-quart containers and label them with names and dates created, and try to use them up within 6 months (though they do tend to last longer). I make stock without a lot of salt and add more after it has thawed for meal prep.

Makes about 2 quarts

One 4-pound (1.8 kg) roasted chicken carcass or a quart-size bag of vegetable scraps (mushrooms, onion ends and skins, fennel fronds, celery hearts, etc.)

1 large yellow onion, peeled and quartered

1 medium carrot, cut into chunks

1 large celery stalk, cut into chunks

3 to 5 large garlic cloves, peeled

1 handful mixed herbs, stems and leaves

1 tablespoon sea salt

1 teaspoon black peppercorns

1. Place all the ingredients in a large soup pot and add enough cold water to cover the ingredients by about 2 inches.

2. Bring to a boil over medium-high heat. Reduce the heat to medium and simmer for 3 hours. Strain the stock into a new pot or bowl, and discard the solids. Let cool to room temperature. If you'd like, skim off any fat that collects at the top of the stock. Store in an airtight container in the fridge for up to 1 week or freeze for up to 6 months.

BEANS FROM SCRATCH

Canned beans do not compare to a big pot of cooked beans that were dried at the perfect time to maintain their flavor sans preservatives. Though I make black beans most frequently, this recipe applies to all types of dried shell beans—chickpeas, pink beans, and even white beans.

Makes about 8 cups

1 pound (454 g) dried black beans

1 bay leaf

5 medium garlic cloves, peeled

6 cups (1.4 L) vegetable stock or water (or a combination)

2 teaspoons sea salt

2 tablespoons roughly chopped fresh soft herbs (like cilantro leaves)

1. Soak the beans in 10 cups of cold water in a very large bowl for at least 8 hours or overnight. Drain and rinse beans.

2. Add the beans, bay leaf, garlic, vegetable stock, and salt to a large pot with a lid. Bring to a boil and then lower the heat to let the beans simmer until tender, 45 to 60 minutes. Put the lid on partially, so more liquid stays in the pot and only some steam is released. Stir occasionally, and add water as needed to keep the beans covered. Taste occasionally to assess how tender they are.

3. When they're as tender as you want them, turn off the heat, remove the bay leaf and garlic cloves, and stir in the herbs. Serve immediately or cool completely before storing in an airtight container in the fridge for up to 1 week. You can also freeze the beans in 1-quart containers for up to 6 months.

PESTO

This dairy-free pesto works on so many foods beyond pasta. Try it on vegetable tacos, a mixed green salad, baked potatoes, or spread it on fish before or after a short roast in a hot oven.

Makes about 1 cup

1 small bunch basil leaves (about 10 sprigs), stems cut and discarded

⅓ cup pine nuts

½ cup (120 ml) extra-virgin olive oil

¼ cup (60 ml) water

2 tablespoons lemon juice (from about 1 medium lemon)

½ teaspoon sea salt

10 twists freshly ground black pepper

Add the basil, nuts, oil, water, lemon juice, salt, and pepper to a powerful blender. Blend until smooth. Add more salt to bring out the flavor, lemon to brighten, or water to loosen, to your taste. Store in an airtight container in the fridge for up to 3 days but bring to room temperature before using. Freeze in an airtight container for up to 6 months.

SANDWICH BREAD

This bread is adapted from a King Arthur Flour recipe. I use rice milk powder instead of standard milk powder (coconut milk powder works well, too). You may need to use a little more water than called for if it is dry where you are.

Makes 1 large loaf (12 to 18 slices)

1 cup plus 2 tablespoons (250 ml) lukewarm water (a little more if dry where you are)

1 tablespoon light honey, like clover

2¼ teaspoons active dry yeast

1¾ teaspoons sea salt

2 tablespoons coconut oil, plus more for greasing

⅓ cup (2½ oz; 70 g) rice milk powder

4 cups (17 oz; 480 g) all-purpose flour

1. Put the water, honey, and yeast in the base of a stand mixer fitted with the dough hook attachment. Stir to combine and let sit for 5 minutes until the yeast foams up.

2. Add the salt, coconut oil, rice milk powder, and flour to the stand mixer. Knead at medium speed to make a smooth dough—this should take about 5 minutes. The dough should feel bouncy and elastic in your hands, not sticky or overly wet.

3. Place the dough in a bowl that is lightly greased with coconut oil. Cover, and let it rise for 60 to 90 minutes, until it's become quite puffy, though not necessarily doubled in size.

4. Gently deflate the dough, and shape it into a fat 9-inch log. Place it in a lightly greased 9- by 5-inch loaf pan, lightly greased with coconut oil.

continued

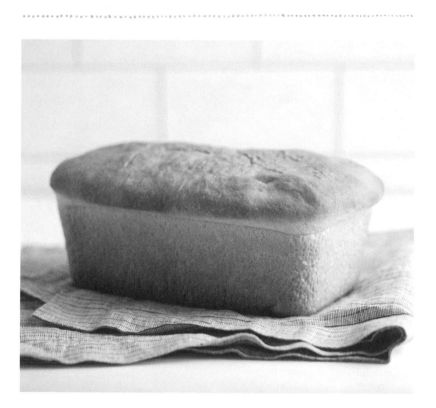

5. Cover the pan, and let the dough rise for 60 to 90 minutes, until it's crowned 1 to 1½ inches over the rim of the pan. Toward the end of the rising time, preheat the oven to 350°F (177°C).

6. Bake the bread for 35 to 40 minutes in total, until golden brown. If it's browning too quickly, tent it lightly with aluminum foil. An instant-read thermometer inserted into the center should read 195°F to 200°F (91–93°C).

7. Remove the bread from the oven, and turn it out onto a wire rack to cool. When completely cool, wrap in plastic and then in aluminum foil, and store at room temperature for up to 1 week. You can also slice and freeze the bread for up to 3 months; toast directly from frozen in a low oven.

SPICY TOMATO SAUCE

More often than not, I add ample red pepper flakes to my classic tomato sauce. It's not intensely spicy but it leaves that sort of warm taste on the back of your tongue that makes you keep spooning it in, especially when you open and heat a jar in the murkiness of winter. I usually can't be bothered to peel tomatoes in the height of New England's very short summer season. Instead, I pile them into a food processor and blitz them until skins and seeds are unrecognizable. If you want to peel your tomatoes first, I won't stand in your way but I may offer you a chilled drink. You'll use this sauce in A Better Bolognese (page 158), in the Pasta with Cauliflower and Capers (page 160), in my Eggs in Tomato Sauce (page 215), and on the Garlicky-Green Pizza (page 223), at the very least.

Makes about 5 cups

5 pounds (2.2 kg) fresh ripe plum tomatoes, cored and chopped into quarters

2 tablespoons extra-virgin olive oil

1 teaspoon red pepper flakes

2 large garlic cloves, peeled and finely diced

1 teaspoon sea salt, plus more to taste

1. Put the tomatoes in a powerful blender or food processor and puree until smooth. You may opt to pass the tomatoes through a food mill, if you want to remove the peels and seeds. Set aside.

2. Heat the oil with the pepper flakes and garlic in a wide shallow pot with a 3-inch side over medium heat until their aroma fills the air around you—and probably the other room. Add the tomatoes and salt. Stir and bring to a low boil. Reduce the heat and simmer until the sauce is reduced by about half, 30 to 40 minutes. The sauce should be thick enough to spread with a spoon, like a soup.

3. Taste and add more salt, as needed. Use immediately or store in an airtight container in the fridge for up to 1 week. You can freeze this sauce brilliantly; it will last up to 6 months in the freezer. Just make sure to thaw it, bring it to a boil again, and reduce it slightly to decrease any extra water.

TOMATO PESTO SAUCE

This sauce is a simple variation on the original. Once you have the Spicy Tomato Sauce made or any other jarred sauce at the ready, stir in pesto until the green flecks dim the red color only slightly and infuse an herbal flavor that feels a little bit wrong but is actually right in so many ways. You're simply adding herbs to sauce. And while I am quite sure my Italian grandmother would pale at the thought, the blend of tomato and pesto is exceptionally satisfying.

Makes about 3½ cups

3 cups Spicy Tomato Sauce (page 35) or any jarred sauce

½ cup Pesto (page 33) or store-bought pesto

¼ teaspoon sea salt, plus more to taste

Add the tomato sauce, pesto, and salt to a medium pot set over medium heat. Stir and heat until the flavors mesh together and the aroma fills the air around you, about 10 minutes. Taste and add more salt, as needed. Use immediately or store in an airtight container in the fridge for up to 1 week. Stir well before using. You can freeze this sauce brilliantly; it will last up to 6 months in the freezer. Just make sure to thaw it, bring it to a boil again, and reduce it slightly to decrease any extra water.

TORTILLAS

This is my basic recipe for bringing homemade tortillas together quickly. Allowing the dough to rest is important as it fully hydrates the masa harina, a flour that can be found in the international foods aisle at most grocery stores. A tortilla press is the best way to go and you can purchase your own for as little as twelve dollars online. Tortillas are best served fresh, and not reheated, so make them in the moment, if you can. In the recipe, I suggest you press all the tortillas before cooking them but once you get familiar with the process, feel free to press and cook as you go. I include a fantastic variation with smoked paprika; the spice lends an earthy flavor to whatever you slide in the tortilla.

Makes 16 tortillas

2 cups masa harina (instant corn masa)

½ teaspoon sea salt

1¼ cups (300 ml) water

1. Combine the masa harina and salt in a large bowl. Pour the water over the dry ingredients and mix with a large spoon or rubber spatula until the dough begins to come together. Using clean hands, work the dough into a smooth ball with no dry bits. Place a damp dish towel over the bowl and let the tortilla mixture rest for 30 minutes.

2. Set out two large clean dish towels on your counter. Set up your tortilla press by cutting a large gallon-size plastic zipper bag to form a greeting card–sized sleeve (cut the top and the two sides off, but keep the folded end). Place the plastic sleeve open on the tortilla press. If you do not have a tortilla press, you can use the same plastic sleeve and a rolling pin but it will likely take you three times as long to roll them out.

continued

3. Cut the tortilla dough in half and again into quarters. Work with one quarter at a time and keep the remaining dough covered with a damp dish towel. Divide each quarter of dough into four equal parts and roll each into a small ball the size of a golf ball.

4. Place one ball in the center of the tortilla press, in between the plastic layers. Close the tortilla press and push down until a tortilla is formed—they should be 5 to 6 inches wide. Flip the plastic-wrapped tortilla and press again to ensure even thickness. Open the press and carefully pull back the plastic to expose the tortilla. Flip it over onto your hand and peel back the other piece of plastic. Lay the tortillas on a clean dish towel, not touching each other, and cover with the other dish towel. Repeat with the remaining dough until you've made enough tortillas for your meal. If you don't want to make them all right now, store the remaining dough in a resealable plastic bag in the fridge and use within 3 days.

5. Place a new dish towel on a plate. Heat a non-stick pan over medium-high heat until very hot. Carefully lift a tortilla into your hand by raising the towel under it and flipping it into your hand. Drop onto the center of the pan and cook for 30 seconds. Flip the tortilla and cook for another 30 seconds. Flip one last time and cook for 30 seconds. Transfer the cooked tortilla to the new dish towel and cover to keep warm. Repeat with all the remaining raw tortillas. Serve the tortillas immediately or store in a resealable plastic bag in the fridge for up to 2 days—but be aware that they will be tougher and firmer when you reheat them.

RECIPE VARIATIONS

Smoked Paprika Tortillas: Dissolve 1 tablespoon of smoked paprika in the water, stirring with a fork until the water takes on a deep orange hue. Proceed with the recipe as described, adding the now-infused water to the masa harina and salt.

Flax Seed Tortillas: Add 4 tablespoons of golden flax seeds to the masa harina. Increase the water by 1 tablespoon. This variation adds a superfood, flax, and a little extra protein to the tortillas.

Creamy Alternatives

I've shifted my pantry to be entirely dairy-free. These rich alternatives provide ample creaminess to everything from a cup of coffee to scones and pancakes. Most of the work involved is in soaking the nuts—after that, blending everything together is a breeze.

ALMOND-DATE MILK

This milk is sweet and light, just the sort of thing to enrich your hot drink, create a satisfying smoothie, or add to a pot of oatmeal.

Makes about 4½ cups

1 cup raw almonds

1 cup (240 ml) tap water

4 cups (960 ml) filtered water

6 Medjool dates, pitted

1. Soak the almonds in the tap water for at least 4 hours or up to overnight. Drain and rinse almonds.

2. Add the almonds and 2 cups of the filtered water to a blender and whiz for 3 minutes until well blitzed.

3. Add the remaining 2 cups filtered water and the dates to the blender. Whiz for 2 minutes.

4. Strain through a nut milk bag or two layers of cheesecloth, pressing the pulp to extract all the milk. Discard the pulp.

5. Store in the fridge and use within 4 days. Shake well before each use.

ALMOND RICOTTA

Growing up in a part Italian-American household, I fell hard and fast for ricotta cheese. We added it to every pasta dish, spread it on toast, and mixed it into big bowls of tomato broth–based soups. I make my own version from almonds now, and mix it into favorite pasta bakes or chop in lots of fresh herbs for an appetizing dip. The key is the soak; soaking for less than 48 hours will yield a grainy ricotta. I promise it's worth the wait.

Makes about 2 cups

2 cups raw skinned almonds, whole or slivered

½ cup (120 ml) filtered water

1 teaspoon sea salt

1 tablespoon plus 2 teaspoons lemon juice (from about ½ medium lemon)

1 teaspoon white miso

1 teaspoon nutritional yeast

1. Put the almonds in a medium bowl, cover with tap water and plastic wrap, and leave to soak for 2 days. Drain and rinse.

2. Add the almonds, filtered water, salt, lemon juice, white miso, and nutritional yeast to a powerful blender. Blend on low speed until a ricotta texture is achieved and no large almond pieces remain. You may need to scrape down the sides of the blender a few times to ensure all the large pieces are blended.

3. Set up a strainer over a bowl and place two layers of cheesecloth in the strainer. Transfer the ricotta to the cheesecloth and strain in the refrigerator for 4 to 6 hours or up to overnight, until some liquid is pulled from the ricotta and the texture is just right.

4. Chill the ricotta before using. Store in an airtight container in the fridge for up to 3 days.

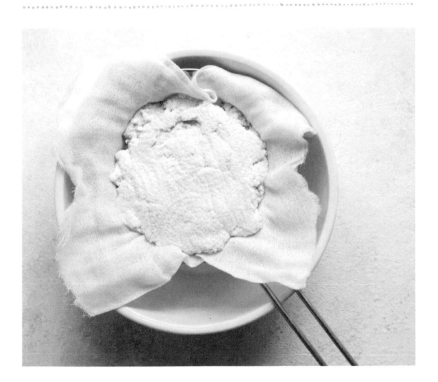

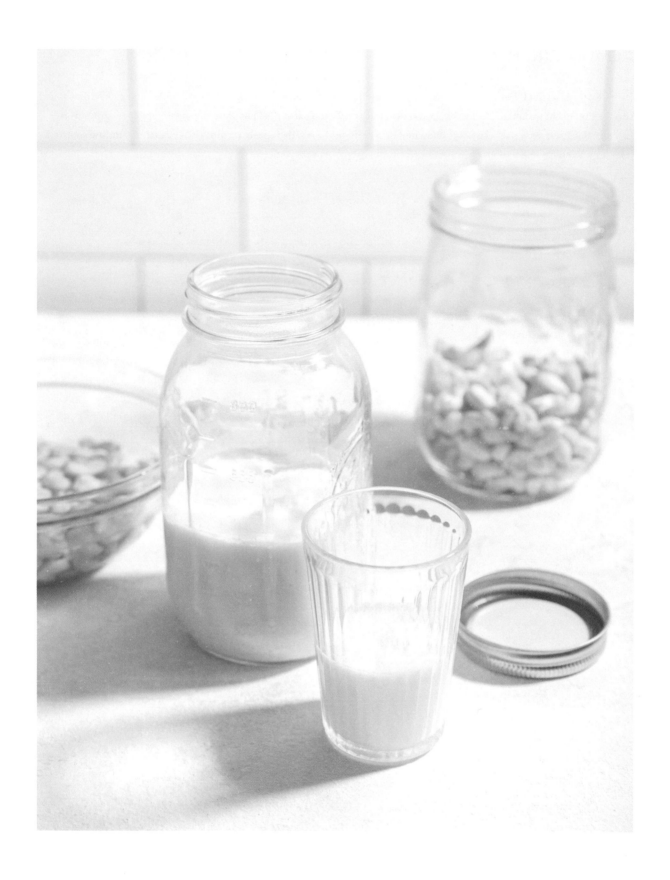

CASHEW MILK

I often alter the method for making cashew milk depending on my available time and intended use. For example, I use a no-fuss recipe in my smoothies; I'll whiz it up for however many minutes I have and then finish the blending with all the smoothie ingredients. The refined variation is way smooth as it's run through a nut milk bag before adding to soups, sauces, or a velvety cocktail. If you have a super powerful blender, you may not need to run the milk through the bag. But if you use a regular blender (and I started this way of eating with an inexpensive ordinary blender), then get a nut milk bag. They're available online for just a few dollars.

The sweet variation, perhaps my favorite, is tempered with a bit of maple syrup, which makes it great in special desserts, over cereal, or just for drinking from a tall glass. Since no binders are used in these recipes, the cashew milk may separate slightly while in the fridge—just shake it well before using.

Makes about 4 cups

1 cup raw whole cashews

1 cup (240 ml) tap water

4 cups (960 ml) filtered water

1. Soak cashews in the tap water for at least 4 hours or up to overnight in a jar or bowl. No need to refrigerate but cover with plastic wrap. Drain and rinse the cashews.

2. Add the cashews and 2 cups of the filtered water to a blender and whiz for 3 minutes until well blitzed.

3. Add the remaining 2 cups filtered water to the blender. Whiz for 1 minute, until smooth. Store in the fridge and use within 4 days. Shake well before each use.

RECIPE VARIATIONS

Refined Cashew Milk: After the final blend, pour the milk through a cheesecloth-lined strainer or through a nut milk bag, discarding the nut pulp. (If you want to reuse the nut pulp, try adding it to the crisp part of my Blueberry Plum Crisp Pie, page 228. Just remember, the pulp is not at all sweet so add a little extra sugar to the crisp mix.) Pour the milk into a container with an airtight lid. Add 1 teaspoon vanilla extract and shake well.

Sweet Cashew Milk: Before the final blend, add 1 tablespoon maple syrup to the blender. Whiz until smooth.

CASHEW YOGURT

Since I've stopped eating animal dairy, I've felt great. But more than all the perfectly smelly cheese in France, I missed yogurt. Especially the super tart kind that is versatile enough to top either a bowl of berries or a bowl of curry. I experimented with a bunch of recipes over the years, only to be let down. This Cashew Yogurt, however, is wonderful. It's based on a version made by holistic nutritionist Sarah Britton of the famed *My New Roots* site. Mine is a medium-thick version—for a thicker yogurt, reduce the water and let the mixture sit longer. My version is also unsweetened and fairly mild, which makes it quite versatile. However, if you'd like a sweeter bowl of yogurt for breakfast or some dessert application, take a look at the variation. Probiotics aren't an inexpensive ingredient but they're so good for you (I pop one daily with a meal to keep my gut healthy), and a thirty-tab bottle (about twenty dollars online) will make thirty batches of homemade yogurt. Make sure to only use a nonmetallic spoon to prepare the yogurt; metal can sometimes react with the probiotics.

Makes about 2 cups

1 cup raw cashews

2 cups (480 ml) tap water

1 cup (240 ml) filtered water

1 tablespoon plus 1 teaspoon lemon juice
    (from about ½ medium lemon)

⅛ teaspoon sea salt

1 probiotic pill (20 billion CFU)

1. Soak the cashews in the tap water for up to 4 to 6 hours or overnight. Drain and rinse the cashews well.

2. Add the cashews, filtered water, lemon juice, and salt to a blender. Blend for 3 minutes until very well blitzed and totally smooth.

3. Add the contents of the probiotic pill (pierce the casing, pour out the grains, and discard the casing) to a clean glass jar. Pour your smooth cashew mixture into the jar and, with a nonmetallic spoon, stir it very well. Place a small square of four layers of cheesecloth or a clean dish towel over the mouth of the jar and secure it in place with a rubber band. Place the jar in a warm, non-drafty part of your kitchen for at least 6 hours or up to 24 hours, until the surface of the yogurt bubbles and it thickens to something luscious that's thicker than heavy cream but still runny. The longer it sits, the thicker it gets.

4. You may use it immediately at room temperature; however, I place an airtight lid on the jar and chill it in the fridge before using. Store in the fridge and use within 4 days. Stir well before each use with a non-metallic spoon.

RECIPE VARIATION

Sweet Cashew Yogurt: Add 1 tablespoon maple syrup plus ½ teaspoon vanilla bean paste or the seeds from a vanilla bean pod to the blender before blitzing. Use immediately or store in an airtight container in the fridge and use within 4 days.

CRÈME FRAÎCHE

This vegan Crème Fraîche might be my favorite recipe. It is heavenly and can be used in a variety of ways like thickening up stews, adding creaminess to sauces, or as a rich condiment in sandwiches. You'll see it referenced throughout my cookbook and I always have a jar in the fridge. It's as useful a condiment as hot sauce and mustard, only made almost entirely from cashews.

Makes about 2 cups

1½ cups raw whole cashews

2 cups (480 ml) tap water

¾ cup (180 ml) filtered water

2 tablespoons lemon juice (from about 1 medium lemon)

½ teaspoon sea salt

1. Soak the cashews in the tap water for at least 4 hours or up to overnight in an uncovered jar or bowl. No need to refrigerate. Drain and rinse cashews.

2. Add the cashews, filtered water, lemon juice, and salt to a blender and puree until thick and creamy.

3. It's ready to use immediately but I suggest you chill it in the fridge before using. Store in an airtight container in the fridge and use within 5 days. Stir well before each use.

RECIPE VARIATION

Lime Crème Fraîche: Mix 1 tablespoon of lime juice with 4 tablespoons of crème fraîche in a small bowl. Use immediately or store in an airtight container in the fridge and use within 5 days.

GHEE

Ghee is clarified butter that you cook for just a bit longer. Essentially, you boil cow's milk butter until all the milk solids and water are removed; what's left is pure, gold fat that is wonderful for high-heat cooking as it doesn't smoke until it reaches 450°F to 475°F (232–246°C). Ghee is not dairy-free (a few trace solids are sometimes left behind) but it does have a pretty long shelf life and can be kept at room temperature. Some high-quality ghee brands are sold in stores nowadays but it's easy to make your own from organic unsalted butter.

Makes about 1½ cups

1 pound (454 g) fresh unsalted butter
(4 sticks)

1. Place the butter in a medium saucepan with straight sides over medium-low heat. As the butter melts slowly, it will separate into layers: the foam will be on top; the clarified butter in the middle; and the milk solids will settle on the bottom of the pan.

2. Let the butter bubble slowly so that the clarified butter becomes golden and the milk solids on the bottom of the pan become lightly toasty. This may take as long as 15 minutes. As this process continues, begin to skim off the foam with a large flat spoon, discarding the foam to a bowl off the heat. Some wait until the end to discard the foam but I prefer to see my clarified butter toast up and removing that foam now helps. Wipe the spoon clean with a paper towel every now and again.

3. Once most of the foam is removed, the milk solids have browned, and the ghee is as golden as a setting sun, turn off the heat and let it sit for a few moments. Set up a strainer lined with cheesecloth over a bowl or large jar. Strain the ghee into the jar, leaving the browned milk solids behind in the pan. If you get a thin layer of foam on top of the ghee, just skim that off one final time. The ghee should cool to room temperature before handling. Store in a jar with an airtight lid at room temperature for up to 1 month.

RECIPE VARIATION

Lime Ghee: Let 4 tablespoons ghee come to room temperature or liquid form. You may need to heat it up slightly. Stir in 1 teaspoon lime zest and ⅛ teaspoon sea salt. Use immediately or store in an airtight container at room temperature for up to 1 month.

TOASTED COCONUT MILK

This creamy and toasty liquid will make any smoothie taste like the tropics. However, if you crave a straight-up tall glass of the stuff, return the Toasted Coconut Milk (once strained) to a blender with a couple of pitted dates, whiz, and drink it down, as is.

Makes about 4 cups

1 cup unsweetened shredded coconut

4 cups (960 ml) filtered water

1. Preheat the oven to 350°F (177°C). Line a rimmed baking sheet with parchment paper.

2. Spread the coconut in a thin layer across the parchment. Toast in the oven for 3 to 5 minutes, until golden brown or your desired color. Toss a couple times to ensure all the coconut gets evenly brown. Remove from the oven and cool for 5 minutes. If it's a little too dark, carefully remove the parchment paper to a counter or kitchen towel so it stops any residual heat from the warm baking sheet.

3. Add the coconut and water to a powerful blender. Blend until pulverized and very smooth, about 3 minutes.

4. Strain the mixture through a nut milk bag or a piece of cheesecloth over a strainer into another bowl. Store in an airtight glass jar in the fridge for up to 4 days. Shake well before each use.

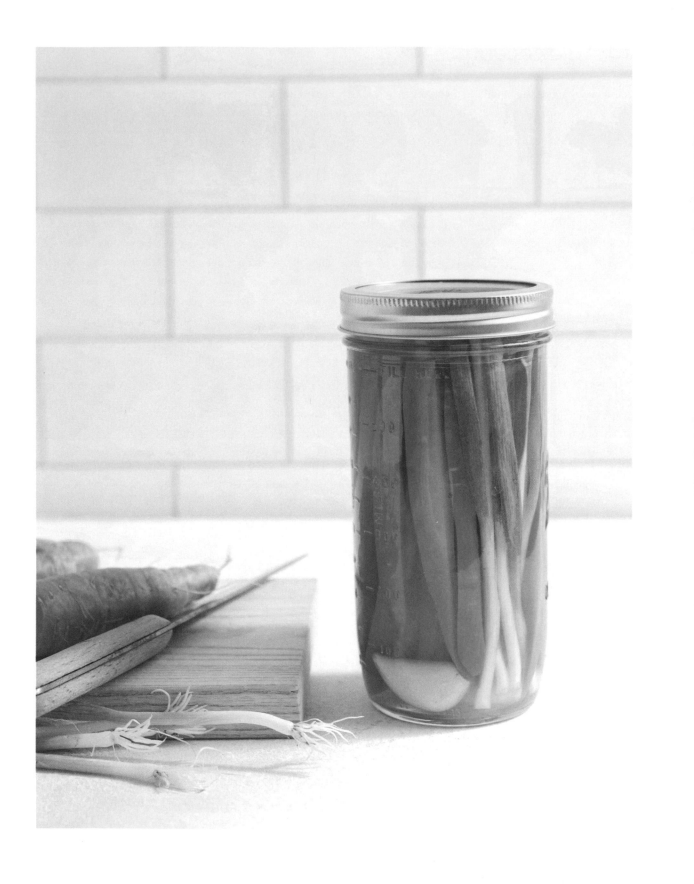

Flavor-Filled Condiments

These homemade condiments add a vibrant smack to everyday recipes, making your basic rice dish or green salad even tastier. You most certainly don't need to stock all of them, but lunches and dinners will be way better with a dollop of several at once. The Herby Yogurt Dressing (page 190) also makes for a great condiment.

CARROT PICKLES

Pickles are the workhorse of my home cooking. They are a surprise and delight on a share board. They provide a wake-me-up tang to deep, soulful stews, soups, and curry bowls. They can be chopped into hummus, dips, and yogurts for a something-special flavor. And, in my home, they're always handy, ready to snap to duty with the quick turn of a lid. My brine is simple and the extra flavoring agents—in this case, garlic and spring onions—are up to you, but I always use garlic as it offers a nice bite. Spring carrots are undeniably good but pour this brine over anything: blanched green beans, cucumber slices, fennel wedges. If the vegetable is exceptionally hard, like carrots, blanch them for 1 to 3 minutes to make them a silkier bite.

Makes one 3-cup jar

12 ounces (340 g) tiny spring carrots, peeled and trimmed to fit in your jar

3 large garlic cloves, peeled and smashed slightly

6 to 8 thin spring onions or scallions, cleaned and trimmed to fit in your jar

1 cup (240 ml) apple cider vinegar

1 cup (240 ml) water

1 tablespoon sea salt

1 tablespoon maple sugar

1. Set up a medium bowl with ice and water. Bring a medium pot of water to a boil. Blanch the carrots by tossing them into the water for 3 minutes, then carefully draining them and shocking them in the bowl of ice water for 3 minutes. Drain and pat dry with a clean towel. Set aside for a moment.

2. Clean a 3-cup wide-mouth jar and lid (or your chosen jar) in hot, soapy water. Sterilize the jar by running it through a dishwasher at the hottest setting or boiling it in a pot on the stove for 10 minutes. Allow to air dry.

3. Place the garlic in the bottom of the jar. Pack the carrots and onions, vertically, into the jar. Put the vinegar, water, salt, and sugar in a medium pot. Bring to a boil, stirring until dissolved, and then carefully pour the hot brine over the carrots, leaving ½ inch of headspace. Wipe the rim and seal the jar with lid and ring. As soon as the jar cools, place it in the refrigerator to rest for 48 hours before eating. Store in the coldest part of your fridge for up to 1 month.

CHIMICHURRI SAUCE

This green sauce is a vibrant staple in my kitchen. It dresses up any grilled food from animal protein to every kind of vegetable. I especially like to serve it with just-boiled or grilled potatoes for a starchy-bright flavor pairing. You can finely chop the ingredients for the sauce but I prefer to blitz them in a food processor when I'm short on time, which is most of the time.

Makes about 1½ cups

1 small bunch parsley (about 8 sprigs),
    stems cut and discarded

1 large bunch cilantro (about 16 sprigs),
    stems cut and discarded

1 small bunch basil (about 6 sprigs),
    stems cut and discarded

2 large garlic cloves, peeled

3 scallions, trimmed and
    roughly chopped

2 tablespoons lime juice (from about
    1 lime)

2 tablespoons apple cider vinegar

¼ cup (60 ml) extra-virgin olive oil

¼ teaspoon sea salt, plus more to taste

Blitz all the ingredients in a powerful blender or food processor until roughly diced and loose, about 20 seconds. Stir it to make sure no big chunks remain. If a big piece of scallion or garlic remains, blitz again. Taste and add more salt, if you like. The flavor intensifies as it sits so feel free to let it rest while you prepare your meal. Store in an airtight container in the fridge for up to 3 days.

CRISPY SHALLOTS AND SHALLOT OIL

These crispy shallots are smoky and salty, like bacon, and come together fast; I use them to top soups, salads, and noodle bowls. The resulting shallot oil is luscious and provides complex smoky flavor to whatever it tops.

Makes about 1 cup

1 cup (240 ml) grape seed or safflower oil

6 medium shallots, peeled and sliced about ⅛-inch thick

Sea salt

1. Put the oil in a small saucepan. Add the shallots and place pot over medium heat. Bring to a simmer. Cook gently, stirring occasionally to keep the shallots under the oil, for about 15 minutes (turn down heat if they seem to be coloring too quickly), until they gradually become golden brown. Keep a close eye on the coloring as they can turn dark brown very quickly.

2. Place a paper towel on a plate. Transfer the shallots to the plate using a slotted spoon, reserving the oil, and let them drain well. Blot shallots to remove any extra oil. They will become crisp as they cool. Sprinkle lightly with salt. Store at room temperature in an airtight container and use within 5 days. Save the oil in a separate bottle and use within 2 weeks.

FERMENTED HOT SAUCE

Hot sauce is an acquired taste and is rarely a love-it or hate-it situation. In fact, hot sauces fall on such a wide spectrum of heat that one person's hot sauce may be another person's candied topping; you just never know. I prefer sauces that mix heat with funk and a little green flavor. My Fermented Hot Sauce recipe has a nice mellow heat that sneaks up on you and it's fermented to develop the healthy probiotics and green flavor. It's exceptionally easy too—just toss all the veg into the jar, fill it up with the briny water, and let it sit until it develops. You'll be able to smell the spice and funk developing if you walk by or hover near the jar. Don't throw away the brine. It's a lighter style of hot liquid that's great added to soups and stews, and just wonderful in a Bloody Mary cocktail. It will also help you form your next batch of hot sauce.

Makes about 4 cups

2 quarts (1.9 L) filtered water, more as needed

4 tablespoons sea salt, plus more as needed

2 pounds (904 g) mixed peppers (mostly cubanelles and garden peppers; just a few jalapeños and serranos to get heat)

1. Clean a very large jar (a half-gallon jar works) and its airtight lid in very hot water and dry with clean towel. To sterilize it, run it through a dishwasher at the hottest setting or boil it in a pot of water for 10 minutes. If using a fermentation crock, clean it in very hot water first and then, to sterilize the crock, scald it with boiling water for at least 30 seconds and allow it to air dry. Find a few small plates that fit into the mouth of your jar and clean, dry, and sterilize those in the same way. Set all aside.

2. Mix the water with the salt, stirring to help dissolve the salt. Set aside to fully dissolve.

continued

½ pound (8 oz; 227 g) cherry tomatoes

5 large garlic cloves, peeled
and smashed

¼ cup (60 ml) brine from a previous
ferment or pickle (like from a jar
of sauerkraut)

3. Remove the stems and caps from the peppers. Cut slits into the tomatoes. Pile all the veg into your jar and place small plates on top to help keep the veg submerged once you add the water. Alternatively, or in addition, you can fill a plastic bag with water and put that on top to aid in keeping the veg submerged. If using a fermentation crock with weights, add the small plates and then the weights to help keep it all submerged. Pour the brine from a previous ferment over the veg.

4. Pour the salted water mixture over the veg mix until the veg are covered by at least 2 inches. Poke any veg that slips through back under the plates. Depending on the size of your large jar, you may need more brine to cover. If you do, start by dissolving 2 tablespoons sea salt in 1 quart filtered water. Add that to the jar until the veg are sufficiently covered.

5. Seal the jar to block out any oxygen. If using a fermentation crock, place the lid on top and add water to the well to block out any oxygen. You'll need to add water to the well every couple of days to keep the oxygen out. Place the jar in a darker nook for 14 days, or until it develops the heat and tang you like. The longer it sits, the more tangy and funky the hot sauce.

6. When you are ready to bottle your hot sauce, open the jar and use tongs to remove the plates and/or fermentation crock weights. Carefully pour the veg and brine through a strainer into a very large bowl and set the brine aside for now. Add the veg to a food processor and whiz for 2 to 3 minutes until the veg is smooth and finely pureed.

7. Add ½ cup of the brine to the food processor and continue whizzing—adding more brine by the tablespoon or two until you until you reach your desired hot sauce consistency (I usually add an extra 4 tablespoons). Bottle it up and store in the back of your fridge. It's ready to use immediately though I like to chill it first. It will keep in an airtight container in the fridge for at least 1 year. Make sure to shake it well before each use, as natural, homemade products often separate.

FERMENTED SPICY CURTIDO

I grew up with tangy cabbage or carrot salads placed on the same plate as a rich dish. I rarely ate these salads because, quite frankly, I was a child who looked at these smelly, funky foods with the sort of contempt reserved for boiled Brussels sprouts, liver and onions, and fresh squid salad. I now know those bright veg scoops were intended to cut the fat of a meaty dish or lighten the entire meal. And to say I love them would be a very accurate understatement. I use this recipe to cut everything—a slice of thick toast with avocado, beside a pile of ghee-roasted wild mushrooms, or alongside that occasional steak. Since fermentations require such precision, please use a scale to weigh everything in this recipe. And don't let the math part scare you; it's a very easy recipe.

You may certainly replace the cabbage with whatever comes from the farm stand, like a big head of kohlrabi, perhaps. If any scum forms on top of the liquid, just scoop it and toss it. The curtido will persevere and be wonderful, still. Remember, however, that if anything smells undesirable or tastes off, toss the whole batch and start again.

Makes about 12 cups

1 large or 2 small cabbages

2 medium yellow bell peppers

4 medium carrots

1 large red onion, peeled

½ jalapeño pepper, seeded and
  finely diced

1 tablespoon red pepper flakes

2 tablespoons fresh oregano leaves

Sea salt

Filtered water

1. Remove the outer leaves of the cabbage, rinse them, and set them aside—you'll need them later. Core and quarter the cabbage and bell peppers.

2. In a food processor or with a boxed grater, grate the cabbage, bell peppers, and carrots to a coarse grind. Thinly slice the red onion. Add the grated veg, red onions, jalapeño, pepper flakes, and oregano to a very large bowl set over a scale. Weigh the ingredients and write down the number. To figure out the amount of salt required to brine this mix, calculate 2 percent of the total weight. The above assortment, for example came to 5 pounds 6½ ounces (2455 g), so 2 percent of 2455 grams is 49 grams. Weigh out 49 grams of sea salt.

3. Sprinkle the salt across the veg mixture, in large pinches, slowly tossing and squeezing the veg mixture to make sure the salt is well distributed and the veg breaks down. Every strand of vegetable should have salt on it. Squeeze and toss for 10 minutes until a brine forms in the bowl.

4. Pack the veg mixture into a large jar which fits another small jar at the top or into a fermentation crock. Press and push until all the veg is packed into the jar or crock with very few to no air pockets. Pour in any remaining brine. Cover the vegetables with 3 or 4 large cabbage leaves and, if using a fermentation crock, add the weights. The brine should cover the veg mixture by about 2 inches. If you need more brine, add it in based on this measurement: dissolve 1 tablespoon sea salt into 2 cups filtered water.

continued

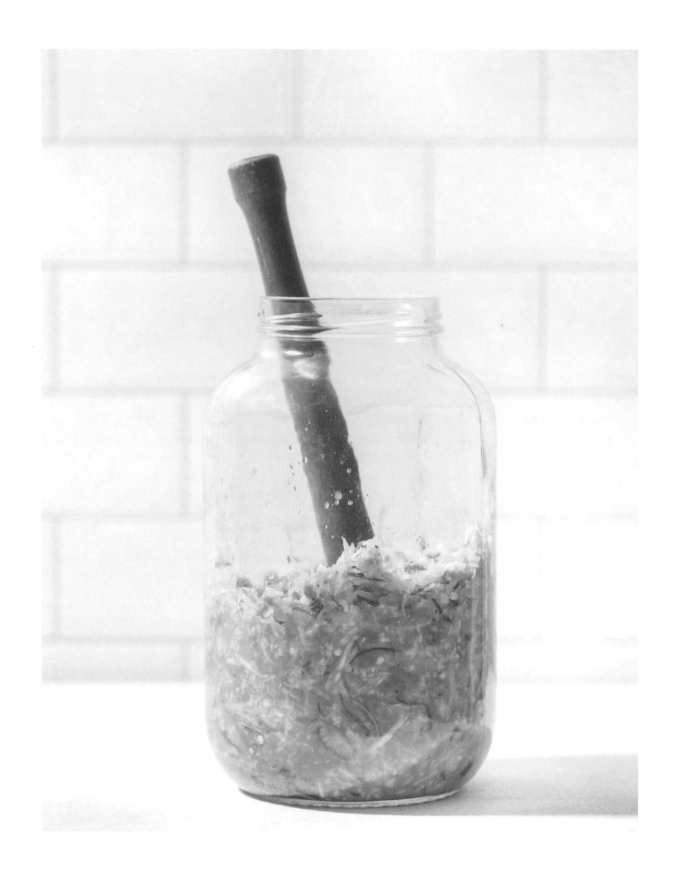

5. Place the small jar inside the large jar. Fill the small jar with a little plain water to hold it in place—this will help keep the veg under the water line. Seal the larger jar with plastic wrap to block out any oxygen. If using a fermentation crock, place the lid on top and add water to the well to block out any oxygen. You'll need to add water to the well every couple of days to keep the oxygen out. Place in a dark nook for 7 to 10 days. The longer it sits, the more tangy the curtido.

6. When you decide to use your curtido, open the jar and remove the interior jar or fermentation crock weights. With tongs, remove the cabbage leaves and discard. Remove the curtido from the jar and pile into a clean jar. Add enough brine to cover the curtido, seal, and store in the coldest part of your fridge. It's ready to eat immediately though I like to chill it first. It will keep in an airtight container in the fridge for up to 3 months.

LEMONY PESTO DRESSING

This dressing is incredibly versatile, so much so that I often double it to use all week. Pour it over everything—a bowl of beans, a pile of pasta, a slab of roasted squash or fish. And if you add a bit more oil and water, it loosens up into a lovely salad dressing.

Makes about ¾ cup

1 small bunch cilantro (about 8 sprigs), stems cut and discarded, plus extra for garnish

1 large bunch basil (about 12 sprigs), stems cut and discarded

2 small garlic cloves, peeled

4 tablespoons lemon juice (from about 2 medium lemons)

3 tablespoons water

½ cup extra-virgin olive oil

½ teaspoon fine sea salt

Add the cilantro leaves, basil leaves, garlic, lemon juice, water, oil, and salt to a powerful blender. Blend until pureed, vivid green, tasty, and bright. Adjust the salt to your taste. Store in an airtight container in the fridge for up to 3 days.

LIME-PICKLED ONIONS

These are super fun and so delicious that you may want to double the recipe for a week's worth of meals. Red onions make a zippier pickle, but there's no shame in using a sweet white onion.

Makes about 1 cup

¼ cup (60 ml) lime juice

¼ cup (60 ml) filtered water

1 tablespoon maple sugar

1 teaspoon sea salt

½ large white or red onion, peeled and
　　sliced ¼-inch thick

1. Combine the lime juice, water, sugar, and salt in a medium bowl and mix until the sugar dissolves.

2. Toss the onion in the pickling liquid a few times until well coated. Let sit for 30 minutes, tossing the onions four or five times while they marinate. Serve with everything. Store in an airtight container in the fridge for up to 3 days.

MUSHROOM POWDER

Mushroom powder is my secret flavor bomb. My recipe takes mere minutes to make so whiz up a big batch for your spice shelf—you can use it in everything that asks to be a bit more savory.

Makes about ⅔ cup

2 ounces (56 g) dried mushrooms
　　(shiitake, porcini, or portobello
　　work well)

1. Clean out your coffee grinder by whizzing up uncooked rice in it twice to remove all coffee granules. In the coffee grinder, whiz up the mushrooms in whatever quantity will fit in your grinder. Grind until all the mushrooms are in powder form. Be sure to clean out your grinder by whizzing up more uncooked rice just after you grind the mushrooms.

2. When ready to funnel into a jar, pour the mixture onto a piece of parchment paper and angle the paper to create a narrow funnel through which the mixture can easily glide into the jar. Store in an airtight jar at room temperature for up to 1 year.

PEACH PICO DE GALLO

My classic Tomato Pico de Gallo is perhaps one of the most asked-about recipes from my first cookbook. It's the sort of family heirloom that no one remembers its exact origin; only that it's always existed and is an important part of my family's story. My version provides the simplest of blueprints for so many ridiculously good produce combinations. This one is filled with ripe peaches and brightens every humdrum dish. You can replace the peaches, if desired, with strawberries, nectarines, or even a mix of dark fruits.

Makes about 2 cups

2 medium red onions, peeled and
    finely diced

2 medium peaches, finely diced

½ jalapeño, seeds and ribs removed,
    finely diced

2 scallions, trimmed and finely diced

3 tablespoons finely chopped
    cilantro leaves

2 tablespoons lime juice
    (from about 1 lime)

2 teaspoons lemon juice
    (from about ½ medium lemon)

½ teaspoon fine sea salt

6 twists freshly ground black pepper

1. Put the onions, peaches, jalapeño, scallions, cilantro, lime juice, lemon juice, salt, and pepper in a medium bowl. Stir to combine well.

2. Refrigerate for 1 to 2 hours to let flavors fully mesh or until ready to use. Store in an airtight container in the fridge for up to 3 days.

RECIPE VARIATION

Tomato Pico de Gallo: For a more classic version, substitute 2 medium finely diced tomatoes for the peach and 1 teaspoon of ketchup.

SMOKY MAYONNAISE

This smoky mayonnaise, made with vegan mayonnaise and a bit of smoked paprika, is wonderful on every sandwich, wrap, and burrito. You may well want to double the recipe and store it in the fridge for the week ahead.

Makes ¼ cup

¼ cup (60 ml) vegan mayonnaise

¼ teaspoon smoked paprika

Mix the mayonnaise with the paprika in a small bowl. Set in the fridge until ready to use.

QUICK PICKLED TURNIPS

This is my go-to quick pickle recipe. I use salad turnips here as they're incredible when just harvested, sweet and crunchy, but you can use this brine with any vegetable.

Makes about ¾ cup

¼ cup (60 ml) rice vinegar

¼ cup (60 ml) apple cider vinegar
  or coconut vinegar

¼ cup (60 ml) water

1 tablespoon maple sugar

1 teaspoon sea salt

2 salad turnips or radishes, julienned

2 large garlic cloves, peeled

Combine the rice vinegar, apple cider vinegar, water, sugar, and salt in a medium bowl and whisk until the sugar dissolves. Add the turnips and garlic and make sure they're submerged in the liquid. Marinate for 20 minutes and use immediately. The turnips get more sour as they sit, though they remain delicious for 1 or 2 days. Store in a sealed jar in the fridge for up to 3 days.

TOMATILLO SALSA VERDE

I put up pounds of tomatillos in the fall, when the local harvest is both bursting and affordable, and make this salsa verde until my stash runs out. Certainly, it's best with fresh tomatillos but you'd be surprised at how thawed tomatillos still taste vibrantly green and ready for amping up warm dishes.

Makes about 2 cups

1 pound (454 g) fresh tomatillos,
  husked, rinsed, and halved

½ medium white onion, peeled and
  roughly chopped

1 large garlic clove, peeled

½ jalapeño, roughly chopped

1 small bunch cilantro (about 10 sprigs),
  stems cut and discarded

1 tablespoon extra-virgin olive oil

1 tablespoon lemon juice
  (from about ½ medium lemon)

1½ teaspoons sea salt, plus more to taste

Put the tomatillos, onion, garlic, jalapeño, cilantro, oil, lemon juice, and salt in a powerful blender and blend, adding 1 or 2 tablespoons of water, if needed, to reach a smooth (but not entirely pureed) consistency. Taste and add more lemon juice or salt, as needed. Store in an airtight container in the fridge for up to 5 days.

Sweet Satisfaction

I haven't given up sweets, preserves, or pie dough in my new way to food. I've simply changed up my versions to make them a bit more wholesome. These recipes satiate a sweet craving in the sort of way that makes me feel A-OK all the time. Also see the Smoky Strawberry Jam (page 185), because that flavor combo changed my sweet world.

HOT HONEY

Honey is a mixed blessing. It's quite clearly sugar and should be consumed in moderation. However, it's lower on the glycemic index than white or brown cane sugar, which makes it more appealing. Honey does have some antioxidant and antibacterial properties, and some say eating a spoonful of local raw honey daily will stave off allergy symptoms. I haven't necessarily found that to be true but it's a lovely thought every time I put a smidge in my tea. This recipe is a blend of my two favorites: honey and hot peppers. If you've never experienced the joy of something that's sweet and truly spicy in one bite, give this honey a go. It's a luxurious condiment for a share board and anything savory, like pizza.

Makes 1 cup

2 Fresno chiles, sliced in half and seeded

2 dried chiles (Thai, Fresno, Arbol, jalapeño), crushed

1 cup (12 oz; 340 g) light honey

1. Clean a jar in hot, soapy water. Sterilize the jar by running it through a dishwasher at the hottest setting or boiling it in a pot on the stove for 10 minutes. Allow to air dry.

2. Place the peppers and honey in a small saucepan set over medium-high heat. Bring to a simmer (tiny bubbles will appear around the edge of the pan) and simmer for 4 to 5 minutes. Remove from the heat and allow to sit at room temperature for 10 minutes.

3. Pour the honey through a strainer to remove (and discard) the peppers. Pour into your desired jar. For the longest shelf life, store in the fridge for up to 4 months but bring to room temperature before each use. The honey will keep for 2 months stored at room temperature.

PIE DOUGH

This is my favorite pie dough, ever. Certainly, it doesn't deliver the flakiness and richness of butter but I've had dairy fanatics tell me this vegan pie crust is even better. And the dough is exceptionally easy to coax into shape and tuck into the pan. This recipe includes spelt flour for added nuttiness and a bit more protein. You can surely use all-white flour, if you prefer.

Makes one 9-inch (23 cm) pie dough

¼ cup plus 2 tablespoons (1 oz; 62 g) coconut oil, solid form

¾ cup (3⅛ oz; 90 g) all-purpose flour

½ cup (1¾ oz; 50 g) whole spelt flour

1 tablespoon maple sugar, clump-free

½ teaspoon sea salt

5 to 6 tablespoons ice-cold water

1. Chill the coconut oil for 10 minutes until fully solid.

2. Pulse together the flours, sugar, and salt in the bowl of a food processor. If making in a regular bowl, mix the dry ingredients together with a large fork or whisk.

3. Add the coconut oil to the dry ingredients and pulse until combined and the flour resembles fine breadcrumbs. Without a food processor, incorporate using a pastry cutter or two forks until the same texture is achieved. Do not use your hands to incorporate the coconut oil as it will melt quickly.

4. Add 4 tablespoons of the water and pulse or mix until the dough begins to resemble coarse breadcrumbs and sticks together when you squeeze it with your hands. Add an additional tablespoon or two of water until the dough sticks together when you pinch it and is not dry. The less water you add, the better.

continued

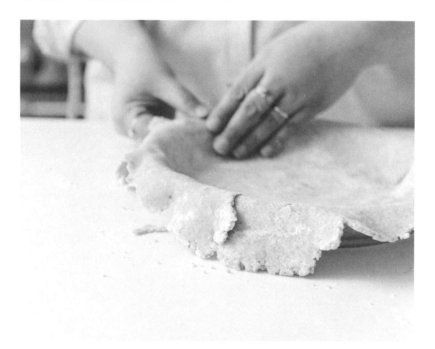

5. Flour a clean part of your counter and transfer the dough to the floured area, using a rubber spatula to get out all the stuck-to-the-bowl bits. Bring the dough together into a disk using well-floured hands. At this point, you can wrap it in plastic wrap and store it in the fridge for 2 days or the freezer for up to 1 month.

6. To use the dough immediately, smear a little coconut oil on the surface of a 9-inch (23 cm) pie plate or foil shell. Re-flour the counter, dough, and a rolling pin. Roll the dough into a thin round large enough to fit the pie plate or foil shell. Once satisfied with the shape, very lightly flour the dough and roll it up on your rolling pin. Transfer the dough to your pie plate by unrolling it gently. Using your hands, make sure the dough sits into all the nooks of the plate. Trim any large overhang and crimp the edge of the dough to your desired design. I prefer to use two fingers on the inside of the dough and one finger on the outside to make a large crimp. Once I've crimped the entire dough, I sometimes crimp again using a fork on the outside of the dough to ensure it stays in place and to make a fork imprint on the exposed dough between crimps. Chill the pie dough for 10 minutes.

7. At this point you may fill and bake the pie to your desired recipe. Cover the edges of the pie crust with foil if they become too brown during that bake.

ORGEAT SYRUP

Orgeat syrup, which I use in the Mai Tai Cocktails (page 233), riffs on a recipe from Teardrop Lounge in Portland, Oregon. Mine uses maple sugar instead of white sugar, to take it down a notch or two on the glycemic index. I also love using an ingredient from closer to home, as maple sugar is from New England.

Makes about 3 cups

3 cups (720 ml) tap water

2 cups raw almonds, sliced or slivered

3 cups (720 ml) filtered water

¼ cup (1⅜ oz; 40 g) lightly packed maple sugar

1 ounce (30 ml) brandy or vodka

¼ teaspoon orange flower water (or Cointreau, in a pinch)

1. Soak the almonds in a bowl with the tap water for 30 minutes.

2. Strain the almonds, discarding the water, and grind them in a food processor until they resemble coarse breadcrumbs.

3. Soak the ground almonds in a bowl with the filtered water for at least 4 hours and not more than 8 hours, stirring occasionally. Strain through cheesecloth into a new clean bottle with an airtight lid.

4. Add the sugar to the bottle. Shake for 10 minutes or so until the sugar is dissolved.

5. Add the brandy, to help lengthen its shelf life, and orange flower water, for amazing flavor. Shake again to combine. Store in an airtight container in the fridge for up to 1 month. Make sure to shake well before each use.

ROASTED STONE FRUIT RHUBARB JAM

In early spring, you may see long, awkward rhubarb stalks at the farm stand; I see my favorite jam. I use rhubarb in every which way—in pie, in savory stews, in cake—but I am most partial to rhubarb jam. In its natural state, rhubarb is a little sweet and a lot tart. To make it more palatable, preservers add pounds of sugar to temper the tart. I, however, just use a mix of fruit and honey. Ripe stone fruit is naturally sweet and honey is just lovely with all the fruit. A long roast in the oven practically caramelizes the fruit and honey, which makes for a very flavorful jam.

Makes 4 to 5 half-pint jars

2½ pounds (1.1 kg) peaches and apricots (fresh or frozen), pitted and diced into 1-inch pieces

½ pound (8 oz; 227 g) rhubarb (fresh or frozen), cut into ½-inch pieces

1 cup (12 oz; 340 g) light honey, like clover

Two vanilla beans, split lengthwise and scraped

1. Preheat the oven to 350°F (177°C). In a roasting dish, spread the stone fruit and rhubarb in a single layer. Drizzle the honey over the fruit and scrape the seeds from the vanilla beans across patches of the fruit, sticking the beans into the dish. Toss with a spatula to distribute the honey and vanilla bean flavor, and roast for 30 minutes (fresh fruit) or closer to 45 minutes (frozen fruit). The fruit is ready when it's easily pierced with a fork.

2. Empty the contents of the roasting dish into a deep and wide skillet over medium-high heat. Cook for 15 minutes until the fruit gets sticky and thick, and any liquid has evaporated.

3. If you're not preserving/canning the jam, allow the mixture to cool and then store in the refrigerator for up to 2 weeks in a sealed container.

4. If you are preserving the jam, bring a large pot of water with a small canning rack in it to boil. The water should be able to cover the jars on the rack by at least 2 inches. To clean the jars, wash them in hot, soapy water; you do not need to sterilize the jars, as they'll be processed for at least 10 minutes. Carefully ladle the hot jam through a regular-mouth funnel into clean jars with new airtight lids, leaving ¼ inch of headspace. Tap the jar a few times to loosen any air bubbles. Wipe the rims and seal carefully, as the jars will be hot. Using canning tongs, place the jars in a single layer in your pot of boiling water. Once the water boils again, process these jars for 15 full minutes. Turn the heat off and remove the jars to a towel on your counter. Let them sit there for 24 hours to fully seal, then store for up to 1 year in a dark pantry.

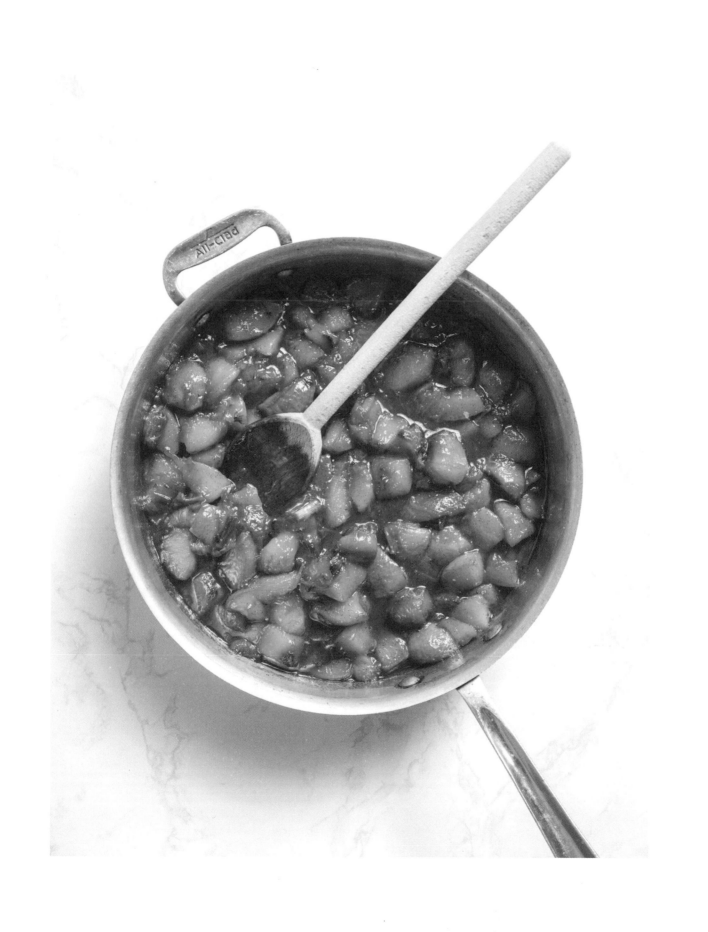

SWEET WHIPPED CREAM

Make this sweet whipped cream in advance, so the flavors and texture have some time to set up in the fridge. Use it on all the desserts.

Makes about 1 cup

¾ cup raw cashews

½ cup (120 ml) filtered water

2 tablespoons coconut cream
(if you can't find coconut cream,
use the solid part from a cold can
of coconut milk)

2 tablespoons maple syrup

¼ teaspoon ground cinnamon

¼ teaspoon sea salt

Add the cashews, water, coconut cream, maple syrup, cinnamon, and salt to a blender and whiz until thick and creamy. Use immediately or, better yet, chill it for a few hours. Store in the fridge and use within 5 days.

VERMOUTH

My sweet vermouth recipe is adapted from a recipe I came across in *Wine Enthusiast Magazine* nearly 10 years ago. The recipe was created by Sebastian Zutant, who at the time was the wine director at Washington, D.C.'s Proof restaurant. (He's since gone on to open his own natural wine bar and bistro, Primrose, with his wife, Lauren.) His base recipe is outstanding but I add a lot more twigs and berries. Some home brewers add the hops after the boil, which means they add it after the wine, the other bitter elements, spices, herbs, and flowers reach a boil. I've tried both ways and while they yield similar taste results, the final vermouth will have a clearer appearance if the hops are added just after the boil. You can sub in dry sherry for the sweet kind listed to get a dry vermouth. I included a sous vide version of this recipe because infusions are often way better in a sous vide machine. But the stovetop version works really well too.

Makes about 3 cups

FOR THE BASE WINE

One 750-ml bottle dry white wine

TO MAKE ON THE STOVETOP

1. Add the wine and all the bitter elements, spices, herbs, and flowers to a medium pot set over medium-high heat. Bring the mixture just to a boil and then turn off the heat. Place the pot on a thick towel on your countertop to cool and infuse for 8 to 12 hours.

continued

FOR THE BITTER ELEMENTS

1 tablespoon dried lemon peel

1 tablespoon dried orange peel

1 scant teaspoon pellet hops—
mild German variety like
Hallertau Blanc

Two 4-inch strips orange zest,
pith removed

2 tablespoons dark toasted wood chips
(optional)

FOR THE SPICES

1 cardamom pod, smashed

½ teaspoon coriander seeds

3 or 4 juniper berries

1 cinnamon stick

1 star anise pod

FOR THE HERBS AND FLOWERS

1 tablespoon dried chamomile flowers

2 or 3 dried culinary rose petal buds

½ teaspoon dried thyme leaves

1 vanilla bean pod, sliced open
lengthwise

FOR THE FINISHING SPIRIT

1 cup (240 ml) cream (sweet) sherry

2. Once infused, strain the solids from the infused wine using a strainer or a coffee filter. Toss the solids and add the infused wine to a clean jar with an airtight lid. Pour the sherry into the jar, seal, and shake. Your vermouth is ready to use immediately. Store it at room temperature for 2 weeks or keep in the back of your fridge for 2 months or longer.

TO MAKE IN A SOUS VIDE

1. Set up your sous vide with no racks inside, and to a temperature of 160°F (71°C).

2. Add the wine and all the bitter elements, spices, herbs, and flowers to a clean, sterilized jar with an airtight seal. Make sure the liquid fills the jar within ½ inch from the rim. Wipe the edge of the jar and seal.

3. Place the jar in the sous vide, very carefully, and place a heavy object on top of it (like a heavy pot) to hold it down. Sous vide the jar for 2 to 4 hours, depending on the desired intensity of your infusion (4 hours is optimal).

4. Just before the infused wine is ready, set up an ice bath nearby.

5. When the time allotted is reached, turn off the sous vide. Remove the jar from the water, very carefully, and sit it on a thick towel on your counter for 2 to 3 minutes. Then, plunge into an ice bath to cool it quickly.

6. Once cool, open the jar, strain the infusion through a strainer or coffee filter, and pour it into a clean glass jar. Pour the sherry into the jar, seal, and shake. Your vermouth is ready to use immediately. Store it at room temperature for 2 weeks or keep in the back of your fridge for 2 months or longer.

A revamped pantry is an ever-changing collection of ingredients, a living-breathing thing that is nurtured from day to day. You run out of some items, you replenish some, you stumble upon brand new ingredients that amp up your pantry further. Use the basics of my revamped pantry as a blueprint for creating your own kind of pantry that is simultaneously wholesome and easy to utilize. I also think a revamped pantry should be kind of exciting—it provides a whole new way to pull together fantastic dishes that nourish and charm both you and your family.

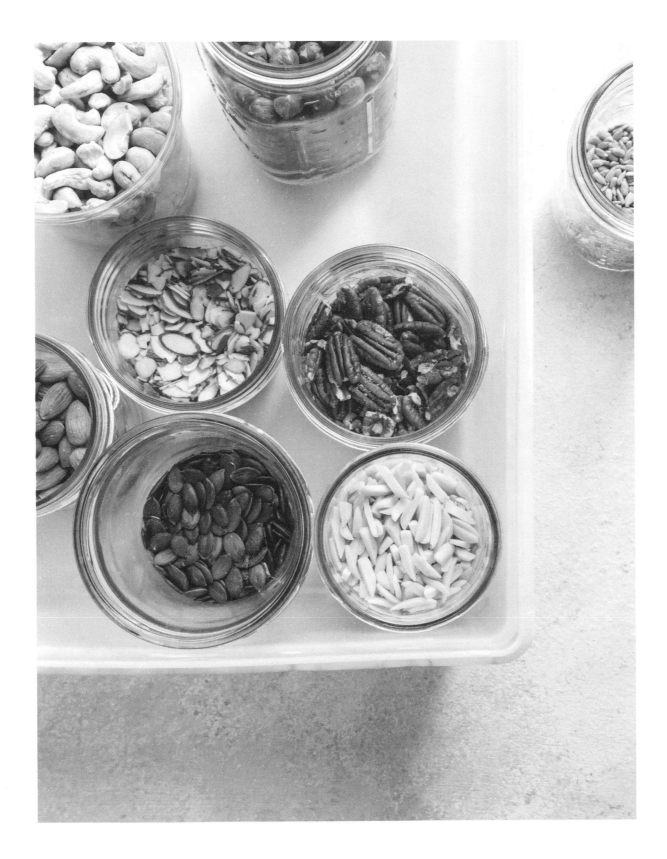

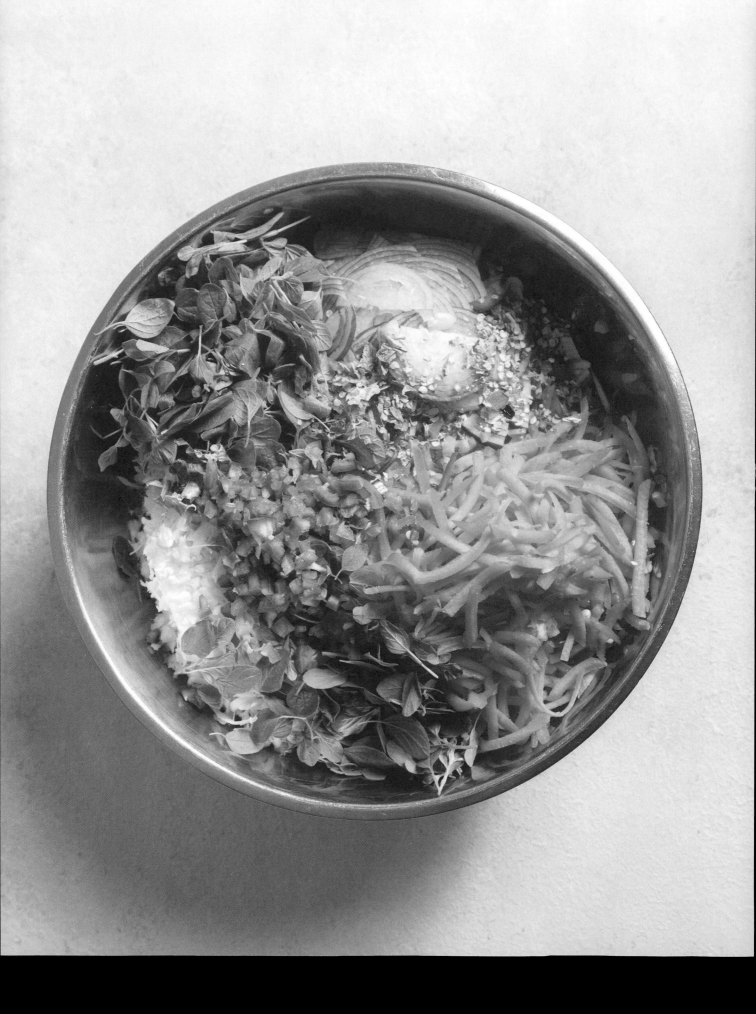

PART TWO

A New Way to Food

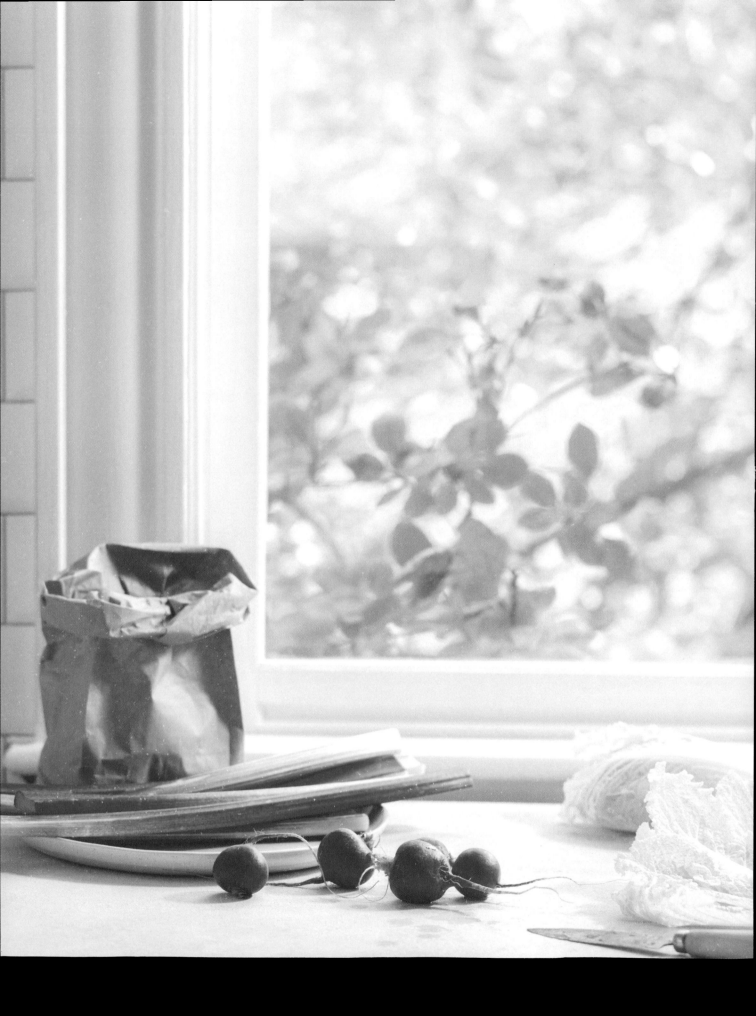

4

LOVE YOUR BODY
Recipes for Active Wellness Mode

It's possible to love yourself and exist in a place of real wellness every single day. Eating like you're worthy of good health is not about restriction or deprivation—quite the opposite; it's about eating all the foods that make you feel strong and healthy. Love your body by honoring it with nourishing foods.

This chapter includes recipes for many of the dishes I ate during my elimination diet and what I eat when I'm in active wellness mode. They include lots of vegetables because produce is really what made me love me. You'll also see recreations of my favorite meals, just with more wholesome ingredients.

Oh, Sherrie

WHEN I MET MY HEALTH COACH, SHERRIE, I didn't really know what to expect. Little did she know, she was my last-ditch effort to getting healthier. In fact, a month prior, a doctor, not my primary care, had suggested that I consider stomach reduction surgery. She said it so matter-of-factly during a routine exam, as if it was such an easy permanent fix—when we all know that any surgery is challenging and that reduction surgery comes with some steep consequences, including not being able to eat certain foods I loved for the rest of my life. In the same breath, she said, "You're not quite at the weight minimum for the surgery but I bet we can figure out some way to get you on the list." I rarely say or write this word because I don't live in the 1700s but I was *flabbergasted*.

That tiny conversation with that doctor made me examine how I cared for myself and, most definitely, the people and systems I chose to look after me from year to year. First, it was *bonkers* (another word I rarely say or write) that a doctor was willing to inflate my size somehow to make a major surgery possible. Second—and it may be *bonkers* that I grabbed on to this takeaway—but if I wasn't big enough for stomach reduction surgery, then perhaps I could still do this without extreme measures (cutting into my body = extreme measures). Perhaps, I could still get healthier and smaller through eating less and moving more.

Sherrie was equally saddened by this story, which proved that she was instantly on my side. And given that my not-so-great health was a lifelong issue, it was hard to find someone, anyone, on my side. Throughout my life, I was the problem. I was doing everything wrong. Thank goodness, recent research has shown that the fat in our bodies is more like a living, breathing organ with a goal to stay alive and present to feed your body whenever you need it. In obese individuals, research shows that fat fights you in weight loss, trying to keep you fat, to keep that fat around in case you need it down the line. Sure, I hadn't made great food choices for much of my life but, in some way, even my own fat wasn't on my side.

Sherrie, however, was really on my side. Sherrie didn't judge me. If anything, she believed that I had been misled or wrongly educated on the crux of my health issues. Gosh, an entire society of people have been misled about fat. Unlike every single nutritionist, health coach, personal trainer, and doctor whom I had worked with over decades, Sherrie didn't see me as the problem. She saw me as the solution. And with the right knowledge, she believed I could get a handle on my health, once and for all.

Sherrie is truly a rad lady who believed in me from the get-go, which makes her one of the dearest people to me forever and ever. But I also believe a big reason that her help actually helped me is because she was a complete stranger. She was a friend of a friend, whom I had never met before. And Sherrie lived halfway across the country, so instead of meeting up in person, all of our meetings were conducted online or over the phone. I believe the distance between us kept her objective. She knew I had tried to lose weight so many times. She knew I was obese. But she gave me permission to see myself as something more than a fat girl. To her, I was a regular girl trying to get help with a problem. And given that her nutritional education was so recent, she had modern-day advice that just made way more sense to me.

THE ELIMINATION DIET

Sherrie suggested I take on a total elimination diet. An elimination diet would involve removing everything that could cause allergies, inflammation, digestive issues, nutritional deficiencies, and, for me, obesity, from my daily food intake. Elimination diets range in terms of what exact foods are allowed and removed, but most cut out gluten, dairy, soy, refined sugar, alcohol, eggs, and processed food. Some also cut out peanuts and corn (although I didn't eliminate those entirely). After getting rid of all these foods, I'd reintroduce everything one at a time to figure out which foods made me feel good and which ones were, well, not supportive of my potentially healthy body.

I had been so reluctant to do an elimination diet in the past because, hello, I love all the foods. But one week later, I was the fat girl opting to only put plants in my mouth and I abruptly stopped all refined sugar, caffeine, animal products, dairy, gluten, certain oils (like bad fats), alcohol, and packaged/processed or fast foods.

The first few days were such a challenge. Let's be honest, they felt impossible. I had a five-day headache from the caffeine withdrawals. Previously, my body lived off ample quantities of sugar, in all its forms, and the withdrawals from that alone forced me to put anything and everything into my mouth to fill the vacancy. Growing up, I was slapped on the hand for fondling (and subsequently eating) olives, nuts, or avocado, but during my first few days of this elimination diet, I consumed them with wild abandon. Giving up alcohol and animal products made me itchy, figuratively, as it was one of the major connection points between my husband, Don, and me. I certainly consulted him, but at the same time, I had to make this decision for me and not anyone else, nor with anyone else.

I decided to go on a plant-based diet mainly because it was Sherrie's area of expertise and, of all the programs I'd tried since I was ten years old, it was the easiest food plan for me to understand. Most importantly, portion control is less of an issue when you're eating only vegetables, fruit, good fats, seeds, nuts, and legumes. And, let's be real, I've always had a problem with authority, especially any sort of authority telling me how much I can eat. After years of everyone telling me what to eat and what not to eat, sometimes keeping it away from my mouth intentionally (more on that in chapter 5), I needed a new way of eating that would not immediately factor in portion control. Rather, portion control would be something to tackle slowly, after I got the good foods into me.

Over time (meaning months), I added eggs, fish, and whole grains back in—though I still keep gluten-free pasta in my pantry because I like the texture in certain dishes. I added in a weekend glass of wine yet continued to steer clear of cocktails because of the unnatural sugars. And after losing seventy pounds over the course of one year, I added in a small portion of grass-fed beef on Saturday nights.

To be clear, I wasn't over-the-top reckless. I did all this active wellness mode stuff in cooperation with my primary care doctor. When I shared my plan, she was supportive, offering up a complementary vitamin regime and ways to get enough nutrients, like protein (i.e., prioritize greens, beans, and eggs) or calcium (i.e., cauliflower, dark greens, broccoli, okra, and tofu).

With this new way of thinking about food, my meals changed dramatically. Most mornings, smoothies loaded with vegetables, fruit, nuts, seeds, and good fats were my breakfast of choice. Lunchtime salads became bigger and more vibrant, filled with a myriad of ingredients versus the same old lettuce leaves and cherry tomato halves. Animal-protein-filled dinner plates were recast as quick bean hashes, veggie sautés, and spiced-up stews. My meals were suddenly invigorating.

Without eating refined sugar, I craved sweets less, opting instead for avocado with a squeeze of lime or a few squares of dark chocolate dipped in almond butter. And instead of complaining about how expensive it is to eat healthfully or even organic, I bought mostly plants and a lot less animal protein and, sure thing, my monthly food budget was halved almost instantly.

I ate all the vegetables, fruits, nuts, seeds, good fats, and whole grains that I wanted, sometimes feeling stuffed from all the goodness in my belly. I ate all I wanted and I lost weight—this was a radical discovery for me. I had spent decades restricting every sort of food and now I could eat anything plant-based, and still lose weight. Radical, indeed. But it wasn't all about the food.

TRACK HOW YOU FEEL

The most critical part of my elimination diet was what I did after eating the food, quite literally. I listened to the gurgling sounds of my stomach and started to feed myself before they got loud. I paid attention to any headaches and noticed that I started having far fewer than ever before. I was aware of every bathroom break, and how I felt afterward. My lifelong sinus issues felt more in control and rarely morphed into full-on bacterial infections. I felt stronger, less tired, and way more alert.

I remember all this because I wrote it all down. After eating, I engaged in a daily journaling ritual that logged the foods that made me feel fit and the ones that didn't. My days went from eating food mostly for comfort to eating food for fuel and—gasp!—to simply feel really darn good. I paid attention to my body, listening to what it craved, what it wanted absolutely nothing to do with, and what made it feel altogether awesome.

The journaling process evolved with me. I started with pencil and paper but eventually I switched to electronic journaling. Each week, I'd start a note in an online application, like Evernote, and jot down the date, the new foods, and how I felt. I liked using an online application because it let me record notes on the go through my mobile phone. I kept it quite short and direct, so as to not give myself an excuse to avoid journaling. I reviewed my notes regularly with Sherrie and she'd offer alternatives or advice based on what I discovered. It became an immensely valuable back-and-forth process that helped me get over humps and not let a particular food reaction discourage me.

Thanks to an elimination diet, thanks to eating a plant-based diet, and thanks to logging all the feelings over the course of a year, my body morphed down to a shape and size I hadn't seen in more than ten years. I was over-the-moon with my progress, mainly because it wasn't just about weight loss. During my elimination diet, I learned to listen to my body, to really listen to whatever was happening inside me, for the first time. I've now created my own way of eating that works for me year-round.

NO LOOKING BACK

If you decide that either an elimination diet or a mostly plant-centric way of eating is worth a go, then first, please, consult your doctor. As I mentioned earlier, my doctor was pretty amazing about it all—and she isn't so enthusiastic about most diets. However, I don't imagine all doctors would feel the same so find someone you trust to offer up their twenty-five cents.

If you opt to do all the hard work to get you to a place of wellness, then do not let anything stand in your way. But also understand humans are not perfect. There will be hiccups. There will be moments when you absolutely feel the need to chomp down on three chocolate bars in one sitting. There will be moments when you don't stick to your chosen plan. Any momentary alterations are way okay, okay?

The fact is, changing the way you eat, the thing you've been taught to do a certain way since birth, is hard. Every major life change is hard. Existing in active wellness mode is hard. Any change to get a bit lighter, a bit stronger, a bit more in tune with your body, a bit healthier, all of the above, is challenging. If you don't stick to your chosen plan over the course of many months, then you may need to reconsider if it's the right plan or the right time for you. However, if you don't stick to your chosen plan once in a while, then please forgive yourself and carry on.

Even now, there are days when I rip open a package of milk chocolate and briskly stuff it into my face, but I quickly accept the moment, forgive myself, and simply say "onward." Please feel free to make a multitude of mishaps and then carry onward because you can do this, I promise you.

Practicing Self-Care, For Real

There seems to be some sort of mass hysteria around prioritizing self-care these days. Certainly, to practice self-care is trendy and of the moment in a way it's really never been before. For example, I don't remember my mother mentioning self-care in the eighties. But in the way busier world that we live in now, it's just plain necessary.

Self-care is critical to a balanced life and if the concept needs to be splashed about in the media for a few more years, I'm totally okay with that. Perhaps the self-care oversaturation will make it so we all really do shift our mindset toward prioritizing our own wellness so we can do our jobs well, take care of our family, and lead somewhat meaningful and satisfying lives (whatever that means to each of us).

The concept of self-care came up in my regular chats with my health coach, Sherrie, who positioned her advice in a way that made self-care seem normal and necessary rather than something extra. Over time, I explored all of the following and figured out what they meant to me in my life:

Lemon water: Every morning, I drink a sixteen-ounce glass of water with a hefty squeeze of fresh lemon juice. This helps cleanse my system and prepare it for all the nutrient-dense food to come that day. I even cart lemons in my luggage on vacation, to make sure I can have my daily lemon water.

Meal maps: Instead of planning out meals one by one, I map out meals for the week. This allows me the opportunity to cook well in advance, typically on Sundays, and plan around any special meals out that involve extra indulgent food. (See chapter 2 for more on this.)

Dry brushing: I engage in a dry brushing ritual each morning before jumping into a warm shower. The dry brushing does two things. First, the brushing sweeps away dead skin cells from the biggest organ of my body, my skin, and stimulates the lymphatic system, the system that collects and transports waste to the blood. Second, the act of brushing my skin requires me to look at every inch of my naked body daily. That process got me to recognize, appreciate, and eventually, love me. I encourage everyone to give it a go.

Skin moisturizer: Putting on moisturizer after a shower just makes sense. I find that using oil versus lotion maximizes the moisturizing benefits and returns all those essential oils stripped from the skin during a shower. In place of store-bought lotions, I apply almond, coconut, or olive oil to my skin daily.

Beauty product clean out: As I got healthier, Sherrie encouraged me to go through all the beauty products in my bathroom and toss any that contained potentially harmful products. Some beauty products contain phthalates and parabens, chemicals that can interfere with the body's hormones and have been found to be associated with certain forms of cancer. My beauty cabinet reduced in size but my peace of mind increased. I now only use beauty products that contain no chemicals known to be harmful to our bodies.

Weighing yourself: While on an elimination diet, I weighed myself daily. This helped me learn which foods lingered longer in the body and which encouraged weight loss. Nowadays, I only weigh myself one or two times per week.

Exercise: It's important to reckon with your take on exercise when you're ready. As I began to feel better, I wanted to walk regularly and would often park my car far away from meeting spots and shop doors to encourage that walking. However, I didn't exercise habitually while on the elimination diet; it is an entirely different beast that I had to conquer separately. I'm finding my way to movement now.

Inspiration everywhere: As I worked my way through that first year, I watched films, read books, and listened to podcasts that supported a healthier lifestyle. I gleaned bits of inspiration from everywhere and found tips to incorporate into my wellness regime.

TEN TIPS TO GET STARTED

While my first year of change was challenging because I was doing so many new-to-me things, it was also dynamic and exciting. I was learning constantly and I was listening to my body for the first time in forever. That year was packed with lessons that I carry with me, wherever I am, wherever I go. Many of them may seem obvious now, years later, but they add up to an entirely different way to think about what goes into my mouth. These are ten tips to consider as you get started.

1. *Forget exercise for now.* If you want to lose an enormous amount of weight, you do not necessarily need to exercise to reach some of your early goals. Sure, every doctor will tell you that regular physical activity provides benefits way beyond just weight loss—it stimulates your brain, reduces anxiety, tones and tightens your body (if that matters to you), and provides quality self-care time. But all you really need to do is change how you eat. Start with that and let exercise work its way into your life when you feel stronger and if you decide it's something you want to do.

2. *Make plants the star of your plate.* There's so much competing data and a billion opinions about what makes a nutritious meal. Ask a farmer, a Food and Drug Administration official, and a holistic nutritionist and you'll get wildly different answers. The winning choice for me was to make a plant the heroine of every dish. (I use the term "plant" broadly to include vegetables, fruits, nuts, legumes, seeds, grains, etc.) Eventually, I added in an egg or small piece of fish here and there as supporting characters, but I continued to make the plant part of the meal compelling and spectacular.

3. *Vegetables have protein.* Don't let anyone declare that vegetables don't have protein. Of course, the protein in a piece of red meat dwarfs the amount of protein in a pile of greens. But greens have about 3 grams of protein per cup and you need to eat several cups in a satisfying meal. Beans have plenty of protein—a cup of pinto beans has about 40 grams of protein—as do nuts (a half-cup portion of whole almonds has about 15 grams). While varying agencies offer different statistics, the average-sized woman who doesn't exercise daily should get anywhere between 45 and 60 grams of protein daily. This is easily possible by eating a variety of vegetables, legumes, nuts, and seeds.

4. *Eat a colorful salad daily.* This is a brilliant way to make sure you're getting ample vegetables into your body. I typically add a salad to whatever I'm eating for lunch or dinner, often just squirting the leaves with lemon juice and a sprinkle of sea salt and freshly ground black pepper. If you're hesitant to cook a completely veg-filled meal, perhaps because your family craves other stuff, begin by adding a salad and seeing how that feels. A big salad nourished me, keeping me fuller longer and giving me the energy I needed to get on with life.

5. *Limit your sugar consumption.* I cut sugar out resolutely during my elimination diet, which helped me stave off my taste for sweets; when I wasn't consuming it, I wasn't craving it. If you do eat sugar, try alternative sweeteners instead. Fruit-based sweeteners like apples, dates, and bananas work great in smoothies, warm cereal and oatmeal, and baked goods. A little maple syrup or coconut sugar is okay too. Whatever you do, steer clear of refined sugars that will spike your blood sugar levels fast and then send you crashing hard. Empty your pantry of them, if you can, and replace them with sweeteners that will do the trick with a little less of a crash.

6. *Eat mindfully.* Whenever I was told to eat mindfully, I would roll my eyes or make a face. I mind people telling me to eat mindfully! But when I pulled my mealtimes away from the television and back to the dining room table, I actually noticed everything I ate and how it made me feel. Sometimes, when I was alone, I would actually say aloud that it was time to eat breakfast now and that momentary pause actually helped me recognize the value in the food before me. It's okay to talk aloud to set yourself up for eating mindfully. Whatever works for you, my friend.

7. *Establish your non-negotiables.* When I engaged in this elimination diet, I decided there were some food rituals that I just couldn't give up, either because they provided some comfort I wasn't ready to release or they bonded me with someone I loved. Figure out your food parameters and let yourself enjoy them.

8. *If you eat animal products, eat the best or not at all.* Not all animal products are created the same way. I realize that this is a difficult issue for some people to confront head-on. In fact, most don't even want to know that some animals are fed industrial-produced grains or pumped full of antibiotics to prevent illness from chemicals in that feed and on farmland. Antibiotics are a problem, people. The more we consume, the less they work.

I get that it's easier to buy cheap meat so you can eat it more frequently. As a society, we've done that for years. However, you can find many ethical farmers who raise cows on grass, who let them roam free in pastures, and who do so using organic methods (meaning no chemicals). This meat is more expensive but if you can't afford to eat quality meat daily, just eat it once a week or twice a month. I buy beef in bulk once or twice a year from a Vermont farmer and freeze the beef parts for year-round meals. It will take a long time to work our way out of buying cheap, chemically laden meat but if everyone ate only the very best a little less frequently, we'd get there.

9. *When you eat something new, write down how you feel.* For some, this may mean keeping a pencil and little diary in their bag for on-the-fly scribbling. For others, like me, this means using an online, note-taking tool. By writing it all down, I could notice patterns like how I felt sick soon after eating massive amounts of very sugary vegetables (beets and carrots) or how it's a little harder for me to digest very fatty animal products (like pork belly). Everybody is different and it's easiest to see patterns when logged.

10. *Don't explain or defend the way you eat.* Certainly, some people in your life—folks who you dine with or who cook for you most frequently—should get a little description of your way of eating. It's a courtesy that lets them support your food choices. That said, I discovered that the less I talked about my way of eating, the less I opened myself up to comments, feedback, advice, and potential insults. This tranquility about my food gave me the confidence to keep doing my thing. It also gave me the wisdom to shut my face about what other people ate because the food they put into their mouths is their business. Unless asked explicitly, any comments I volunteered, however well intentioned, could be taken as offensive. Outside of writing this cookbook, because I did have to lay a stake in the ground on what I eat, I avoid judging what you eat and, in turn, I hope you avoid passing judgment on what I eat, okay? Okay.

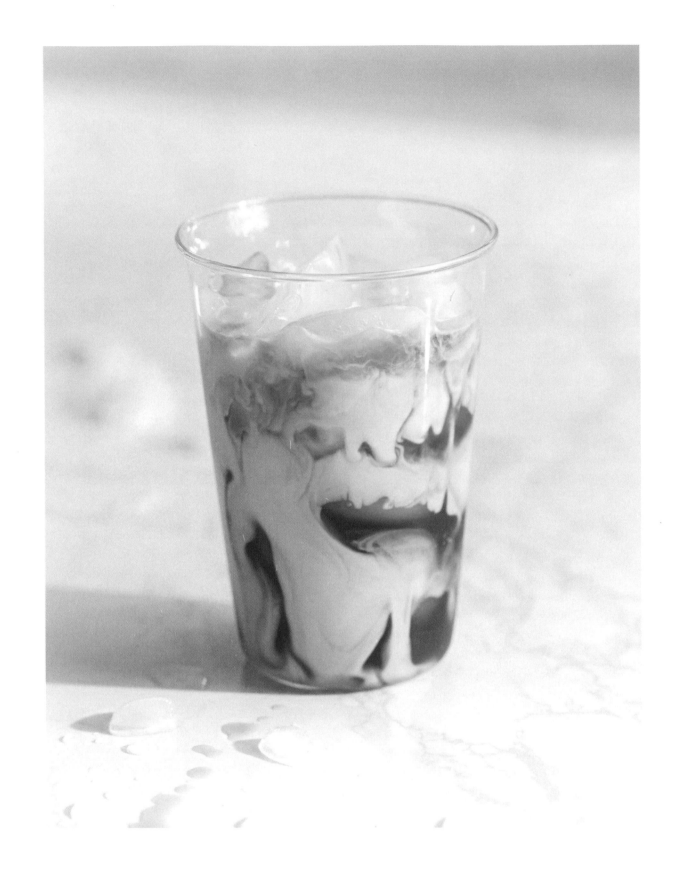

Iced CAFÉ AU LAIT

When I'm in active wellness mode, I often start my day with an extra-tall glass of water with a little lemon juice. After I sip that down, I'll brew a cup of decaffeinated black coffee if I need to get out the door quickly. But when I work from home or want a drink that's a bit more toothsome and buttery, this is what I'll make. I prefer this drink with a Bialetti-style serving of espresso or a French press full of very dark, decaffeinated coffee (because I've got enough energy for the both of us), but use whatever method or equipment you prefer.

Makes 1 drink

FREQUENCY: *Almost every day*

FOOD PREFERENCES: *DF, GF, RSF, V*

HANDS-ON TIME: *5 minutes*

TOTAL TIME: *5 minutes*

1 cup (240 ml) Almond-Date Milk
    (page 38) or plain, unsweetened
    plant milk

Ice

1 teaspoon maple syrup (optional)

1 cup (240 ml) freshly made,
    strong coffee

Add the milk and a handful of ice to a tall 16-ounce glass. If you are using unsweetened plant milk, add the maple syrup, if desired. Slowly pour in the coffee, leaving ample room at the top to add more ice, if you like. Enjoy immediately.

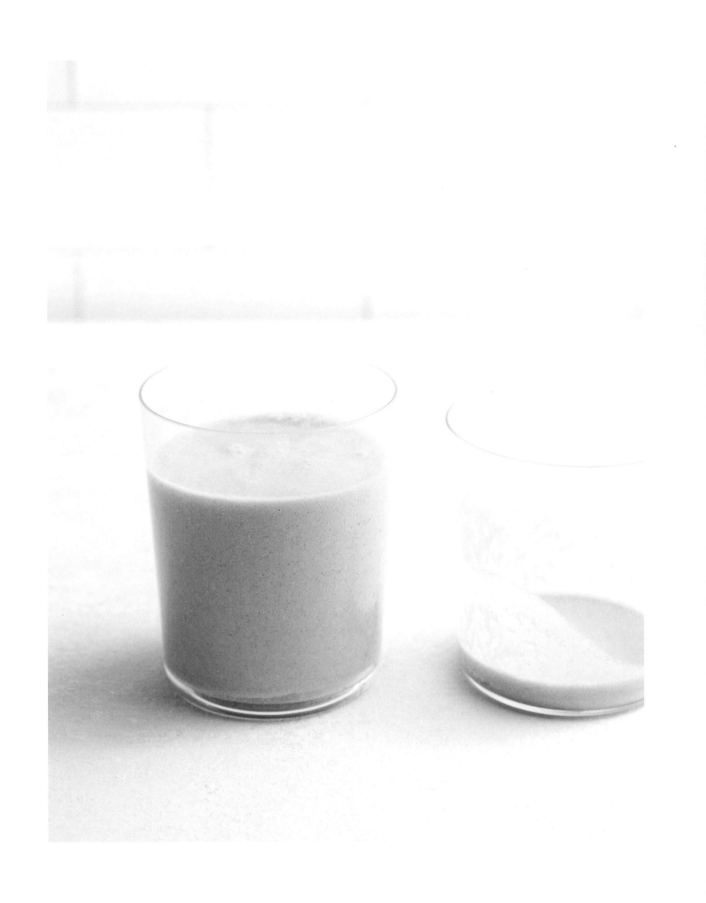

EVERYTHING GREEN *Smoothie*

It feels so strange to love smoothies. It's like I've come to the dark side as some sort of health geek who craves pureed produce with delicately sliced fruit and perfectly placed granola pieces on top. That's so not me, people. But this smoothie (and the two that follow) are just easy, fresh ways to nourish my body and feel full for much of the morning.

My go-to smoothie is a mix of green veg and green fruit, a few add-ins for richness, and both plant milk and water. You may most certainly do all plant milk but, eventually, you won't need it. The water, lime juice, and ice make this smoothie way more refreshing and less dessert-like. I use refined coconut oil in most of my recipes, as it doesn't taste so obviously of coconut flesh. If you prefer the taste of coconut, go unrefined, all the way.

In all of these recipes, I recommend that you sip your smoothie slowly. This was a suggestion from my health coach, Sherrie, and it has made such a difference in my life. Sipping slowly gives my stomach time to fill up and my taste buds time to feel the full impact of all the flavors. In turn, I appreciate the food, even celebrate and savor it.

Makes about 2 cups

FREQUENCY: *Almost every day*

FOOD PREFERENCES: *DF, GF, RSF, V*

HANDS-ON TIME: *7 minutes*

TOTAL TIME: *7 minutes*

. . . .

1 cup cleaned, roughly chopped, tightly packed greens (such as swiss chard, kale, spinach)

One 2-inch stub of cucumber, unpeeled, cleaned

1 small green apple, stem and core removed

2 tablespoons protein or superfood (such as rolled oats, black chia seeds, flax seeds, hemp seeds, protein powder)

1 tablespoon refined coconut oil

2 teaspoons maple syrup, more or less as you prefer

Pinch of sea salt

2 tablespoons lime juice (from about 1 lime)

½ cup (120 ml) Cashew Milk (page 41) or other unsweetened plant milk

½ cup (120 ml) water

4 to 6 small ice cubes

Add all the ingredients in the order listed to a powerful blender. Blend on high (or on the smoothie setting, if you have one) until smooth and cold, adding more water if your blender stalls. Enjoy immediately but sip slowly.

CHOCOLATE ZUCCHINI *Smoothie*

While the Everything Green Smoothie is garden-fresh, this smoothie is everything velvety rich and chocolatey. It's totally good for you but also feels a bit more easygoing, closer in flavor to a traditional chocolate shake. If the other smoothie recipes scream, "let's get fit," this smoothie says, "let's just chill a little and go with the flow."

When I'm in active wellness mode, I drink a full two-cup smoothie as a meal for breakfast or lunch. Sometimes, I add a smoothie onto a meal for vitamins, nourishment, or just because it tastes good. At those times, I drink half a cup to one cup alongside a salad or as an afternoon snack, saving the remainder for the next day. If you store it in an airtight container in the fridge overnight, the flavor will remain unchanged. If you want that icy cold feeling on day two, blend the remaining smoothie with a few ice cubes and enjoy immediately, but drink slowly to savor it.

Makes about 2 cups

FREQUENCY: *Almost every day*

FOOD PREFERENCES: *DF, GF, RSF, V*

HANDS-ON TIME: *7 minutes*

TOTAL TIME: *7 minutes*

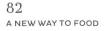

1 heaping cup shredded zucchini, fresh or frozen (about ½ small zucchini)

½ medium banana, fresh or frozen

2 tablespoons raw cacao powder

2 tablespoons protein or superfood (such as rolled oats, black chia seeds, flax seeds, hemp seeds, protein powder)

1 tablespoon coconut oil

2 teaspoons maple syrup, more or less as you prefer

⅛ teaspoon ground cinnamon

Pinch of sea salt

½ cup (120 ml) Cashew Milk (page 41) or other unsweetened plant milk

½ cup (120 ml) water

4 to 6 small ice cubes (optional, useful if zucchini is fresh)

Add all the ingredients in the order listed to a powerful blender. Blend on high (or on the smoothie setting, if you have one) until smooth and cold, adding more water if your blender stalls. Enjoy immediately but sip slowly.

TROPICAL *Smoothie*

This smoothie makes a Monday feel like a Saturday spent in the sand, surrounded by palm trees and plastic cups touched with tiny umbrellas. It's the Toasted Coconut Milk that makes all the difference. You may certainly use the store-bought, non-toasted stuff, but just once, give the full version a go.

Makes about 3 cups

FREQUENCY: *Almost every day*

FOOD PREFERENCES: *DF, GF, NF, RSF, V*

HANDS-ON TIME: *7 minutes*

TOTAL TIME: *20 minutes*

· ·

1 cup cleaned, roughly chopped, tightly packed greens (such as swiss chard, kale, spinach)

½ medium banana, fresh or frozen

1 large celery stalk

½ large fresh mango, chopped, or ⅔ cup frozen mango

2 tablespoons protein or superfood (such as rolled oats, black chia seeds, flax seeds, hemp seeds, protein powder)

1 tablespoon coconut oil

1 tablespoon maple syrup, more or less as you prefer

Pinch of sea salt

3 tablespoons lime juice

¾ cup (180 ml) Toasted Coconut Milk (page 45) or unsweetened plant milk

4 to 6 small ice cubes

Add all the ingredients in the order listed to a powerful blender. Blend on high (or on the smoothie setting, if you have one) until smooth and cold. Enjoy immediately but sip slowly.

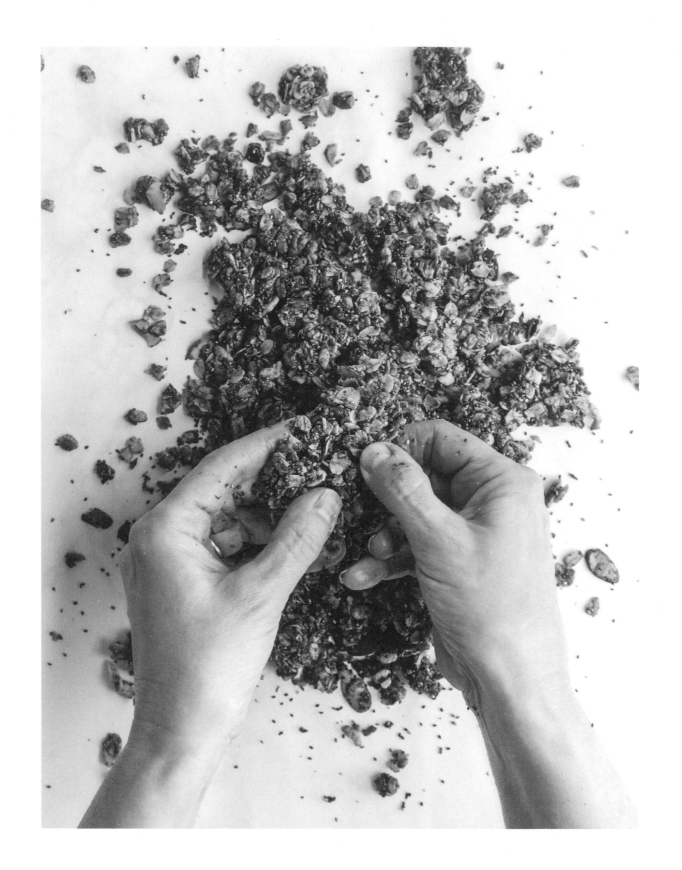

Cacao-Coffee GRANOLA

While tossing my Cacao-Coffee Granola with yogurt or piling it on top of a smoothie is totally suitable, I unabashedly stuff handfuls straight into my mouth. I don't try to be pretty about this because it's too good to worry about how I look eating it. It does make a fairly nourishing and filling snack, too. And if you bake it into cookies, well, then you'll stuff those into your mouth as well. However you decide to enjoy it is most definitely up to you.

Use whatever nuts you like, just make sure to chop them a bit so they're not too far off in size from the oats. Sometimes, I substitute rye flakes for half of the oats; they add a nice flavor nuance, different nutrients, and good texture. If you want to make this gluten-free, make sure to find gluten-free oats.

Makes about 3½ cups

FREQUENCY: *Almost every day*

FOOD PREFERENCES: *DF, GF, RSF, V*

HANDS-ON TIME: *10 minutes*

TOTAL TIME: *40 minutes*

- -

2 cups old-fashioned rolled oats
    or gluten-free oats

1 cup mixed chopped raw nuts
    (I use sliced almonds and
    chopped pecans)

½ cup black chia seeds

½ cup unsweetened shredded coconut

1 cup unsweetened crispy
    brown rice cereal

½ cup (120 ml) extra-virgin olive oil

½ cup (120 ml) maple syrup

2 tablespoons roughly ground coffee
    (regular or decaffeinated)

2 tablespoons raw cacao powder

¼ teaspoon sea salt

1. Preheat the oven to 350ºF (177°C). Line a rimmed baking sheet with parchment paper.

2. Add the oats, nuts, chia seeds, coconut, and cereal to a large bowl and toss together. Spread into a thin layer on the lined baking sheet. Roast in the oven for 8 to 10 minutes, turning the pan once.

3. Add the oil, maple syrup, ground coffee, cacao powder, and salt to a medium pot over medium heat. Stir while you bring it to a simmer. Simmer until everything blends together, about 3 minutes. Remove from the heat and strain through a fine-mesh colander or cheesecloth to remove the coffee grounds.

4. Remove the granola mix from the oven and, using the parchment paper, carefully slide the warmed granola back into a large bowl, returning the parchment back to the baking sheet. Pour the warm liquid over the granola and stir until every bit is touched by the liquid.

5. Spread the granola into a thin layer on the lined baking sheet. Roast in the oven for 12 minutes, turning the pan once. Remove from the oven and let it sit on the range for 10 minutes. Break into bite-sized pieces (or your preferred size) and let cool completely. Store in an airtight container at room temperature for up to 1 week.

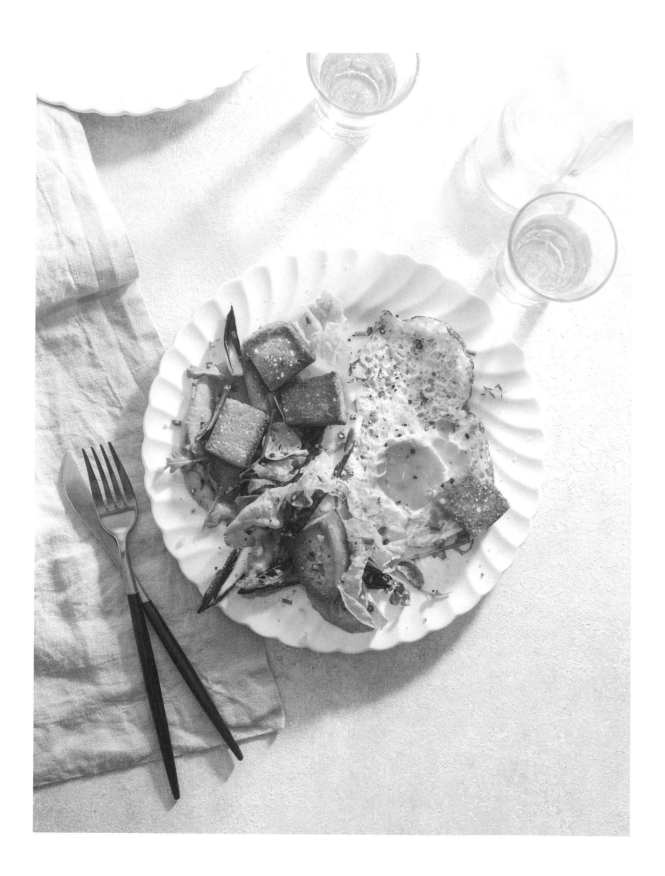

BREAKFAST TOAST SALAD *with a Fried Egg*

Soon into my health turnaround, I noticed that when I ate vegetables first thing in the morning, I felt fuller longer and way more energetic. After a produce-filled smoothie, I was ready to go, go, go, and after this crisp salad, I felt lighter on my feet, ready to get into the ring and tear up the day.

This is something of a quickie salad—just use lemon, lime, or vinegar in the dressing, and whatever leaves you have in your fridge. I often buy a bagful of butter lettuce, spinach, or green chard leaves early in the week to use just for breakfast. The toast is entirely up to your taste and while a dark seedy loaf would be so nourishing, I love using Sandwich Bread (page 34) expressly for this salad. You can further hearty-up this dish, or share it, with two eggs versus one.

Serves 1

FREQUENCY: *Almost every day*

FOOD PREFERENCES: *DF, NF, RSF*

HANDS-ON TIME: *15 minutes*

TOTAL TIME: *15 minutes*

· ·

2 teaspoons coconut vinegar or
    white wine vinegar

1 teaspoon lemon juice (from about
    ½ medium lemon)

3 tablespoons extra-virgin olive oil

¼ teaspoon sea salt, plus more
    for seasoning

6 twists freshly ground black pepper,
    plus more for seasoning

½ small head butter lettuce, leaves
    cleaned and torn into small pieces

1 slice sourdough bread, cut into
    1-inch squares

1 egg

Hot sauce, to serve (optional)

1. Add the vinegar, lemon juice, 1 tablespoon of the oil, the salt, and black pepper to a jar. Shake until well combined and set aside.

2. Put the lettuce in a medium bowl and pour over the dressing. Toss a few times to ensure the leaves are well coated in dressing. Place the salad on a serving plate.

3. Warm 1 tablespoon of the oil in a frying pan set over medium-high heat. Toss the bread squares into the warm oil and fry until golden brown, 4 to 5 minutes. Make sure to turn or toss the bread a few times to get an even color. Season and toss with a pinch of salt and pepper. Pour the bread over the salad.

4. In the same frying pan set over medium-high heat, warm the remaining 1 tablespoon oil. Crack the egg into the pan and fry until the white part is set and the yellow part is still just a touch wobbly (sunny side up) or until how you prefer your egg. Turn the heat off.

5. Slide the egg on top of the salad. Sprinkle the entire dish with extra salt or pepper, to taste. Add a little hot sauce to the egg, if you'd like. Serve immediately.

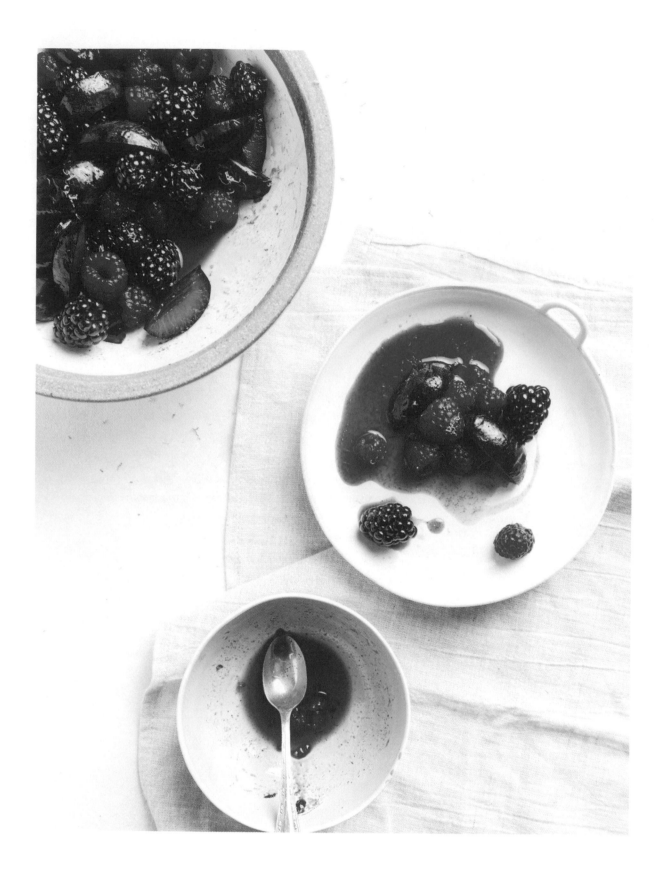

Smoked RED FRUIT SALAD

This recipe is what saved fruit salad for me. I grew up eating tins filled with syrupy sweet peaches in little plastic cups of tutti-frutti mix studded with candied cherries; those styles made me run fast from every kind of fruit salad. But well into my reintroduction to fresh produce, I noticed I was avoiding fruit. That gave me pause. The actual fruit wasn't the villain, only the cloying sauce that often took on a perfumed, almost unnatural taste of its own.

Since my tastes had changed as an adult, leaning savory versus sweet, I sprinkled a little smoked paprika on some fruit and, phew, fruit was instantly saved. Now I don't sprinkle spices on all of my fruit but if there's a red fruit in sight, it gets smoked paprika. It also gets a little lime and, if the fruit is super tart, a splash of maple syrup. This is medium-smoky and not over the top. If you want a smokier taste, just add more smoked paprika.

Serves 4 to 6

FREQUENCY: *Almost every day*

FOOD PREFERENCES: *DF, GF, NF, RSF, V*

HANDS-ON TIME: *20 minutes*

TOTAL TIME: *20 minutes*

. . . .

1 cup blackberries

3 to 5 purple or red plums, thinly sliced

2 cups sweet cherries, pitted, or black raspberries

¼ teaspoon smoked paprika

1 tablespoon lime juice (from about ½ lime), plus more to taste

1 tablespoon maple syrup (optional)

½ teaspoon lime zest (from about 1 lime), for garnish

1. Add the blackberries, plums, and cherries to a medium bowl. If you'd like, slice some of the cherries in half to show their intense color. Don't toss the fruit together just yet, as it's delicate.

2. Sprinkle the smoked paprika over the fruit. Add the lime juice and maple syrup, if using. With a larger dinner spoon, carefully toss the fruit together, coating all the fruit in spices and juice.

3. Taste and add more spice or syrup, to your preference. Let sit for a few minutes for the flavors to meld. Before serving, garnish with lime zest.

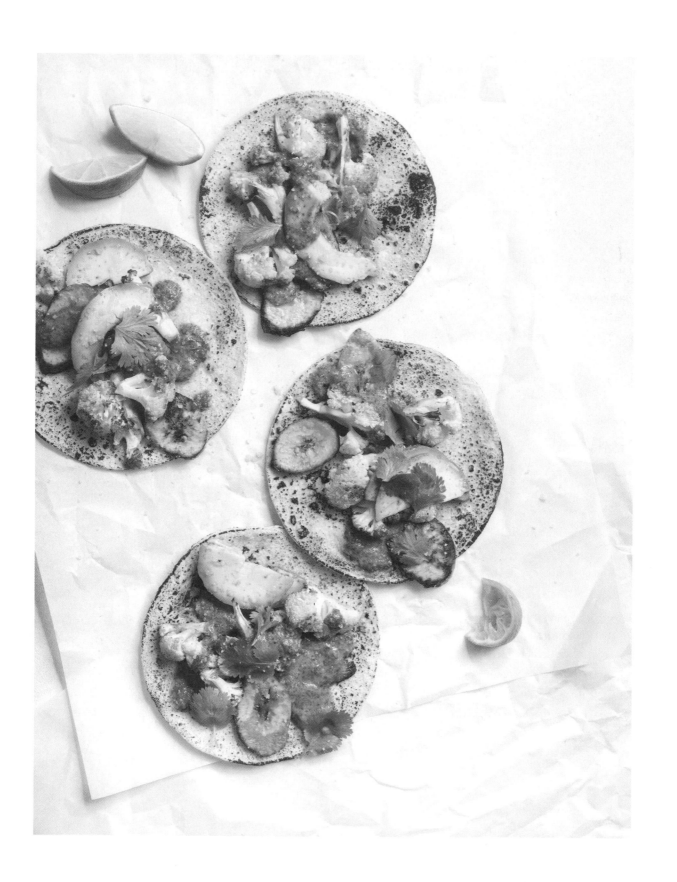

CAULIFLOWER AND PLANTAIN TACOS
with Lemony Pesto Dressing

The magic of this weeknight meal is the mix of sweet plantain with savory cauliflower—it's a fabulous combination. With the creamy avocado and bright, tangy pesto dressing, the entire taco is a real winner. Don't let the fact that I use two baking sheets to roast the veg stop you from giving this recipe a try. If you want, use one very large sheet and keep the vegetables separated so you can scoop either one off the sheet easily the moment it's ready.

Instead of cauliflower, you may opt for broccoli or even thickly sliced cabbage wedges—just slice the core of the cabbage out after it roasts and before you assemble the tacos. Plantains are starchy and slightly sweet, which I likely adore because they were the early morning breakfast candy of my childhood. But if you don't want to mess with them for any reason, a white yam works beautifully too. It delivers the same texture and taste sensation.

Buy an avocado about two days in advance so it ripens in time. If you opt to buy versus make your tortillas, please scrutinize the ingredients on your tortilla packaging. Most tortillas sold everywhere (even at the natural grocers) contain sugar. Search for an all-natural version that only uses corn, water, and lime. Save your sugar for dessert.

Serves 2

FREQUENCY: *Almost every day*

FOOD PREFERENCES: *DF, GF, NF, RSF, V*

HANDS-ON TIME: *20 minutes*

TOTAL TIME: *40 minutes*

. . . .

1 small head cauliflower, broken into small florets

2 tablespoons extra-virgin olive oil, divided

¼ teaspoon smoked paprika

½ teaspoon sea salt, divided

1 large ripe plantain or 1 small white yam, peeled and sliced into coins

4 Tortillas, homemade (page 36) or any natural, sugar-free corn tortillas

¾ cup Lemony Pesto Dressing (page 53)

1 avocado, pitted, peeled, and thinly sliced (optional)

1 small bunch cilantro (about 10 sprigs), stems cut and discarded (optional)

1. Preheat the oven to 350°F (177°C). Line two baking sheets with parchment paper.

2. On one baking sheet, toss the cauliflower with 1 tablespoon of the oil, the smoked paprika, and ¼ teaspoon of the salt. On the other baking sheet, toss the plantain with the remaining 1 tablespoon oil and remaining ¼ teaspoon salt. Make sure everything is well coated. Roast both baking sheets for about 20 minutes, until the veg is fork tender and begins to pick up a little golden color.

3. Heat a non-stick pan over medium-high heat. Cook each tortilla for 30 seconds to 1 minute on each side. Store within a clean kitchen towel to keep warm.

4. To serve, divide the veg between the tortillas. Drizzle 1 or 2 tablespoons of dressing on each pile of veg and garnish with avocado and cilantro leaves, if desired. Serve immediately or store in the fridge for up to 3 days, assembling meals as needed.

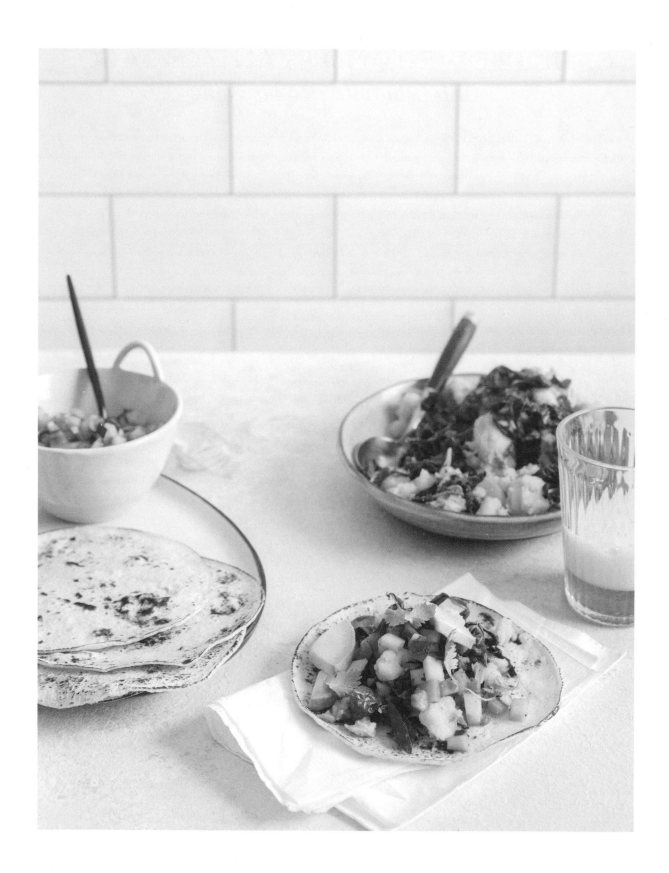

SMASHED POTATOES AND GREENS TACOS *with Pico de Gallo*

I made these tacos frequently during my elimination diet. Potatoes were often withheld from me as a child so it was such a joy to eat them freely, without all the nonsense, as an adult. My husband has also never met a mashed potato he didn't instantly adore; stick it into a tortilla and the Irish-Latin connection is real, people. Tomato Pico de Gallo (homemade or a store-bought version) is the classic topping, but if it's the middle of summer and you're loaded with peaches, the Peach Pico de Gallo is a delicious combination.

Serves 2

FREQUENCY: *Almost every day*
FOOD PREFERENCES: *DF, GF, RSF, V*
HANDS-ON TIME: *30 minutes*
TOTAL TIME: *1 hour 30 minutes*

· ·

2 thin-skinned Yukon Gold potatoes

1½ teaspoons sea salt, divided, plus more for seasoning

2 tablespoons extra-virgin olive oil, divided

3 cups mixed greens (like kale, chard, or spinach), tightly packed

2 small garlic cloves, peeled and thinly sliced

½ teaspoon cumin

1 teaspoon coconut vinegar or apple cider vinegar

2 tablespoons plain, unsweetened plant milk

4 Tortillas, homemade (page 36) or any natural, sugar-free tortillas

Tomato Pico de Gallo or Peach Pico de Gallo (page 55) or a natural store-bought version, for serving

1 avocado, pitted, peeled, and thinly sliced (optional)

5 or 6 cilantro sprigs, stems cut and discarded (optional)

1. Chop the potatoes into large 2-inch chunks. Place them in a medium pot with enough water to cover them and bring the water to a boil. Once the water boils, lower the heat to a rolling boil. Add 1 teaspoon of the salt and cook for about 12 minutes or until the potatoes are fork tender. Drain and place in a large bowl. Set aside to cool.

2. Warm 1 tablespoon of the oil in a large skillet set over medium heat. Add the greens, garlic, cumin, and remaining ½ teaspoon salt. Toss a few times with tongs while they sizzle and lower the heat to medium low, letting them wilt slowly over 2 to 3 minutes. Turn the heat off and stir in the vinegar.

3. With a large fork, mash your potatoes until they resemble not quite mashed potatoes and mix in the milk. Add the remaining 1 tablespoon oil, a heavy sprinkle of salt, and the cooked greens. Stir everything together until the greens and potatoes are well meshed.

4. Heat a non-stick pan over medium-high heat. Cook each tortilla for 30 seconds to 1 minute on each side. Store covered by a clean kitchen towel to keep warm.

5. To serve, divide the veg between the tortillas. Scoop 1 or 2 tablespoons of pico de gallo on the veg and garnish with avocado and cilantro leaves, if desired. Serve immediately or store in the fridge for up to 3 days, assembling for meals as needed.

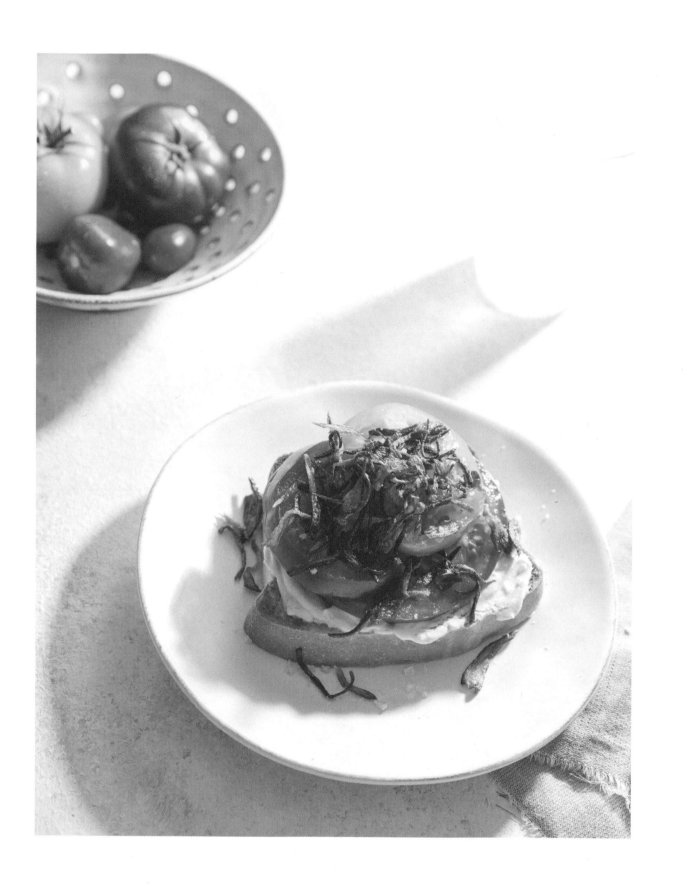

A New TOMATO SANDWICH

I realize this recipe may appear to be a lot of work for something as simple as a tomato sandwich. I also understand that slapping store-bought mayo and a tomato wedge on store-bought white bread would be "easier," but it's not easier for all of us. I don't eat dairy, and finding a supple white bread sans dairy is hard. Some of us restrict mayonnaise and the store-bought alternatives are mostly oil. And many of us avoid bacon, not because it's not delicious, but because we limit saturated fats or the amount of cholesterol in our life or both. My New Tomato Sandwich is a few recipes dressed up into one stellar sandwich.

Makes 1 open-faced sandwich

FREQUENCY: *Once per week*

FOOD PREFERENCES: *DF, GF, RSF, Veg*

HANDS-ON TIME: *10 minutes*

TOTAL TIME: *15 minutes*

. . . .

1 large ripe tomato, sliced into
  ½-inch thick slices

Flaky sea salt, for sprinkling

2 slices Sandwich Bread, homemade
  (page 34) or store-bought bread,
  sliced to suit

2 tablespoons Crème Fraîche (page 43)

¼ cup Crispy Shallots (page 49)

1. Preheat the oven to 325°F (163°C).

2. Place the tomato slices in a single layer on a plate or cutting board. Sprinkle with salt, to taste, and let sit while you toast your bread.

3. Place the sandwich bread slices on a baking sheet and toast in the oven, flipping once, for 5 minutes or until a shade of light gold brown and crispy. Remove and cool briefly.

4. Spread 1 tablespoon of crème fraîche on one side of each piece of toast. Pile a tomato slice or two on top of the crème fraîche. Divide the crispy shallots between each slice of toast, sprinkling them on top of the tomatoes. Serve with extra salt, if desired.

SPRING ROLL *Salad*

This raw tangle of vegetables, noodles, and a barely-there dressing is my upgrade on a fresh spring roll but in salad format. The only work is getting the ingredients prepped and in their place before tossing everything together; you'll end up with about a pound of prepared vegetables. This dressing recipe is best made in a powerful blender or food processor (as it breaks down the ginger nicely) and makes enough dressing for the first pass at the salad and enough for a second pass the next day. The whole mess is quite refreshing and zingy but as comforting as the inside of a fresh spring roll.

Serves 4

FREQUENCY: *Almost every day*

FOOD PREFERENCES: *DF, GF, NF, RSF, V*

HANDS-ON TIME: *20 minutes*

TOTAL TIME: *45 minutes*

4 scallions, trimmed and thinly sliced

One 1½-ounce (43 g) pack rice vermicelli noodles

1 yellow pepper, cored and very thinly sliced

2 medium carrots, very thinly sliced lengthwise

1 quarter head Napa cabbage, very thinly sliced

1 medium fennel bulb, cored, stalks removed, and very thinly sliced, or 1 watermelon radish, thinly sliced

1 large bunch cilantro (about 20 sprigs), stems cut and discarded

5 full sprigs fresh mint, stems removed and discarded, leaves torn into quarter-size pieces

ingredients continued

1. Put the scallions into a bowl of water for 20 minutes to crisp up; drain and set aside.

2. Cook your noodles according to the package instructions or as follows. Place the noodles in a deep bowl and pour boiling water over them to cover. Let sit for 3 minutes. Drain, rinse, and cut into short lengths (about 2-in) with kitchen scissors. Transfer the noodles to a shallow bowl of cold water to cool while you assemble the rest of the salad.

3. Combine the pepper, carrots, cabbage, fennel, cilantro, and mint in a large bowl. Toss until it looks like pretty confetti. Add the noodles and the reserved scallions, and toss again.

4. Blend the ginger, lime juice, sriracha, honey, soy sauce, and sesame oil together in a powerful blender or food processor. This makes about ⅔ cup dressing. Spoon 6 tablespoons of the dressing over the veg and noodles. Gently toss with your clean hands until the dressing is well dispersed. Taste and add more dressing or salt, as you desire. Serve with extra dressing, Crispy Shallots (for a nice crunch and added salt), and chile slices, if desired.

One 4-inch knob ginger, peeled
    and minced

4 tablespoons lime juice (from about
    2 limes)

2 teaspoons sriracha sauce

1 tablespoon light honey, like clover

2 tablespoons soy sauce

6 tablespoons toasted sesame oil

Sea salt

3 tablespoons Crispy Shallots
    (page 49), for garnish

1 red Thai chile, thinly sliced,
    for garnish (optional)

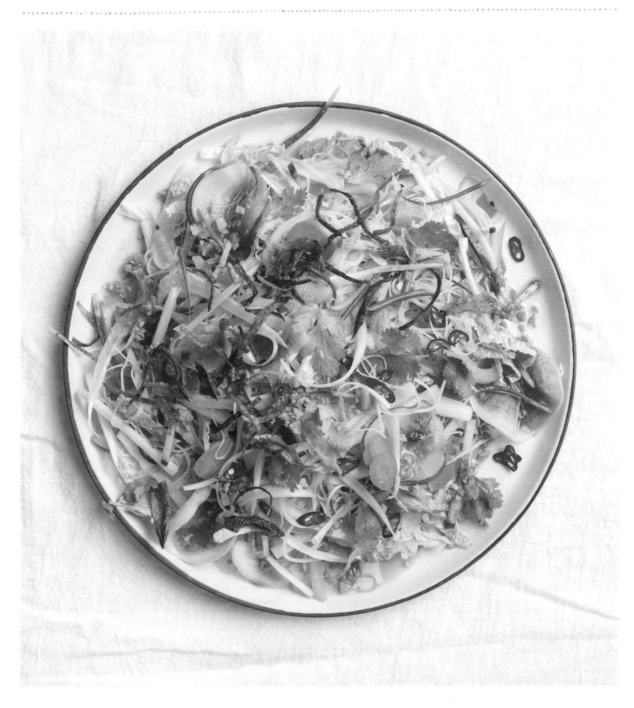

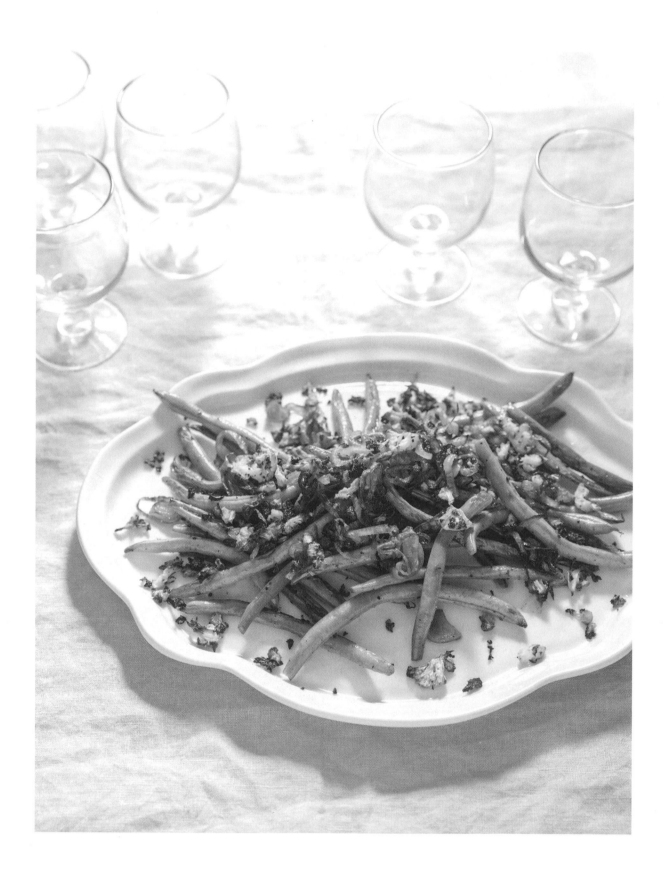

Ode to a GREEN BEAN CASSEROLE

This is not a traditional green bean casserole. It's a surprisingly satisfying vegan dish to take to a celebratory potluck or serve at a weeknight dinner party. The green beans form a savory, umami-ish base, the sautéed shallots are a sweet and tangy layer, and the crispy cauliflower crumbs stand in for breadcrumbs. I've served this dish just from the oven and after a spell at room temperature, and it holds up both ways. I've even set this casserole out during cocktail hour and noticed guests tossing beans back with a bit of bubbly. So serve it however you want—but don't skip the final sprinkle of salt and pepper.

Serves 4 to 6

FREQUENCY: *Once per week*

FOOD PREFERENCES: *DF, GF, RSF, V*

HANDS-ON TIME: *25 minutes*

TOTAL TIME: *1 hour 5 minutes*

· · · · · · · · · · · · · · · · · · · ·

1 small head cauliflower

6 tablespoons extra-virgin olive oil, divided, plus more for garnish

Sea salt

2 medium shallots, thinly sliced

2 tablespoons apple cider vinegar

1 pound (454 g) green beans, cleaned and stems trimmed

Freshly ground black pepper

1. Preheat the oven to 375°F (191°C). Line a baking sheet with parchment paper.

2. Chop the cauliflower into small cranberry-size pieces. Transfer to the lined baking sheet and toss with 2 tablespoons of the oil and a sprinkle of salt. Roast for 30 to 40 minutes, tossing and stirring regularly, until the cauliflower takes on the color of dark breadcrumbs. Remove from the oven and cool.

3. While the cauliflower is roasting, drizzle 2 tablespoons of the oil in a pan over medium-high heat. Add the shallots and coat in the olive oil. Lower the heat to medium-low and cook until the shallots become translucent and only slightly caramelized, 12 to 15 minutes. Carefully add the vinegar and cook until most of the vinegar evaporates, leaving a bright flavor, 1 to 2 minutes. Remove the shallots from the pan and let cool.

4. Add the remaining 2 tablespoons oil to the same pan. Toss in the green beans and cook, stirring every so often to cook all sides, until wilted slightly but still crisp, 5 to 7 minutes.

5. To assemble, place the green beans on a serving platter. Top with the caramelized shallots and then the cauliflower crumbs. Serve hot or at room temperature with an extra drizzle of olive oil, and salt and pepper to taste.

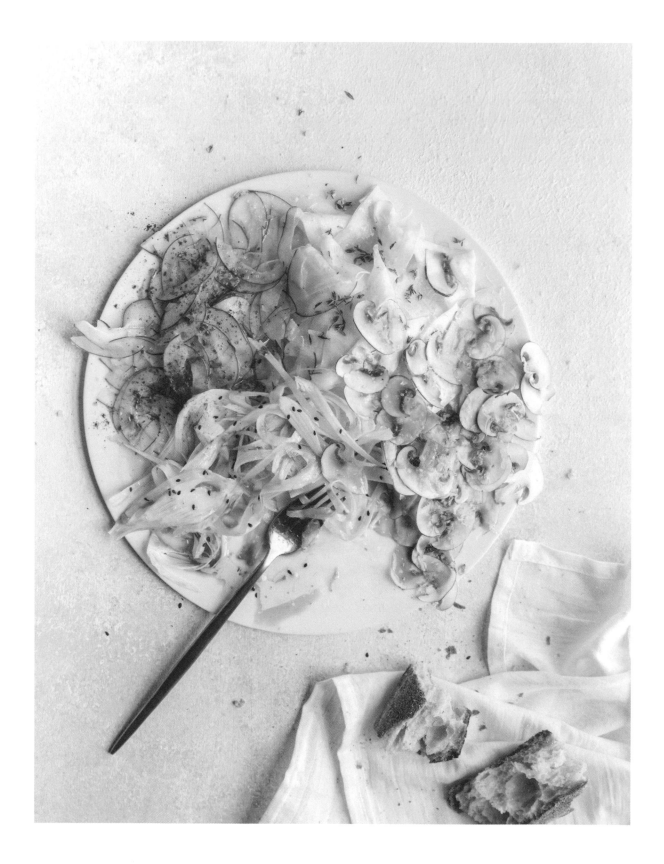

Carpaccio-Style VEGETABLE FEAST

This is what I want to eat every day: fresh, in-season produce, thinly sliced and dressed with really good olive oil and citrus juice. You choose the vegetable; just make sure it's sturdy and enjoyable raw. This recipe consists of a basic formula for putting together a single carpaccio plate as well as several example ingredient combinations that impress every time. They feed one or two people as a side dish, appetizer, or salad, but put four or five combinations in front of two of you, and that's a full meal.

Season the entire dish well with salt to help bring out the sweet vegetal flavor. And, if you like spice, play around with smoked paprika on zucchini or chili powder on cucumber.

An inexpensive mandoline, available online for twenty dollars or less, will make the slicing easy work. After devouring all the vegetables, don't forget to mop up the liquid on the bottom of the plate with a chunk of bread. It's definitely a cook's treat.

Serves 1 to 2

FREQUENCY: *Almost everyday*

FOOD PREFERENCES: *DF, GF, NF, RSF, V*

HANDS-ON TIME: *5 minutes*

TOTAL TIME: *15 minutes*

1 solid vegetable, cleaned and dried (like fennel, summer squash, or cucumber)

2 tablespoons extra-virgin olive oil

2 tablespoons lemon or lime juice (from about 1 medium lemon or 1 lime)

1 teaspoon lemon or lime zest (from about ½ medium fruit)

¼ teaspoon sea salt

1 baguette, sliced, for serving (optional)

1. Using a mandoline and finger guard, carefully shave your vegetable over a cutting board. Arrange the vegetable slices on a flat plate.

2. Drizzle the oil and citrus juice over the vegetables, then sprinkle with zest and salt. Wait 10 minutes and serve with baguette slices, if desired.

RECIPE VARIATIONS

Mushrooms, Lemon, Sea Salt

4 or 5 large button mushrooms, cleaned and dried

2 tablespoons extra-virgin olive oil

2 tablespoons lemon juice (from about 1 medium lemon)

1 teaspoon lemon zest (from about ½ medium lemon)

¼ teaspoon sea salt

1 baguette, sliced, for serving (optional)

continued

Zucchini, Smoked Paprika, Lime

2 small zucchinis, cleaned and dried

2 tablespoons extra-virgin olive oil

2 tablespoons lime juice (from about
    1 lime)

1 teaspoon smoked paprika

¼ teaspoon sea salt

1 baguette, sliced, for serving
    (optional)

Summer Squash, Lemon, Thyme Leaves

2 small summer squash, cleaned
    and dried

2 tablespoons extra-virgin olive oil

2 tablespoons lemon juice (from about
    1 medium lemon)

1 teaspoon fresh thyme leaves

¼ teaspoon sea salt

1 baguette, sliced, for serving
    (optional)

Fennel, Orange, Black Sesame Seeds

1 large fennel bulb, stalks and core
    removed, cleaned and dried

2 tablespoons extra-virgin olive oil

2 tablespoons orange juice (from about
    ½ orange)

¼ teaspoon black sesame seeds

¼ teaspoon sea salt

1 baguette, sliced, for serving
    (optional)

Cucumber, Lime, Chili Powder

1 large cucumber, cleaned and dried,
    seed core removed

2 tablespoons extra-virgin olive oil

2 tablespoons lime juice (from about
    1 lime)

½ teaspoon chili powder

¼ teaspoon sea salt

1 baguette, sliced, for serving
    (optional)

GRAPEFRUIT SODA *and Bitters*

Most nights, I drink a little something to aid the day's digestion. It varies, depending on my mood and just how much digestion I need to aid. Sometimes, I'll sip from a cup of ginger tea with lemon right before bed. The lemon is like a palate cleanser for the day, getting me ready for a good night's sleep.

While I did pay close attention to eating well while in active wellness mode, I didn't give up everything, especially very important food rituals. Every few weeks, my husband and I indulged in spicy Sichuan cuisine from our local spot. Sure, I stuck to fish and vegetables, but the food sometimes swims in hot chili oil (my favorite thing). On those nights, I'd need some extra digestion help. Sometimes, the bartenders would make me a bitter-filled non-alcoholic cocktail to enjoy while I was eating. Once home, a few drops of bitters mixed in flat or sparkling water always did the trick.

This recipe uses two types of bitters but do whatever you like—sometimes I swap in maple bitters or grapefruit bitters. The rosemary garnish is known to aid digestion, among other things. It's a nice complement.

Makes 1 drink

FREQUENCY: *Almost everyday*

FOOD PREFERENCES: *DF, GF, NF, RSF, V*

HANDS-ON TIME: *5 minutes*

TOTAL TIME: *5 minutes*

. . . .

½ teaspoon Peychaud's bitters

½ teaspoon orange bitters

1 cup (240 ml) cold unsweetened grapefruit soda water (I prefer LaCroix Sparkling Water)

One 3-inch rosemary sprig, for garnish

Add both bitters to a glass. Pour the soda over the bitters. Smack the rosemary in the palm of your hand a few times to release some of the oils before garnishing the drink.

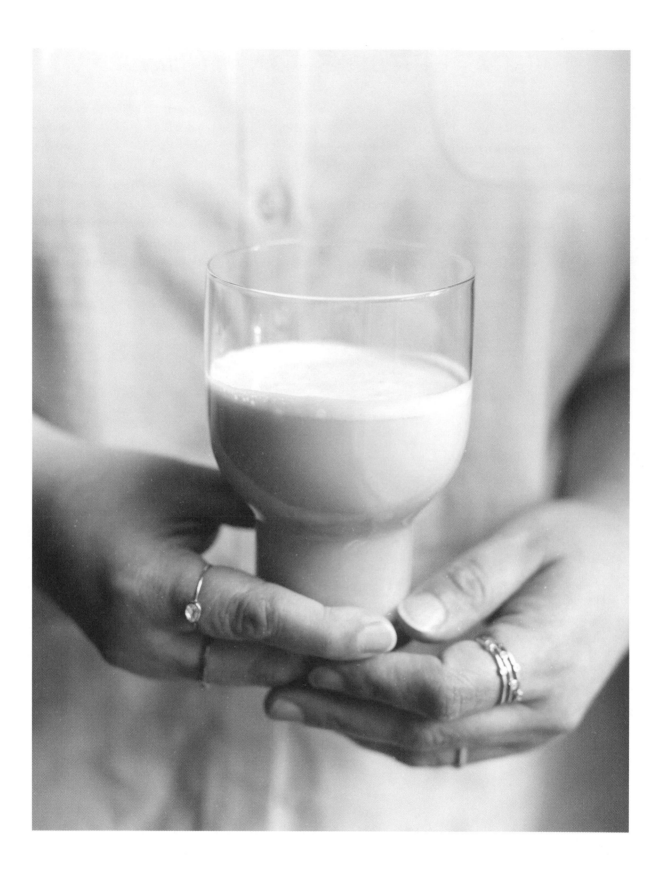

TURMERIC *Milk*

Consider this like a warming eggnog, just without dairy and eggs. I make this when I crave a semi-sweet treat that's rich and nourishing. Although the tart and spicy taste of turmeric is not for everyone, it's worth trying for the health benefits alone: a few pinches of turmeric can help reduce inflammation in the body. The ghee adds a certain richness and has been used in Ayurvedic cooking for centuries.

Makes about 1 cup

FREQUENCY: *A couple times per month*

FOOD PREFERENCES: *RSF*

HANDS-ON TIME: *5 minutes*

TOTAL TIME: *5 minutes*

1 cup (240 ml) Almond-Date Milk (page 38) or other unsweetened plant milk

¾ teaspoon ground turmeric

1 teaspoon light honey, like clover, plus more to taste

1 teaspoon Ghee (page 44)

1. Warm the milk until hot but not boiling in a small pot set over medium heat.

2. Add the milk, turmeric, honey, and ghee to a powerful blender. Blend on high for 1 to 2 minutes until everything is well combined. Serve immediately and sip slowly.

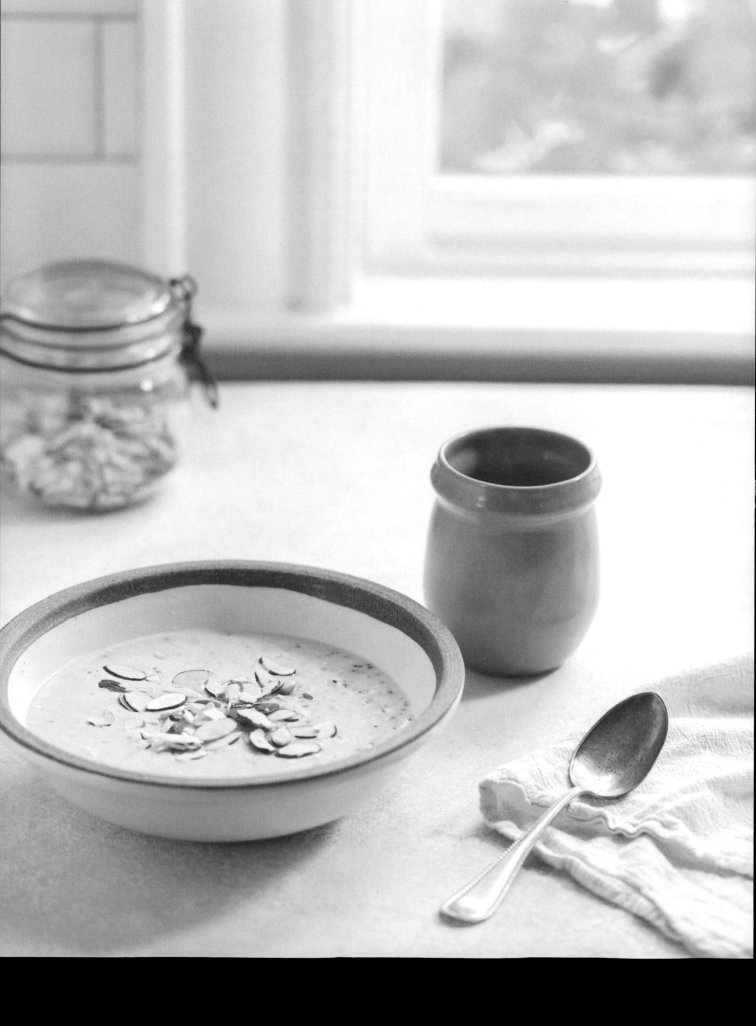

5

LOVE YOURSELF

Recipes for Reckoning with Your Past

It's not possible to change your body without also changing your thoughts. As you get started on your health journey, it's essential to take stock of your history. Many of our food issues travel with us from childhood. Real change occurs only after facing your food habits and investigating your relationship to how and what you eat.

The recipes in this chapter are inspired by my childhood, some even lifted straight from my mother's stove or my memory of that stove, anyway. In some cases, I revamped the ingredients or techniques so I could keep eating them regularly. A few, however, just taste better the way they were made decades ago. In those cases, I made tiny tweaks but left the crux of the dish just as it was intended. I encourage you to take a closer look at your family food traditions to create updated versions of the foods that bring you comfort and remind you of home.

The Very Beginning

IT'S DIFFICULT TO WRITE ABOUT the beginning. Not because it was bad, but because my childhood was big. It was glorious and complicated and so lovely that my heart hurts a little from remembering.

As the decade turned toward the 1970s, a Vietnam vet from a noisy Italian family was finally home. Fresh off his tour of duty, my father noticed my mother, an aspiring singer from the mountains of rural Honduras, dressed in a tight groovy dress, strutting down the street. He followed her home and charmed her into a date. Shortly thereafter, they married and moved into a tiny, two-family home. Nine people squeezed into that thousand-square-foot house and lived a typical immigrant-like life. Eventually, my parents, my sister, and I would live in three different parts of the country.

My dad, an accountant, would take on a side gig running a mail-order bookstore. My mother would work as a caregiver, as there were always kids to watch everywhere. We even moved to the south so my father could work at that era's version of a start-up company (it was a failure). For me, however, the years I remember most fondly were squeezed into that tiny New Jersey home.

I was the eldest child and surprisingly introverted for a straight-A student with such strong opinions. I was big, too. My father was overweight so I figured I was just the manifestation of his unfortunate genetics. But living deep within two exceedingly generous cultures of food (Italian and Honduran), and with a mother and a father who were really winging parenthood the best they could, you wouldn't have been too surprised either.

A CULTURE OF FOOD AND DRINK

In our tiny, outdated kitchen, meals were a mixed bag. One day, we'd devour a gooey baked ziti made completely from scratch, including the pasta, by my Italian grandmother. And, the next, we'd suffer through frozen veg cooked into a watery mess, courtesy of my mother, ceaselessly trying to be a dreamed-up version of the perfect American housewife. This was mainly given to the fact that my dad's family never really approved of her. She was constantly striving to feel welcomed. She'd bake up frozen dinners during the week, as they seemed to make my dad happy (and if he was happy, his mother was happy enough). He was particularly fond of the frozen stuffed clams that came in a box and were ready in 30 minutes, maybe less. They were topped with breadcrumbs and dried parsley flakes and maybe even a few clams made it into the shell. I loved them too.

My mother was better at making Latin dishes, though she'd be the very first to tell you she wasn't a great cook. Still, she always had a pot of orange-tinted rice and another of black beans, usually with poached eggs adrift in the soupy liquid, on the back burners. She'd make homemade candy from just whole milk and white sugar with ease. While all the other kids ran to the corner store for packaged chocolate bars and hard ten-cent candy, I'd park my big-little-girl body in front of the homemade candy plate and slice off thin slivers with a dull knife.

When mealtime was more leisurely, the ladies of the house would fry up ripe plantains and sprinkle them with Parmesan cheese, serving them alongside refried beans and over-easy eggs. My mother would sometimes present them with slices carved from a large ball of whole milk mozzarella from Nicolo's Italian Bakery & Deli, always sprinkled with regular table salt. That food memory alone makes me instantly miss that small home on Chestnut Street.

We forgave her cooking abilities because my mother's real talent was at popping up parties. Between Saturday breakfasts and Sunday dinners, a permanent party materialized most weekends, with Saturday nights as the peak of celebration. With all that food and all those parties, my childhood felt so very big and so very wonderful. And, perhaps, a little bit sad—but I didn't really see it in my youngest years.

THE WITHHOLDING OF FOOD

My father was more intellectual and, generally, not very much in the weeds with my sister or me when we were young. He worked, brought home a paycheck, watched television, read books, ate whatever he wanted (off his plates and ours—he'd snatch crispy bacon right off my sister's plate weekly), and let my mother do much of the parenting.

She was squarely focused on two somewhat opposing elements: caring for others and caring for her own appearance. In Honduras, she had received her college degree in social work and, in the States, she did so much through our local church and other agencies to help those who had less or were less capable of taking care of themselves.

Perhaps more important than charity, my mother's appearance was paramount. She was a former model, appearing in photographs in her homeland, often representing au courant hats or dresses, and that model mentality followed her through life. She persistently prepared for a photo shoot every moment of the day, compact mirror and hairbrush never too far away. Curvy but thin, my mother crafted a closet full of the prototypical body-skimming clothes of the seventies. She didn't find many occasions to wear most of these fairly alluring pieces, what with the running after children day and night, but she stocked them nonetheless. That closet both amazed and frightened me.

As a big child, about twenty pounds overweight and growing steadily, I was generally nervous about my appearance all the time—and my mother's fastidious focus on her own image just made it more challenging. My mother styled herself as much as ten times per day, up until and including the many years she wore wigs after going through treatment for ovarian cancer. And men always noticed how good she looked—even well into her seventies, men approached her at the local coffee shop. Unfortunately, the only person who noticed how I looked during my younger years was my mother.

Sure, I cared about looking clean and current but tight clothes weren't my thing—in fact, the looser the garment, the better. That didn't sit well with my mother, who much preferred to see me in skirts and dresses over the brown-paper-bag style of clothing I embraced. Like every young girl, I brushed my hair once in the morning but, after years living with such a fastidious groomer, I convinced myself to get a perm for most of the eighties. She also wished I wore makeup; when a friend had some on, my mother would perennially ask why I didn't make my face up in the same way. I think she wanted me to look like my made-up friends, all glittering and glamorous.

I do remember the moment I first felt too big. A local playground had just had a seesaw installed and many area children were thrilled to give it a go. After waiting in line, I grabbed one end of the seesaw and another girl grabbed the other end. We giddily hopped on and—thud—I briskly plopped to the ground. She hung overhead, legs moving like wings flapping through the air to push downward. Eventually, she cried and an adult helped her off. Other girls tried to get on but when it was clear that my body mass was the downer in this up-and-down situation, I shuffled off, mortified.

The story got back to my beautiful mother. First the cookies and candy disappeared, often tucked away in high cabinets out of my reach. Then the rice and pasta were curtailed, portioned out mindfully, always resulting in an argument if I wanted a second or third serving. Fruit also got a bad rap and my orange juice consumption was closely monitored until I went off to college. But the more these foods were suppressed, the more I craved them. Eventually, a few sweets found their way back into the kitchen but they all had two words written on the package: fat-free. Those foods were so filled with fake sweeteners, chemicals, and preservatives that it would have been far healthier for me to just mainline straight cane sugar. Plus, fat-free sandwich cookies were never as satisfying as the real stuff.

Listen, I know my mother practiced food stashing to help her overweight daughter and she did it from personal experience. I remember stories she shared of her fuller-figured days. She was an overweight child too and, somehow, whether through insults or encouragement from her family and teachers, she finally shed the pounds, so much so that she became the sort of woman who appeared in fashion photography. If she could do it, maybe she could help me do it. I bet that's what she thought. And my father just followed her lead.

Twenty or thirty extra pounds isn't so much on an adult but it's enormously life altering on a little girl's frame. And while my parents thought they were helping, I grew up with the basic understanding that everything that was delicious had to be kept as far away from my lips as possible, even if that meant locking it in an upper cabinet, hiding food in unexpected places like file cabinets or under a bed, and punishing me for using my wisdom to suss it all out somehow.

I found the withholding of food quite troublesome, but it was, for the most part, a private battle with my parents and within myself. It was impossible, however, to avoid the coarse realities of how the rest of the world would handle my size.

COMPLIMENTS ARE SOMETIMES INSULTS

Many children grow up hearing about their good qualities, almost universally, as if expected. Think about it: the moment you see a baby or child, you say to yourself and sometimes aloud, "he's so cute" or "she's so pretty." I heard many of those things too; only many of my compliments were caveated, given how big I was. Yes, seriously. I heard every one of the following compliments, dozens of times, during my adolescence:

> *"You're so beautiful and such a* big *girl."*
> *"You're so pretty,* if *only you'd lose a little weight."*
> *"You have such a pretty* face.*"*
> "Good thing *you're so smart."*
> "Thank goodness, *you're smart."*

No matter the words chosen, the moment the outside world began acknowledging my appearance and, inadvertently, how big I was, I began to think something was wrong with me. Not just a little wrong with me, a lot wrong with me. My sister, cousins, and young girlfriends never received compliments that had these sorts of caveats or unsaid references in my presence. And my mother, ever the most beautiful one in a room, was constantly fawned upon in front of me, never with any conditions.

As I got into my teens, I realized these stipulations were insults and sometimes the insult didn't even have words. Expert sleuths don't need words to express their discontent, do they? Hugs were so hard for me—and that could be why I bestow them so liberally today. When I did get hugs, almost exclusively from my mother, I don't doubt that she was lavishing love upon me. But in real life, those hugs morphed into pat downs. Like a detective trying to spot any extra weight, my mother would literally pet and squeeze my sides. This happened up until my thirties when I finally had had my very last pat down and tried to calmly explain that I knew her game. Calmly may have involved shouting and crying. I did my best. She did her best, too.

However unintentionally these compliments and hugs were doled out, they were still slights and ultimately comments on my big body. And as I endured them from day to day, year to year, I began to believe them. Certainly, I believed I had a problem but, more than that, I began to believe the problem had me. Instead of just being overweight, my mind believed that I was big and that being big was who I was. The problem shifted from my body to my mind. And in my mind, I became forever a fat girl.

I'M A PARENTIFIED CHILD

I was a pretty driven kid, eager to learn, a bit like my father. I completed my homework daily and recorded exceptional grades; learning was just super natural to me. An overachiever, however, doesn't always get rewarded. As I got older and continued to excel, my parents eventually felt ill-equipped to help me with any of my schoolwork. And, let's be honest, my dad was simply too exhausted when he came home from his twelve-hour job to help me with my homework. As well, my mother's first language was Spanish so she was in no position to help me work through my writing, let alone help me calculate complicated division problems. I believe that my mother was, in many ways, much smarter than my father, more capable of handling the curveballs of life, but the language barrier made it close to impossible for her to help her little kid learn from classic schoolbooks.

Essentially, the only person who could help me learn was me, so I had no choice but to become self-sufficient. Already the eldest child, I simply figured stuff out on my own. Ultimately, I became the designated parental stand-in who helped my sister with tough homework—

and, naturally, I gave her and my parents a tough time about it. But I didn't ask too many questions of others because I didn't want to appear too vulnerable. Helplessness wasn't acknowledged in our small nuclear family. Sure, if you fell down and scraped your knee, my mother might wipe the tears and give you a hug (maybe with a pat down, too). But if my father was around, he'd force you to get right up, demand you stop crying, and remind you of his good friends that were violently killed in Vietnam right before his eyes. His sort of conditioning encouraged you to just get on with it and take care of yourself, stat.

However, when you're a child who appears to be fairly capable, responsible, and smart, some adults start to think of you as more than a child. My parents began to think that I could handle more adult-like stuff, and started to rely on me more and more. It was nuanced, at first. Perhaps a few extra chores got tossed my way, and that's okay. Maybe they'd raise my allowance if I helped my sister with her homework or if I watched her while they were out, and I suppose that made sense. But as I got older, the expectations changed a bit.

I got my first real job when I was fourteen. I was so excited to get out of the house and earn my own money. But times weren't always easy and my paycheck sometimes got folded in to help with household expenses rather than go into my much-needed college fund. Once I learned how to drive, I was sent on household errands. And as I got older, my father and mother began discussing tough stuff with me, individually. Instead of having meaningful conversations with each other, which they did less and less frequently, my father would discuss news of the day with me. He'd comment on our household finances and how my mother spent his money. My mother, passionate about politics until days before her death, would quite frequently talk politics with me versus my father, as they'd just end up in disagreement or one person calling the other "stupid."

Ultimately, as I reached adulthood, probably way sooner than I should have, my parents, two adults who never really figured out how to communicate with each other or handle all the problems of adulthood collaboratively, eventually started to use me more as confidant or mediator. I grew up rarely feeling the freedom of childhood and mostly feeling some underlying responsibility for a family that had no strong direction. I couldn't get to college fast enough.

I also grew up with the unfailing opinion that my parents had no business being married and should separate at the first opportunity. When they finally did after thirty-one years of marriage, I didn't have the emotional intelligence to really stand behind that youthful opinion. I struggled through their separation, often as go-between for their fewer and fewer conversations. I never really learned how to deal with all of that discomfort; the only solution I could come up with was to eat it.

FOOD BECOMES MY COMFORT

To review, I grew up in a culture of food and drink. All the delicious foods were withheld from me because I was a fat girl. No matter how smart or attractive I may have been, comments about my fat-girl size were constantly hurled at me during the first eighteen years of my life. And, as a parentified child, I was regularly responsible for something or someone, and quite often felt like a substitute for a mother or a father. Since I didn't experience adequate time to really develop ideal coping strategies for all this discomfort, I did what so many humans do. I found my perfect way to self-soothe: I ate anything I wanted all of the time.

Without sweets in my life on the regular, I found my way to have them. As a very young girl, I'd just gorge on them at the homes of my girlfriends. I knew which girlfriends had those famously delectable chocolate sandwich cookies and I arranged to spend time at their houses. After-school snacks at my home were invariably boring and often good for me. But at a girlfriend's house, they were consistently cookies.

At school lunch, I could eat without supervision and often filled up on chocolate milk and French fries because why not. As I started an endless stream of after-school jobs in my teens, my extra money went toward one of two causes: my family's household expenses or my food habit. I'd purchase individually packaged chocolate-covered snack cakes and practiced the fine art of food hiding. I'd put chocolate cakes under my bed, in desk drawers, in my backpack, and even in unexpected places like deep in my closet or in boxes of books. After all, I had learned from the best.

I wish I could say it all stopped once I moved out on my own but that'd be a lie. In fact, living free from my parent's gaze gave me full sovereignty over the food that passed through my lips. I consumed all I wanted in my college cafeteria, rarely going for the good-for-you stuff. And, once out in the working world, I rewarded a day of hard work with a burger and fries or a big ice cream sundae, because I could. And if the workday was bad, the food order only doubled.

Whatever my age, when shit hit the wall, food never failed me. It filled me up and created this very warm feeling inside my belly. It was a feeling I hadn't really felt before at any other time in my life. I felt full, satisfied, and complete in some way. I felt nurtured and nourished. And while whatever I ate didn't give me the energy to get through long periods of time, it certainly gave me a warm rush for an hour or two. My cheeks would get flushed. The hairs on my arms would stand at attention. I might perspire a bit from the tingling inside. It was a feeling I only felt when I filled my belly up with all the food.

Perhaps that infusion of delicious food, that likely contained a lot of sugar, was a euphoric high, similar to the sort of high you feel after taking an enormously powerful drug. As a right-thinking adult today, I acknowledge that. I now know a food rush is similar to a rush from a drug. But in the moment when I was eating whatever I wanted as quickly as possible, as if someone might interrupt me or yank it from my hands, I knew this warm feeling as something else. I knew this feeling as love. I fell in love with food on a daily basis. I loved the delirious feeling I got from eating anything I wanted. I loved food and it loved me back.

Naturally, once I met and fell in love with my husband, I reassessed this food-rush feeling. It was love but not romantic love. It was the kind of love that provided comfort. At some point, I realized that I didn't get all the kinds of love I needed in my youth, and, sadly, I didn't learn the essential skills to self-love. I do think I felt moments of love—I really do—but I generally felt anxious and worried most of the time, only eager to anticipate the tough moments before they happened. Because of this, I sought refuge, relief, and respite from food every single day. And, let me be clear, unlike my parents, food never failed to provide that feeling. That feeling was so powerful that it did, however, mask the fact that by the time I was forty, I was teetering close to three hundred pounds.

Subconsciously, I suppose I needed comfort more than I needed my good health. It is okay that all of this happened to me. I know my parents loved me and I also know that they didn't have the resources or experience to raise a well-adjusted fat kid. I have come to terms with all this and continue to reckon with it on a daily basis.

It is also okay that one day I decided that I needed good health more than I needed this artificial comfort. I decided to get uncomfortable, and that's the best part of this story.

EVENTUALLY, I BECAME MY COMFORT

It was New Year's Day 2015, the most frightful day of the year for this fat girl. Slumped in front of the television overeating absolutely nothing memorable, I was about to become the very first cliché of yet another new year. For the thousandth time, I committed to figuring out my health situation, whispering it to myself aloud, "I will prioritize my health, and I will lose weight." I commit to losing weight on the first day of every New Year. You know the drill. It's a thing. It's definitely my thing. It may be your thing, too.

But on this New Year's Day, in between big gulps of red wine, the whispers stuck. The very next day, I reached out to Sherrie, a nutritionist and health coach, and with her objective guidance, I started on my path to a new way to food. The moment I made it through week one of a hardcore elimination diet successfully was the moment I started to see me as in control of me. I had done it, alone, without my parents coaxing me into yet another new diet, without my friends guilting me into a gym membership that I didn't want, and without my husband because my health wasn't about him. All of this was about me, finding my way on my own, getting help only when I needed it, and finding new ways to comfort me.

The original elimination diet was a three-week challenge to myself. When I got through those three weeks, I extended it another month. After two months, I added another month. After about three months, I added cage-free eggs, sustainable fish, and whole grains to my home cooking but stayed on this restrictive elimination diet for close to a year.

As my body started to feel better, my brain was grappling with some of the painful memories I've shared already, memories that I didn't quite understand yet. I wondered why I binged privately but ate fairly conservatively when out in public. It was difficult for me to reckon how if I ate the same amount of food as my very slim girlfriend, my stomach would clamor for more, making grumbly noises until it was filled with way more food than it needed. I struggled with why I kept shoveling food into my mouth, even when I felt sick from the overeating. And I ultimately thought that real love from someone else would fix me, like some wild fairy tale. Once my Prince Charming showed up, it was all going to be okay, right? So not true. No one could fix me but me.

Ultimately, I dealt with each of these issues one by one. I walked through them like user experience cases— a field I had worked in while at various technology start-ups—and asked myself hard questions.

That first year of my new way of eating I questioned everything: how I felt after every dose of plant-based food, how I had eaten all my life, and how I got here: to this place of total indifference to self-care. Questions led to answers. Answers led to wisdom. In fact, each answer proved to be a point in some invisible diagram; the diagram became an informal map that helped me finally reach better health.

I didn't do all of this on my own. After about a year on my path, I engaged a therapist and she provided the much-needed support to explore all these questions. Certainly, she didn't have all the answers, but by meeting with her weekly, I felt encouraged and bolstered to continue to seek out both answers and some sort of understanding with myself. I now understand how I got here. I get why I ate to feel comfort. I finally cozied up into a much better place, a place from which I could comfort myself now.

Let's be clear, though. While finding a way to comfort and love me has given me the gift of much better health, I'm not skinny and I didn't write this cookbook to make you skinny. I think of myself as a regular person, with all her flaws and scars. I'm a regular girl who weighs less but I'm still curvy and soft on the outside and I'm trying daily to be a lot less tough on the inside. I prioritize me above everyone else, not in a selfish way but in a way that I can be totally present and available to myself and everyone else around me. I wrote this cookbook to help you get there, too.

NINE STEPS TO LOVE YOURSELF

I promise you that learning to love yourself is worth it. I don't mean the kind of love that makes you so proud to hug yourself every day, though I have now learned more about that specific asana in yoga. I also don't mean the kind of love that lets you give yourself a pass for any careless behavior, whether it's eating an ice cream sundae ten days in a row or shouting at a server for forgetting the cherry on top. It's important to be a kind human, you know. This isn't about being selfish.

When I say I love myself, now, I mean, I understand my past, I appreciate my present, and I am enthusiastic for my future; I mean, it's okay to eat however I want here or there, for very good reasons, and it's okay to pause first and say, "What is this food going to do for my health today?"; I mean, I don't need to explain myself or toss out excuses for my behavior, I simply need to be kind to myself and to others.

This process isn't easy. But as the saying goes, nothing worth doing is ever easy. For real, this is worth doing and it doesn't just work for someone like me with suitcases full of food baggage. There are so many ways in which you may avoid loving yourself. Perhaps you drink a little too much booze to feel better. Perhaps you think you aren't pretty enough, good enough, strong enough, or smart enough to finally figure out what's standing between you and self-love. Don't let any of those demons stop you from taking good care of yourself. Please believe me, if I can change my world, you can change yours.

To help you find your path to loving yourself, I've summarized everything I did to get there. Remember, I am not a psychologist or even really trained in learning self-love. I am sharing all of this 100 percent from personal experience. Some of it may help and you may choose to skip some of it. Whatever path you take, just take it.

1. *Reflect on your past.* Engage in a mindset that is open to exploring your past. Think about positive memories (moments full of happiness) and any negative events (moments that left you bewildered, upset, angry, or disappointed). This reflective phase isn't a moment; it's a process of thoughtful consideration that may last weeks or months. My reflective time has lasted years and I still consider myself in a time of reflection. I reflect on my past consistently; it's a mindset I have never really left even when I am very much living in the moment.

2. *Write down the demons* that emerge from this reflection time. The pain begins to feel addressable when you write it down. When you write, be explicit. Once you have an exhaustive list, go back through it and ask yourself "why" for each one. For example, if you wrote down "I overeat," ask yourself "why" until you reach as solid of an answer as you can. This may take you into reflective mode or it may just provide a very common sense cause.

3. *Own your demons.* Whatever pain, anger, or disappointment you feel around any of these demons you've described, take responsibility for how you feel about it all today. If you've been an overeater all of your life, you can't change that you ate too much when you were younger. Move past any blame and take control of it now. For example, my parents did not make me a fat girl. They did the best they could with what they knew at the time. I have taken responsibility for feeling like a fat girl and I have given myself the power to break that long-held belief. Before you can break anything, however, you have to own it fully.

4. *Decide which demons you want to crush.* Learning to love yourself doesn't happen in a day or two.

Perhaps the decision happens in a moment, but the real work takes time and focus. Pick a demon or two that you'd like to reflect on further, explore in depth, and work to crush or minimize. It can be overwhelming to tackle them all at once. For example, I couldn't figure out a new way to eat and a new way to exercise at the same time. It was just too much. A few years after my elimination diet helped me find a new way to food, I am only now beginning to explore movement (to feel good and not necessarily to lose weight).

5. *Build positive relationships.* To tackle some of my demons, I needed help. I engaged with a total stranger to coach me toward putting good food in my mouth. I found a therapist who helped explore some of the demons from my childhood. I deprioritized demanding relationships that weren't giving me much in terms of love, understanding, and support. I elevated my relationships with women who understood my struggles, who shared objective advice, who didn't judge me, who just enjoyed my company and friendship. Seek these relationships outside of your partner or spouse. I certainly consulted my husband, but I didn't rely on him as my sole positive relationship.

6. *Seek beneficial inspiration.* I read self-help books, of course, but I also read books that explored some of the hard topics of my life, like the mechanics of how fat works in our bodies; how to learn to love others the way they want to be loved; and ways to calm my brain and find mindfulness. However, in today's world, it's about more than books. I surrounded myself with all sorts of motivating and encouraging stimuli. I started following health-focused folks on social media. I subscribed to a couple new periodicals that got my brain jazzed about what was going on in the world. I listened to brand-new podcasts, including ones about love and business, and even ones created by athletes, people who I thought were so unlike me, but in reality, their struggles are similar and their methods are exciting.

7. *Be mindful of everything.* When I say mindful, I mean, pay close attention to every single action you take. If you want to eat, pause and really take in that feeling before eating. If you want to drink, pause and ask yourself why before you do. By all means, do the things you want to do. However, it's important in this process to understand why you do them before you do. There may, in fact, be an opportunity to learn or heal or love in that moment. You don't want to miss it.

8. *Forgive yourself and your past.* I hated myself for so long for, one, letting myself get so enormous and, two, thinking that I wasn't worthy of good health. In my youth, I definitely blamed everyone else but myself for my body predicament. Over time, I found so much compassion for myself. The only way to love me was to acknowledge my past and my demons and then let it all go. I don't forget—that would be impossible—but I do forgive my parents and all those who hurled insults at me. Most of all, I forgive myself for letting life get so impossibly difficult. Saying the words "I understand and it's okay" aloud has proven to be such a life preserver. Those words help me stay afloat, for real.

9. *Love yourself, even if you don't yet.* You need to take the action to love yourself long before you feel that love deep within. Loving yourself is not a feeling you summon. You can't whisper, "I love myself" and then you just feel it. I wish it worked that way. For me, I had to physically take action to love myself in order to finally feel real love for myself. It's as if the little actions, all added up on top of each other, builds that bridge to real self-love.

If you want to love yourself enough to look at your naked body in a mirror, don't wait. Just look at your naked body in a mirror. I started the process of dry brushing my skin each morning before a shower. Not only was it a little abrasive but it was also painful to look at all my nooks and crannies. After doing it every day for a year, I started to appreciate my thick thighs and often rubbed my puffy belly. By looking at my body, I found so much gratitude for every part and, eventually, loved taking care of those parts. My thighs are still thick. My belly is still puffy. But I love them so much for carrying me through this world the best they can and that's really all I can hope for them. And for me, really.

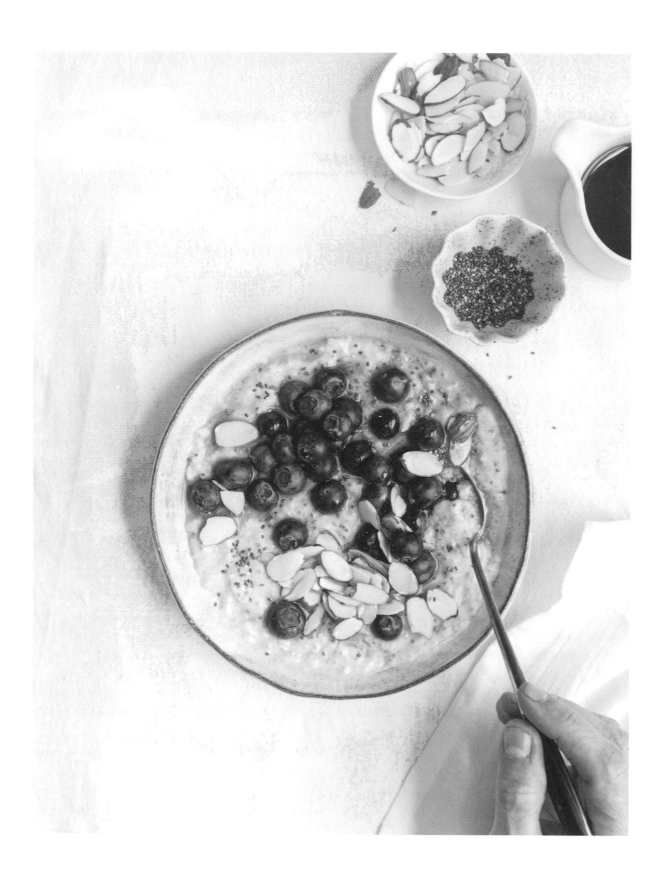

My Special OATMEAL

Early life breakfasts included two types of oatmeal. On most days, my mother would rip open a package of oats and mix the contents with boiling water, perhaps sprinkling a little sugar on top to make them more palatable—but quite often, leaving off the sugar for her big-little girl. Almost as amends, every other weekend or so, she'd whisk a pot of creamy special oatmeal. Her version was looser in consistency, like a velvety vichyssoise, only steaming hot, rich, and so sweet. And, she infused her special oatmeal with two flavors that, together, always taste like the ultimate comfort food: vanilla and cinnamon.

While I wouldn't dream of changing her flavors or the soupy texture, I've spiked this version with chia seeds for more protein, and a mix of cashew milk and water for a less caloric but more balanced bowl. Just as it is, I'd eat this entire serving for a super filling breakfast. Alternatively, you can stretch several meals from this, especially when paired with a dense smoothie; serve leftovers cold or quickly reheat with extra plant milk or water. It's also easy to make this gluten-free by simply sourcing gluten-free oats.

Makes about 2 cups

FREQUENCY: *Almost everyday*

FOOD PREFERENCES: *DF, GF, RSF, V*

HANDS-ON TIME: *15 minutes*

TOTAL TIME: *15 minutes*

. . . .

⅓ cup old-fashioned rolled oats or
    gluten-free oats

1 tablespoon black chia seeds

⅛ teaspoon sea salt

1 cup (240 ml) water

1 cup (240 ml) Cashew Milk (page 41)
    or other unsweetened plant milk

½ teaspoon vanilla extract

1 tablespoon maple syrup

¼ teaspoon cinnamon

Slivered almonds, blueberries or
    banana, chocolate chips, extra maple
    syrup, to garnish (optional)

1. Add the oats, chia, salt, water, cashew milk, vanilla, and maple syrup to a medium pot set over medium-high heat. Stir and bring to a low boil and simmer for about 5 minutes to soften the oats. Stir in the cinnamon. Simmer for 1 to 2 minutes longer just to mesh the flavors.

2. Pour the oatmeal into one or two shallow bowls and top with your favorite garnishes.

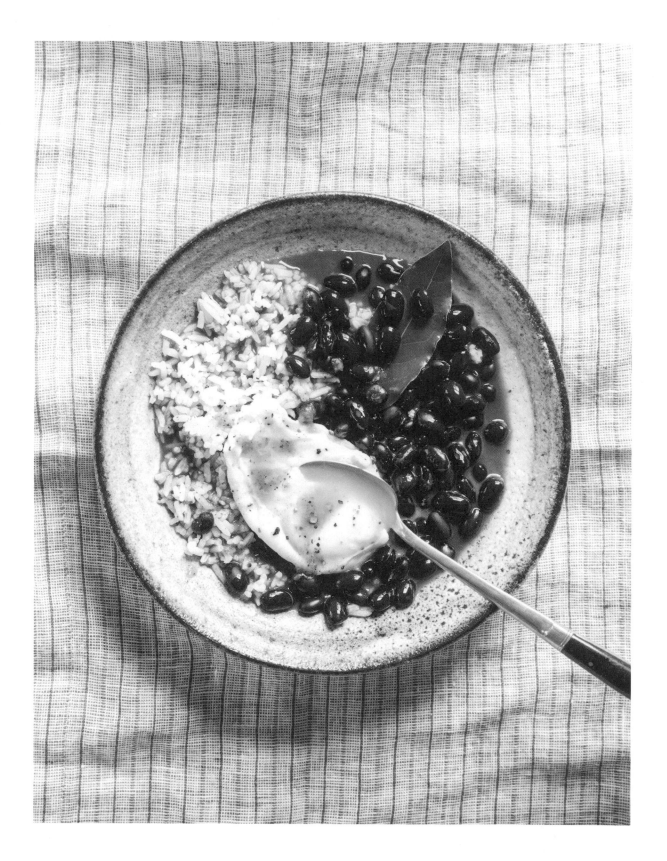

BLACK BEANS, POACHED EGG, RICE

This dish, as recounted by my mother, was one of the meals she missed most from growing up in rural Honduras. I always startled at that detail, as she invariably had a pot of black beans simmering on our kitchen stove and continued to eat this regularly as an adult. But, I suppose, there's something quite poignant and memorable about her grandmother, my great-grandmother, quick-poaching an egg in the bean liquid and sneaking her a bowl before all the farmers came in from the fields for their bowl. Nowadays, I eat this for breakfast, lunch, dinner, or just as an anytime snack. It offers a surge of long-lasting protein as well as a bit of comfort that only a hearty, sentimental meal can provide.

I highly encourage you to make the beans from scratch, but you may opt to use black beans from a can to save yourself a bit of time. The flavor is a little less satisfying but it certainly does the trick. Just make sure to use the bean liquid, as well as extra water, to create a broth.

Serves 1

FREQUENCY: *Almost everyday*

FOOD PREFERENCES: *DF, GF, RSF*

HANDS-ON TIME: *10 minutes*

TOTAL TIME: *10 minutes*

. . . .

1 cup Beans from Scratch (page 33)
    in the broth they were cooked in,
    plus ¼ cup extra broth

1 egg

1 cup Spanish Turmeric Rice (page 127)
    or any cooked rice, warmed

Fermented Hot Sauce (page 49)
    or any hot sauce, to garnish

Cilantro leaves, to garnish

1. Warm up the black beans in their extra broth in a medium pot set over medium heat until slightly bubbly. Make a small well in the center and break the egg into the well. Lower the heat to allow the egg to simmer in the broth until poached, 3 to 4 minutes. To push it along, spoon bean broth over the top of the egg.

2. To serve, spoon the cooked rice into one side of the bowl. Pour the beans with broth into the other side of the bowl. Gently spoon the egg on top. Serve with hot sauce and cilantro.

PUMPKIN BLACK BEAN ENCHILADAS
with Lime Ghee

The only time we had enchiladas growing up was when we visited any of the lackluster Mexican restaurants dotted across northern New Jersey. While the saffron rice was barely passable and the salsa was good enough, I was consistently impressed by restaurant-style enchiladas, and, I imagine, it was due to all that gooey cheese that covered up any shortfall in flavor.

These days, I don't eat dairy. However, my enchilada cravings have not diminished altogether and, when I need my fix, pumpkin comes to the rescue. This recipe is flavorful and so lush that I don't miss the cheese. But if you need cheese, go ahead and add a little.

The sauce recipe is spicy because that's how I prefer it. Omit the peppers to keep the dish mild, especially for the little ones. The recipe provides enough sauce for two batches of enchiladas; save half for a future meal. And while cilantro leaves are lovely on top, providing a green flavor punch that tempers the spice, the addition of lime ghee is luscious. Try a little drizzle for another layer of richness.

Serves 2

FREQUENCY: *Once per week*

FOOD PREFERENCES: *DF, GF, NF, RSF, Veg*

HANDS-ON TIME: *30 minutes*

TOTAL TIME: *1 hour 20 minutes*

FOR THE PUMPKIN ENCHILADA SAUCE

½ ounce (14 g) dried pasilla chiles,
    stems and caps removed

1 pound (454 g) tomatillos,
    husks removed, cut into quarters

1 tablespoon safflower oil or other
    flavorless oil

1¼ teaspoons sea salt, divided

One 15-ounce (425 g) can pumpkin
    puree or 2 cups roasted pumpkin,
    peeled and seeded

3 large garlic cloves, peeled

1 teaspoon ground cumin

1 teaspoon dried oregano

MAKE THE PUMPKIN ENCHILADA SAUCE

1. Preheat the oven to 400°F (204°C). Line a baking sheet with parchment paper.

2. Place the chiles in a shallow bowl and pour boiling water over top, totally submerging them. Cover the bowl with a plate and allow to rehydrate for 30 minutes.

3. Put the tomatillos on the lined baking sheet. Drizzle with safflower oil and sprinkle with ¼ teaspoon of the salt. Toss with clean hands until the fruit is well covered with oil. Roast in the oven for about 30 minutes until soft, shriveled, golden brown, and a little charred in spots. Remove from oven and cool briefly.

4. Remove the rehydrated chiles from the liquid and discard the liquid. Slice open and discard the seeds.

5. Add the chiles, tomatillos, remaining 1 teaspoon salt, pumpkin, garlic, cumin, oregano, olive oil, and broth to a food processor or powerful blender. Whiz until pureed and smooth. Pour the enchilada sauce into a pot and simmer over medium heat for 5 minutes to help further blend and smooth out the flavors.

6. Measure out 2½ cups of sauce (for one batch of enchiladas), and freeze the remaining sauce in an airtight container for up to 3 months. Defrost in the refrigerator overnight before reheating and using.

continued

3 tablespoons extra-virgin olive oil

2 cups (480 ml) vegetable broth

FOR THE PUMPKIN BLACK BEAN ENCHILADAS

1 tablespoon safflower oil or other flavorless oil

2 medium shallots, chopped

One 15-ounce (425 g) can black beans, drained and rinsed

3 cups greens (spinach, radish tops, cilantro), chopped

¼ teaspoon sea salt

2½ cups (600 ml) Pumpkin Enchilada Sauce

Four 8-inch natural, sugar-free corn tortillas

Cilantro leaves, for garnish

2 tablespoons Lime Ghee (page 44), melted and drizzled over top (optional)

MAKE THE PUMPKIN BLACK BEAN ENCHILADAS

1. Preheat the oven to 350°F (177°C). In a shallow frying pan, warm the safflower oil over medium heat. Sauté the shallots until translucent and a little golden. Add the beans, pushing them around a few times to heat through. Toss in the greens and the salt, and cook just until the greens wilt. Turn off the heat.

2. Pour 1 cup of the sauce in an 8- by 8-inch baking dish, spreading it out with the back of a spoon. In each tortilla, spread one quarter of the black bean mix and drizzle 2 tablespoons of the enchilada sauce. Roll each up and place it seam side down into the baking dish. When all the tortillas are filled and placed, pour the remaining enchilada sauce over the top. Bake for 20 minutes or until the enchiladas are warmed through, the sauce is bubbling, and the edges of the tortillas have crisped up slightly. Remove from the oven and cool slightly before serving.

3. Serve warm with cilantro leaves and a drizzle of ghee.

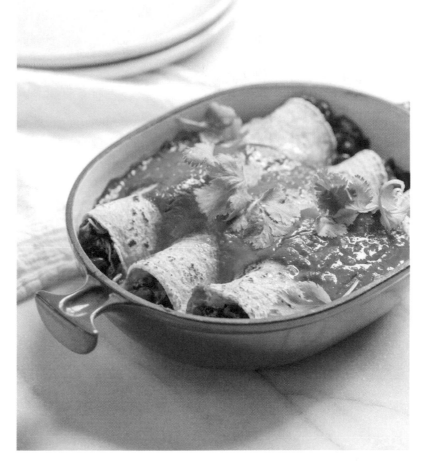

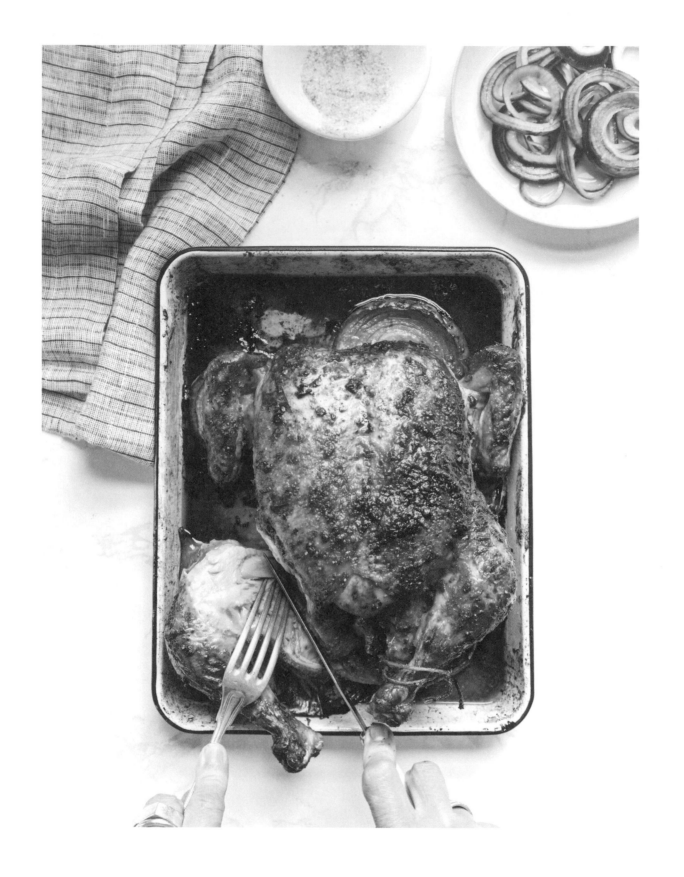

Roasted CHIPOTLE CHICKEN

My family's pantry was filled with piles of red ground spices that were used often, rubbed all over our thrice-weekly chicken. In fact, the shelves were stained with the spices that had fallen out of the jars, powdery messes that were fun to drag a finger through, writing messages to the pantry gods or just to my mother. I learned rather quickly to never put a finger in my mouth after tracing through the spices; they could be quite mild or they could be . . . cayenne pepper!

There are no such powders in this recipe; the spicy chipotle pepper paste is made with just a few ingredients. Make sure to rub the entire chicken and don't skip getting underneath the skin; the red flavor needs to be everywhere. Store the extra adobo sauce in the fridge and add a teaspoon to a pot of beans, any stew that needs spice, a batch of hummus, or even to grains like rice or couscous.

Serves 2 to 4 (with accompaniments)

FREQUENCY: *Almost everyday*

FOOD PREFERENCES: *DF, GF, NF, RSF*

HANDS-ON TIME: *20 minutes*

TOTAL TIME: *3 hours 35 minutes*

. . . .

One 4-pound (1.8 kg) whole chicken, innards reserved for another use or discarded

2 chipotle peppers plus 2 tablespoons sauce from a can of chipotle in adobo sauce

3 tablespoons extra-virgin olive oil

1 tablespoon sea salt

Lime-Pickled Onions (page 54), for serving

Spanish Turmeric Rice (page 127), for serving

1. Put the whole chicken onto a plate and place it uncovered in the fridge for 2 to 4 hours. This will help dry out the skin a little and get it crispier.

2. Preheat the oven to 450°F (232°C).

3. Add the chipotle peppers, adobo sauce, and oil to a small food processor and blitz until blended together, about 30 seconds. Alternatively, finely dice the chipotle pepper and use a mortar and pestle to mash it with the sauce and oil.

4. Place the chicken on a roasting rack in a roasting pan. Loosen the skin from around the breasts and rub the chipotle mixture underneath the skin and all over the chicken, including inside the cavity. Sprinkle with the salt. Truss (or tie) the legs together with kitchen twine. Turn the wings under each breast—you may need to break a joint to do this.

5. Roast in the oven for 15 minutes. Turn the heat down to 300°F (177°C) and roast for 60 to 75 minutes, until a meat thermometer inserted into the thickest part of the chicken registers at 165°F (74°C) or the juices run clear at a small cut in the thickest part of the thigh.

6. Remove from the oven and let rest 10 minutes before carving. Serve warm with the pickled onions and rice. Reserve the carcass for making chicken stock (page 32).

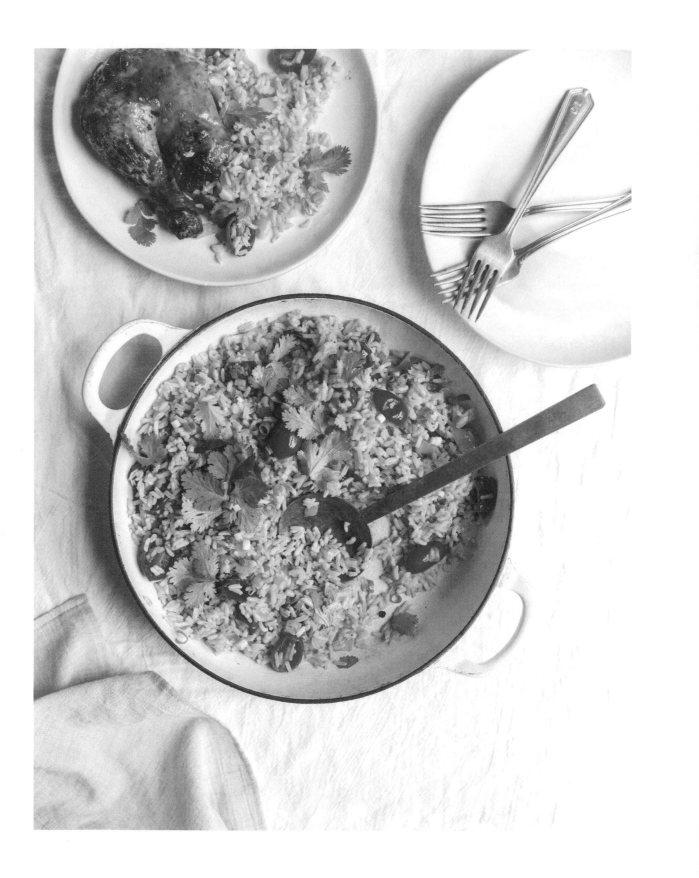

Spanish TURMERIC RICE

Someone far more educated than me could write an entire book that chronicles the adventures of Spanish rice across the world. Every region, every village, and every family has their own recipe that's the absolute most perfect version on the planet. We had a fairly mild version in our family, too, and it made an appearance at every single dinner. Rather than being an occasional guest on the plate, like any side dish should, rice was consistently the main event. To be honest, I grew tired of eating rice every day of my youth.

This new recipe most certainly helped me rediscover my love for orange-tinted rice. Instead of achiote powder or even saffron, the former used most regularly and the latter used only when we found it cheap, turmeric is the star of this dish. With the sliced cherry tomatoes for sweetness and the scallions and cilantro for green flavor, this rice is now on regular rotation in my home. If you enjoy non-plant-based broths, substituting turkey or chicken broth would further pump up the fat content and, naturally, the flavor.

Makes about 8 cups

FREQUENCY: *Once per week*

FOOD PREFERENCES: *DF, GF, NF, RSF, V*

HANDS-ON TIME: *20 minutes*

TOTAL TIME: *20 minutes*

2 tablespoons extra-virgin olive oil

1 large white onion, peeled and diced

3 large garlic cloves, peeled and finely diced

2 cups long grain white rice

1½ teaspoons ground turmeric

12 twists freshly ground black pepper

3 cups (720 ml) vegetable stock

1 pint (9¾ oz; 275 g) cherry tomatoes, halved

1 teaspoon sea salt, plus more to taste

5 scallions, trimmed and finely diced

1 large bunch cilantro (about 16 sprigs), stems cut and discarded

1. Warm the oil over medium heat in a heavy-bottom pot with a tight-fitting lid. Add the onion and sauté until translucent, about 4 minutes. Add the garlic and sauté for 1 minute more. Stir in the rice, turmeric, and pepper. Toss and sauté until the rice is well coated in oil and the onions and garlic are dispersed, about 2 minutes. Stir in the stock, the tomatoes, and the salt. After the initial stir, let it be. Raise the heat to medium-high and allow the mixture come to a boil. Once boiling, lower the heat, cover, and simmer the rice about 20 minutes or until cooked through. Do not stir the rice again.

2. Uncover and remove the pot from the heat. Fluff the rice with a fork. Top with scallions and cilantro, and fluff them into the rice a bit, just before serving. The rice will keep in an airtight container in the fridge for up to 1 week.

SCALLION-MARINATED SKIRT STEAK,
Homemade Tortillas, and Spicy Greens with Basil

Steak was not a regular thing at all when I was a kid. It was expensive, even the low-quality sort, and served only occasionally. It's most likely that my parents were simply trying to save dollars but I like to wear my paprika-colored glasses when I say they were purposefully preserving steak as an exceptional treat, as I believe it should be. When we had a reason to celebrate, my mother served skirt steak. She'd rub it with garlic, lemon, cilantro, and oil, and, after a brief sit, it would be grilled just barely to keep a pretty pink center and proper meaty flavor.

I serve steak once per week tops, sometimes only twice per month, in my household today. And while a proper rib-eye is magnificent, this skirt steak is memorable. It reminds me of my mother's version, only amped up to be more modern and green (the scallion marinade is a stunning shade). Served with homemade tortillas and spicy greens, this steak is a touch more wholesome but still celebratory. Share it with the ones you love.

The greens are inspired by a dish I had at ABCV, a Jean-Georges restaurant in New York City. I promise that these greens are a crowd-pleaser so if you are serving more than two, just double or triple the recipe. If you prefer a less spicy dish, remove the seeds from the jalapeño pepper and finely dice before adding to the pan. You can most certainly chiffonade the basil but the vegetal hit of full basil leaves counters the spice well.

Serves 4

FREQUENCY: *Once a season*

FOOD PREFERENCES: *DF, GF, NF, RSF*

HANDS-ON TIME: *25 minutes*

TOTAL TIME: *7 hours 25 minutes*

···

FOR THE SCALLION-MARINATED SKIRT STEAK

10 scallions, trimmed

One 2-inch knob ginger, peeled

1 tablespoon coriander seeds

3 medium garlic cloves, peeled

1 tablespoon coconut vinegar or
    apple cider vinegar

1 tablespoon sea salt, plus more to taste

½ cup (120 ml) extra-virgin olive oil

⅓ cup (80 ml) filtered water

One 2½-pound (1.1 kg) skirt steak,
    or several smaller pieces to the
    total weight

MAKE THE SCALLION-MARINATED SKIRT STEAK

1. Toast the scallions, ginger, coriander seeds, and garlic in a dry frying pan (meaning, with no oil added) over medium-high heat just until everything picks up a little golden color, 3 to 4 minutes. The scallions will char up a touch but do not burn the ginger, coriander, or garlic. We're just trying to activate the oils and develop an aroma. Remove to a plate and let cool.

2. Put the toasted aromatics in a powerful blender. Add the vinegar, salt, oil, and water to the blender. Blitz until a smooth paste comes together, about 30 seconds.

3. Place the skirt steak in a large casserole dish or other shallow bowl or even a resealable plastic bag that will hold the entire steak. Slather the entire contents of the blender all over both sides of the skirt steak. Cover with plastic wrap and refrigerate for 6 to 12 hours. Remove from the fridge 1 hour before cooking.

continued

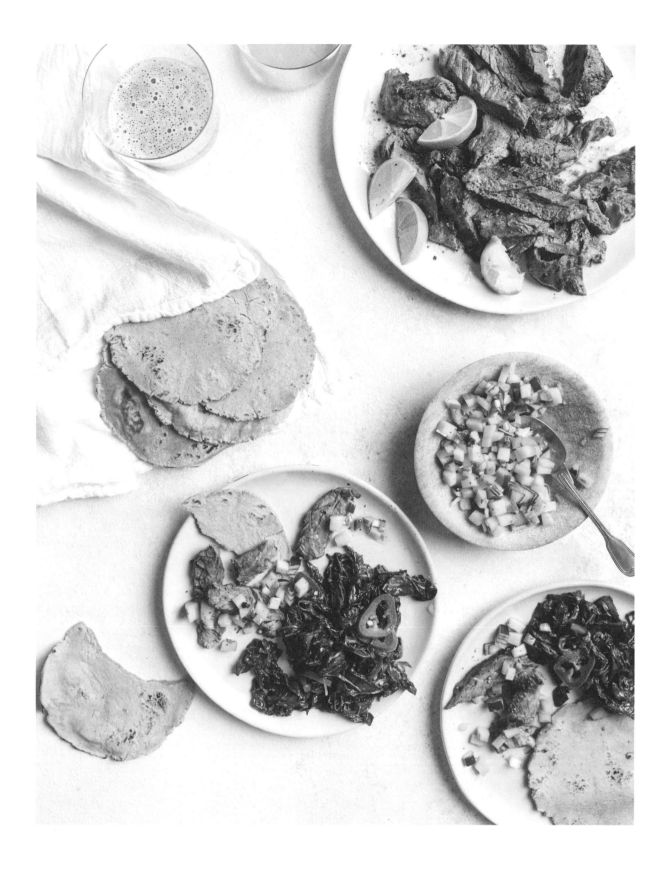

FOR THE SPICY GREENS
WITH BASIL

1 large bunch Swiss chard (about
    10 stalks), cleaned, stems reserved
    for smoothies

2 tablespoons coconut oil

½ cup (120 ml) liquid (water, red or
    white wine, or broth)

½ jalapeño pepper, thinly sliced

2 tablespoons apple cider vinegar
    or coconut vinegar

1 small bunch basil (about 10 sprigs),
    stems cut and discarded

¼ teaspoon sea salt, plus more to taste

TO SERVE

4 Tortillas, homemade (page 36)
    or any natural, sugar-free
    corn tortillas

4. Set a grill to 400°F to 450°F (204 to 232°C) or a grill pan on the stove to medium-high heat. Oil the grates or the pan. (You can also use a cast iron skillet, just trim the steak into a few pieces to fit.) Remove the excess marinade from the steak and discard. Grill the steak for 3 to 4 minutes per side for medium rare or until the center of the thickest part registers 125°F (52°C). Turn the steak once to avoid any flare-ups, but don't move it around a lot. Once cooked to your preferred degree of doneness, remove the steak to a plate and cover loosely with foil to rest for 10 minutes. After the rest, slice on the diagonal, against the grain and into thin strips, with a sharp knife and serve immediately.

MAKE THE SPICY GREENS WITH BASIL

1. Roll up the Swiss chard leaves and slice them into 2-inch-thick ribbons.

2. Melt the coconut oil in a non-stick pan with a lid set over medium-high heat. When the pan has warmed sufficiently, add the Swiss chard and sauté until it begins to wilt, 2 to 3 minutes.

3. Add the liquid and jalapeño to the pan. It will bubble up for a second. Lower the heat to medium and cover the pan, letting it cook in its liquid for 2 to 3 minutes.

4. Remove the lid and let the remaining liquid evaporate or burn off over the course of 3 to 4 minutes. Stir in the vinegar and let that mesh with the greens for 1 minute. Turn the heat off and stir in the basil and salt. Serve immediately.

TO ASSEMBLE THE DISH

1. Place a new dish towel on a plate. Heat a non-stick pan over medium-high heat until very hot. Cook each of the tortillas for 30 seconds to 1 minute on either side. Store within a clean kitchen towel to keep warm.

2. Serve the steak alongside the greens on a plate. Place wrapped tortillas on the table and pull tortillas from the dish towel, as needed. Fill a tortilla with steak and eat with the greens.

MANGO-LIME *Soda*

I remember lemonade stands from my childhood. Kids would gather tables, signs, and their mother's latest batch of lemonade to sell for ten cents per glass. In some Latin neighborhoods, the stands are run by adults and the drinks are way more tropical in nature. This straightforward refreshing soda is inspired by the folks, strangers to me but also familiar, who exposed me to mango, papaya, pineapple, and every other good tropical fruit when I was young. This soda is not fancy or over the top. It's versatile though, so go ahead and use pineapple. And if you'd like a dose of booze, add it an ounce at a time. I like it with a tablespoon or two of red wine floated over the top, too; it's a quick hack for sangria that comes together in a flash.

Makes 4 drinks

FREQUENCY: *A couple times per month*

FOOD PREFERENCES: *DF, GF, NF, RSF, V*

HANDS-ON TIME: *10 minutes*

TOTAL TIME: *10 minutes*

- -

8 ounces (227 g) fresh or frozen mango chunks

¼ cup (60 ml) lime juice (from about 2 medium limes)

3 tablespoons maple syrup

½ cup (120 ml) filtered water

24 small ice cubes, for serving

2 cups (480 ml) sparkling water

1. Add the mango, lime juice, maple syrup, and water to a powerful blender. Blend until combined and smooth. This makes about 1½ cups mango mix.

2. Pour 2 tablespoons of the mango mix into four 8-ounce glasses. Add 6 small ice cubes and 4 ounces of sparkling water to each glass. Stir with a spoon and enjoy.

3. Store the mango mix in an airtight jar in the fridge for up to 3 days.

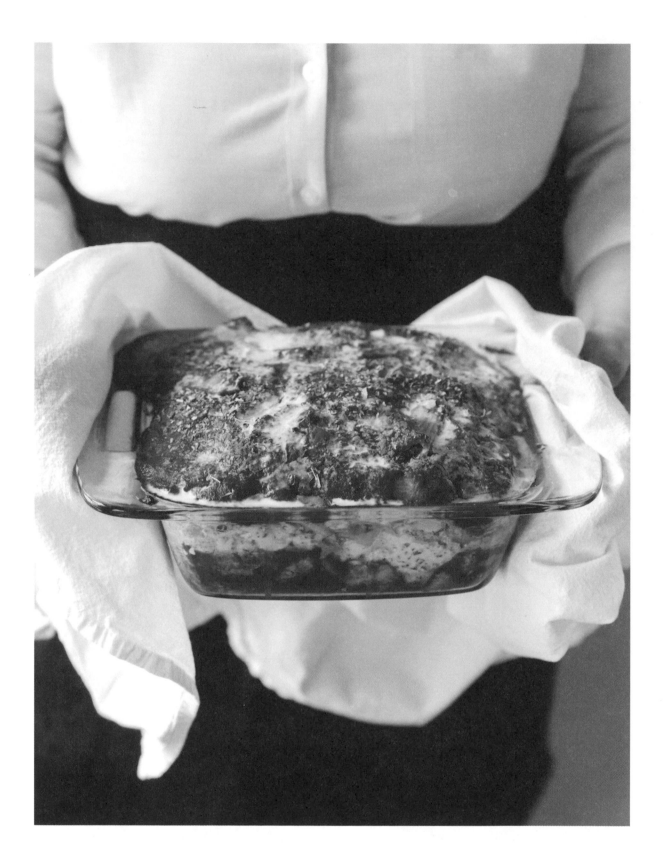

Gooey BAKED ZITI

My childhood was filled with every sort of pasta, almost always homemade by my Italian grandmother. I clearly remember her short clean arms digging deep into a huge bowl of ricotta, herbs, and eggs, mixing it by hand to transform individual ingredients into one smooth filling. Hers was the very best ziti and one I've wanted to re-create since switching up how I eat.

Filled with almond ricotta, this baked ziti is remarkably close to the cheesy kind. Many dairy lovers have given it rave reviews. The recipe is also easy to pull together on a weeknight—just be sure to factor in the 48-hour soaking time for the almonds for the ricotta.

Serves 4 to 6

FREQUENCY: *A couple times per month*
FOOD PREFERENCES: *DF, NF, RSF, V*
HANDS-ON TIME: *15 minutes*
TOTAL TIME: *40 minutes*

. . . .

1 teaspoon sea salt, plus more for pasta water

1 pound (454 g) penne-shaped pasta

1 tablespoon extra-virgin olive oil, plus more for drizzling

2 cups (480 ml) Almond Ricotta (page 39)

4 tablespoons minced parsley

3 tablespoons dry Italian seasoning herbs, divided

3 tablespoons nutritional yeast, divided

2 eggs, lightly beaten

7 tablespoons Cashew Milk (page 41) or other unsweetened plant milk, divided

4 cups (960 ml) Spicy Tomato Sauce (page 35) or any preferred tomato sauce, at room temperature

2 tablespoons Ghee (page 44), melted

1. Preheat the oven to 350°F (177°C).

2. Heat 4 quarts of water in a large pot over medium-high heat. Once it comes to a boil, add a big handful of salt (at least 3 tablespoons). Add the pasta and cook according to your pasta package directions. Drain the pasta, drizzle with oil to coat, and let cool to room temperature. Don't begin assembling the casserole until the pasta is cooled.

3. Add the salt, ricotta, parsley, 2 tablespoons of the Italian seasoning, 2 tablespoons of the nutritional yeast, eggs, and 4 tablespoons of the cashew milk to a large bowl. Mix until well combined. Add in the cooked pasta and mix until the pasta is evenly coated.

4. Spread 1 cup of tomato sauce across the bottom of a 8- by 8-inch (for a taller baked ziti) or 9- by 11-inch (for a shorter baked ziti) casserole dish. Add all of the coated pasta into the dish and spread to fit the entire dish. Spread the remaining sauce evenly across the top of the pasta. Drizzle the remaining 3 tablespoons cashew milk and the ghee across the top of the pasta, evenly. Sprinkle the remaining 1 tablespoon Italian seasoning and 1 tablespoon nutritional yeast across the top of the pasta evenly. Bake in the oven for 25 to 30 minutes until bubbly and hot. Remove the baked ziti from the oven and cool for a few minutes before serving.

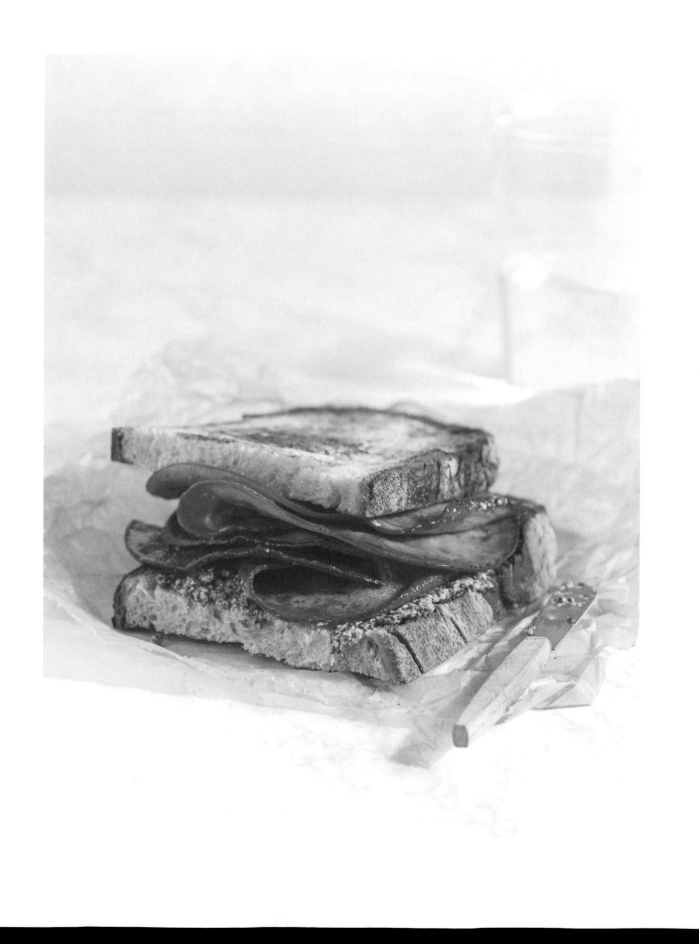

Fried MORTADELLA SANDWICH

This was my elementary school lunch most days and there's no reinventing it as a wholesome dish, ever. It's fatty, full of sodium, and most types of mortadella contain nitrates. It's absolutely delicious, too, and one of those dishes that will always remind me of those innocent moments when my mother loved me with food. Why she considered mortadella healthier for me than cookies is beyond me. That said, about once per year, I love myself by eating this dish and I'm totally okay with that.

Makes 1 sandwich

FREQUENCY: *Once per year, really*

FOOD PREFERENCES: *DF, NF, RSF*

HANDS-ON TIME: *10 minutes*

TOTAL TIME: *10 minutes*

. . . .

2 slices wheat bread

4 slices mortadella or bologna, sliced thin (but not shaved)

1 or 2 teaspoons whole grain mustard

1. Preheat the oven to 325°F (163°C). Line a plate with a sheet of paper towel.

2. Place the bread slices on a rimmed baking sheet. Toast the bread for 5 to 10 minutes, flipping once, until the toast is as golden brown as you like it.

3. Place a non-stick pan over medium heat. When the pan has warmed up, put the mortadella slices in the pan, making sure they're not touching. If your pan is small, cook in two batches. Fry the mortadella, flipping once, until both sides have a golden brown glow, about 5 minutes. Remove to the paper-towel-lined plate.

4. Spread as much mustard as you like on one side of one or both pieces of toast. Pile the mortadella slices on one piece of toast. Place the other slice of toast on top. Slice, if you like, and serve immediately.

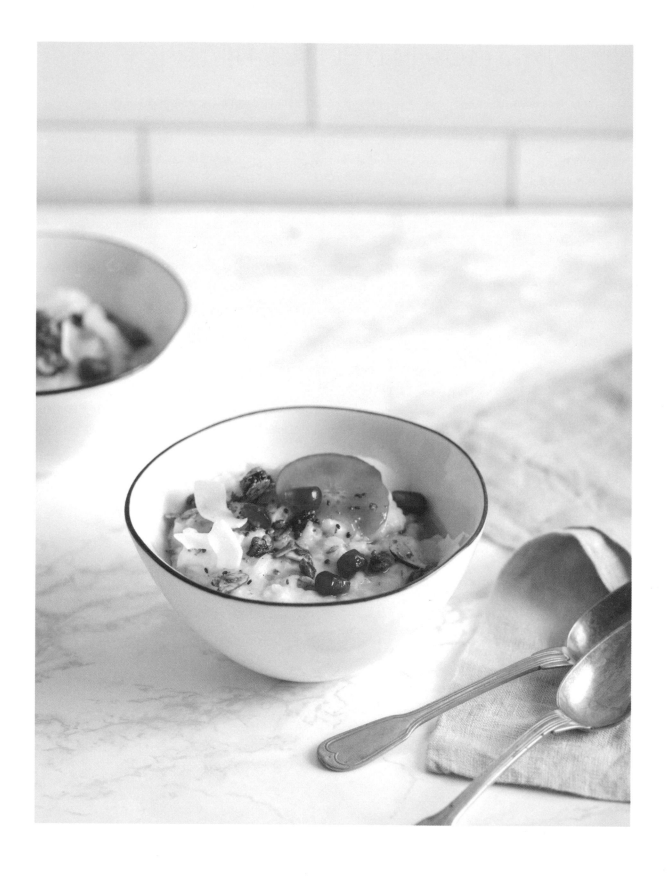

Takeout RICE PUDDING

There was plenty of rice in my childhood kitchen, the long-grain kind, the orange-tinted variety, and all the brown rice, too. When my mother had a sweet craving, which was fairly often, she'd pull together a bowl of rice pudding from leftover white or brown rice. She said that her mother and grandmother would do the same when she was a little one.

During my whole health transformation, I didn't keep too many sweets in the house. I did, however, keep a few food traditions. One day, I found myself in the kitchen, making this semi-sweet dish from memory and now I make it whenever a craving for something sweet and comforting hits.

This rice pudding is not overly sweet; it has just a touch of maple sugar. It is, however, perfectly tuned to taming my sweet tooth. Keep a close eye on the pot or set a timer after it comes to a simmer, as it will begin to stick to the bottom of the pan around the 8-minute mark.

Makes about 2½ cups

FREQUENCY: *A couple times per month*

FOOD PREFERENCES: *DF, GF, RSF, Veg*

HANDS-ON TIME: *15 minutes*

TOTAL TIME: *20 minutes*

. . . .

2 cups leftover cooked Chinese restaurant rice, tightly packed

3 cups (720 ml) plain unsweetened almond milk or other plant-based milk

¼ cup (1⅜ oz; 40 g) lightly packed maple sugar

One cinnamon stick, or ¼ teaspoon ground cinnamon

One vanilla bean, sliced open

¼ teaspoon sea salt, plus more for serving

Toasted coconut flakes, for serving

Honey, for serving

1. Add the rice, milk, sugar, cinnamon, vanilla bean, and salt to a pot set over medium heat. Bring to a simmer and then lower the heat to medium-low. Cook until most of the liquid evaporates, 10 to 15 minutes, stirring occasionally, especially near the end of the cooking time. The rice will become soft and gooey and may stick slightly to the bottom of the pan, so stir consistently to avoid any sticking. Let for cool about 5 minutes.

2. Serve the rice pudding in small bowls or glasses immediately. Top with coconut flakes (toasted for 10 minutes in a 350°F/177°C oven, if you like), a touch of honey, a sprinkle of sea salt, or all of the above.

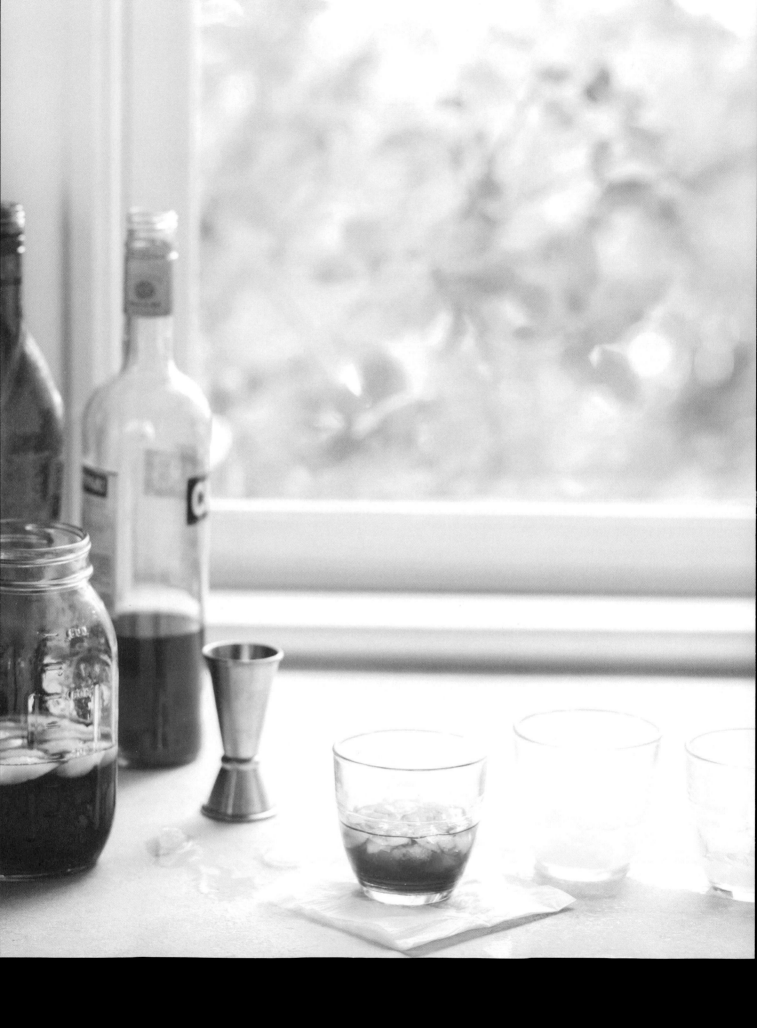

6

STAY CONNECTED

Recipes for Getting Healthy in a Couple

If you have a partner—or even a strong circle of friends and family—your meals and eating habits are often about more than just you. And during a wellness transformation, some real conflict can come into play there. It's important for you to focus on your own well-being—to be your own advocate and to be concerned with your own health—while also maintaining connection to and honoring those you love.

This chapter includes recipes inspired by new rituals with my partner, including fresh recreations of a few traditionally indulgent dishes, a few desserts, and a stunning, bubbly semi-homemade cocktail that's made for celebrating with your favorite people.

Transforming within a Twosome

I WAS RAISED THINKING you were supposed to go on diets with other people. When my mother curbed my sweets at any given time, she'd often curb those sweets herself. She liked to point out that she was on a diet with me; that we were losing weight together. In real life, it never really worked out that way—I stayed big and she stayed beautiful—but it was a little less painful to think we were in it together.

As I got older, girlfriends were often on diets together, too, especially in college, and they usually worked out or walked together. I had several different "walking buddies" over the years—they were at the same moment my cheerleader and my nemesis, because girls get mean when they want you to work out. If I rolled over and pulled the blanket up over myself in my college dorm bed, refusing to move a muscle, that cheerleader could turn into a monster in five seconds flat. I've had music blasted, dirty clothes tossed on me, and water poured on my head—on repeat.

Losing weight with my mother or getting healthy with girlfriends never worked for me. Those situations always left me feeling behind, as I rarely lost as many pounds as everyone else and I could never lift ample weight or walk fast enough (let alone, run). But I felt deep in my bones that the final solution would come when I had ample dollars to do what fancy folks and celebrities do: hire a personal trainer. If Oprah could lose all that weight (the first time) with a trainer, then perhaps I could, too.

When I began earning real money from a full-time job, I allocated the funds to hook up with a personal trainer. I've spent lots of money on trainers over the years and here's what I have to say about them: personal trainers may be able to help but only after you've first helped yourself. Just saying the words "I'm ready to get well" won't make you ready to get well. You've got to dig through your trenches first.

Personally, I had to do the hard mental work to get to a place where my transformation could finally stick. I had to reflect and cry and talk it all out until I understood how I got here because I now know I wasn't close to 300 pounds simply because I put food in my mouth. I wasn't big because I hated exercise. There were about a million reasons why I was so heavy and as I continue to work to understand each one, I secure my position in wellness for life.

During my transformation, I had a lot of help and guidance. My coach, Sherrie, was an angel, sent to me at the perfect moment. I have a few girlfriends who listened, really listened; who didn't push me to exercise or follow their example in anyway; who just let me learn and evolve on my own. And, I most definitely consulted and shared all the ups and downs with my husband, Don. He's been my husband for many years and has rooted for me from day one. He's also struggled with wellness in his own way. In fact, our struggles were very similar and we felt a fairly instant bond when we met years ago. It's so hard to be big in a world that's constantly broadcasting that you must be skinny, and he just gets what that feels like. He gets me.

When I embarked on the elimination diet that helped me begin to love me, at last, I had already been on numerous diets with Don. We ate piles of bacon during the Atkins days; counted points and weighed in during the Weight Watchers days; and restricted every kind of food together for a long, long time. You know what we had to show for it all? Even larger frames, further distorted views of our bodies, and odd, contrived responsibilities for the other's health issues.

We had tried to embrace wellness and fallen short several times together. Each time it didn't work out, we'd cozy up and agree to try again sometime. To be honest, I was surprised by our failures. Sure, I never got healthy with a family member or a girlfriend, but once the man of my dreams arrived, I was certain that I'd conquer this weight issue once and forever. Yeah, no.

This time around, after my fairy-tale bubble had been burst numerous times, I only asked two questions of Don when I decided to give an elimination diet a go. One, I wanted to know if he felt okay if I gave it a try on my own. (The answer was: "Of course.") Two, I asked whether he minded if we ate the way I was eating for the meals we enjoyed together, mainly dinner, so I didn't have to cook two meals each evening. (The answer was: "Sure, I'll give it a go.") That was it.

With that easy consultation, I moved ahead, generally on my own, but not necessarily alone. It felt very different this time around. I was focused on my body and not our bodies. I monitored my weight each week, which was going down quicker than it had in the past. I woke up with lots of energy on most mornings, and made sure to drink a glass of water with lemon before eating any food to cleanse my system, preparing it to absorb all those nutritious vegetables. I tracked the foods that made me feel good and stopped eating the ones that felt not-so-great. I let any of those reflections guide our shared meals but I kept my overall concern to my body, not our bodies.

I did listen to his take on the foods we ate and changed up the dishes I made because I totally respect the fact that he's not into, say, lentils. But I didn't describe my process in gross detail on a daily basis. I didn't take responsibility for how he ate at any given moment. I didn't feel mortified if he lost more weight than me and, generally, I didn't ask about his process too much.

You see, I am only responsible for my health. I worked hard to genuinely distance myself from Don's health journey and remain focused on my own. Sometimes I shared my successes and sometimes I shared confusing moments, but mostly I wrote it all down, discussed it with Sherrie, and moved ahead on my own. And, this time around, it worked. It worked because I was getting healthy for me and with me. I wasn't getting healthy with him, the person who meant the world to me, because tying our successes and failures together wasn't going to help me understand my body and my issues. I needed to focus on *my* feelings, not worry about *his* feelings. I needed to understand why I put all the foods in *my* mouth, and not take responsibility for why he put all the foods in *his* mouth.

Now sometimes this new way of eating was a fit for Don and sometimes it just didn't vibe with his life at a given time. That's okay. However, to make sure we stayed connected, I did keep some of the food rituals from before the elimination diet and I believe that has made this solo path possible, for both of us.

RITUALS THAT BIND US

When I met my husband, we had both lived outside of our family homes for close to ten years. We had had a little time to grow up, to explore and develop our individual interests. We quickly discovered our shared passions for food and celebrations. On our first date, we reveled in a spread of some of the best Italian food in the city—piles of pasta, a wide antipasti platter, and *fritto misto* (my favorite). On our second date, we trimmed a holiday tree together, running around to cut the tree down, picking up white lights and fresh ornaments, and grabbing a small assortment of picnic food to enjoy post-decorating. After that second date, I was hooked.

Once we moved in together, we were one of a handful of couples in our extended circle of friends who jumped on the opportunity to host everyone at our place. We loved everything about entertaining: figuring out what we wanted to serve, exploring new foods to share with friends, shifting into mixologist mode with new drink recipes, cleaning and decorating, you name it. We just fell into cultivating mini-celebrations; it became one of our things.

To feel adequately smart about food and drink for these weekend parties, we dined out quite frequently. We loved stumbling onto hidden food gems, wherever they may be; discovering new ingredients, flavor combinations, and cocktails really made us happy. At the time, I was building up my professional interest in food and laying the foundation for morphing into a cookbook author and food writer. Don was growing into an expert on amateur barbecue, all things pizza, and Irish whiskey. As well, he loved learning about the cuisines of my childhood and, as he'll tell you, he fell for Spanish rice like I fell for his family's Irish potatoes: instantly.

With all this youthful food love between us, it was so easy for me to do what I do best: find comfort with food. Naturally, I bulked up—though it took years for me to notice that part. I was simply having so much fun, exploring the thing I loved more than anything in the world, the thing that provided me so much comfort, with the person I loved more than anything in the world. It felt a little too good, almost destined in some way, and, gosh, now I know that it was. If I hadn't met him and continued to explore comfort through food, I don't think I would have gained a lot of weight, lost a lot of weight, and, ultimately, written this cookbook. I do consider the way this all played out a blessing, *I really do*. But let's get back to the food.

One of the places we've visited quite frequently was a local Sichuan joint that served really good spicy dishes and amazing cocktails. In fact, the bartenders have won awards for being some of the best in the world. The place is run by a father and son team, a family, who always smiled or hugged it out when you arrived.

Don and I slid up to the restaurant's bar on a weekly basis. We'd order fragrant and fiery dishes cooked in the back kitchen in a hot second and sip exquisite cocktails, often adorned extravagantly with tropical fruit, citrus wedges, booze-infused cherries, and other funky garnishes. Our favorite dishes were an intensely spiced soup filled with sliced duck and pork dumplings that floated in a bowl of hot chili oil. When we had that food and those drinks before us, it's as if we were home.

When I set out to change the way I ate, both cocktails and meat were off my menu. Sadly, cocktails are often just glasses of (deliciously indulgent) sugar plus booze. And duck and pork just weren't my thing at the time. Once we stopped visiting our special place and any of the other restaurants we hit up regularly, our relationship suffered a bit. That Sichuan place was where we were able to let off a little steam and find instant happiness, and once it was off menu, we were left scattered, looking for something fun to continue to connect us.

Once I realized that stopping Sichuan food had made us a little sad, I sought out Sherrie for advice. She explained that it was important to keep a food ritual or two between partners, something special that bonded us, in order to not feel that weird emptiness and remain connected to the things you love, mainly each other. Shortly thereafter, Don and I discussed an alternative menu for Sichuan food nights: instead of our usual, we'd switch to a spicy fish soup, white rice, and green vegetables. He enjoyed cocktails but I stuck to my no-processed-sugar rule and allowed myself a single glass of white wine. Once we informed our restaurant family of my dietary changes, they were all in with us and even created a bubbly, no-alcohol, bitter tonic in order to put a pretty drink before me, but also to help my digestion of all the rich food.

Our connection rebounded instantly. We kept a meaningful food ritual between us and I still stayed on my plan—and found my way to begin to incorporate fish into my new style of eating. Instead of going out to eat elsewhere or eating more of the food that made me fat, I thought up an idea to stay connected around food, but in a new way.

FRIDAY NIGHT PICNICS

Rather than order takeout or visit lackluster restaurants (both of which couldn't always accommodate our distinct food preferences) on the weekend, I craved alternative approaches to a fun Friday night. We were already going on date nights for Sichuan food once every couple of weeks. We had found a secure place to unwind over our favorite healthy-ish dishes, a spot where we could connect with each other and our extended bar family. I wanted that warm feeling way more frequently.

I don't remember who developed the core idea but instead of going out, we decided to dine in on Friday nights. After all, with a long day of work behind us, it felt cozy to snug up amid familiar objects and the sort of food we wanted to eat. But instead of cooking dishes to enjoy at the dining room table, I got into child-mode and spread it all out on a picnic blanket. Set squarely on the living room floor, we placed a few blankets, various pillows, a stack of cookbooks as a tabletop, and candles. This picnic setup became our deluxe restaurant for the evening.

Don focused on the drink, shaking himself up a cocktail or opening a beer. And, on most Fridays, he'd pour me a single glass of a favorite white or red wine. With beverages in hand, we'd toss off our shoes and sit on the floor to recap the day and really reconnect. A few sips in, I'd run off into the kitchen to finish making our wholesome dish.

The dishes were generally full of vegetables but crafted with comfort in mind. I wanted us to feel free to place this food on the floor and dig in with one hand or simple utensils, never a knife. With extra napkins on hand, we'd graze over whatever was before us, savor some strong refreshments, and relate in a new way. Several hours later, our connection had been reestablished, albeit from a slightly different perspective.

Eventually, I felt secure enough in me and disciplined in my new way of eating—since I was dropping weight and that kept me inspired—to add a dessert or two to our Friday night repertoire. I also felt okay adding in an occasional favorite cocktail.

COOKING TOGETHER

Since we're a couple who is bonded by, among other things, food and celebration, we returned to cooking together pretty quickly after my weight loss. You see, if this plant-centric way of eating was the sort of thing that was sticking around for a while or forever, then I wanted to involve my partner in the actual cooking, in whatever way felt most comfy.

Since I generally planned our dinners, we'd divvy up a recipe on any given night. If we made the Spicy Zucchini Spaghetti (page 167)—which we've made many, many times—he'd focus on filling the pot with several quarts of water and getting it to a rolling boil. I'd sauté the garlic, shred the zucchini, and generally bring the sauce to life.

After adding a heavy hand of salt to the boiling water, Don would add the pasta, stir it gently, and test each strand as the minutes went on, until it was cooked to just before al dente. He'd ask if I needed starchy water from the pot before he drained the pasta into a colander and hand it off to me.

I'd sauté the garlic and add the thin zucchini noodles. I'd tumble the cooked pasta into the pan, add a little starchy pasta water, and toss a glossy sauce to life. I'd carefully twist the pasta into individual bowls, sprinkle in browned garlic slices and sea salt, and we'd fork piles between our lips. If eating this on a weekend night, we might add a glass of wine and a couple of lit tea lights. However the table was set, we made the whole meal together, with a lot of kindness and consideration.

Cooking together made the meal ours, not mine or his. And whether you're on some new wellness path or just want to share some of the work, finding a way to make a meal together in collaboration, almost dance-like in nature, is something you won't regret.

New Ways to Connect

Though I do love to stuff food into my face, I endeavored to find new ways to pass my fun time and, naturally, to do all the fun things together. I'm only too pleased to venture to a winery or brewery on the weekend, maybe stop for a pizza, and then head home to chill with a film. But my new way of eating got me thinking about non-food ways to do fun stuff together. Plus, I didn't do all the hard work to understand why I comforted myself with food just to stick to the same old eating-oriented pastimes. Here are five new things we rotated into our day dates and date nights:

Café time: Cafés are these glorious little spots that get you gabbing. While this still involves drinking something, it's not exactly the same as dining out in a restaurant. Instead, you order a coffee (for him) or a tea (for me), find a cushy table with a little good light, and talk for hours. We added café dates into our fun time as it offered a low-key, low-impact way to enjoy each other's company without being tied to ordering a complete meal. It also got us out of our home life routine, giving us a new setting in which to amuse ourselves and each other.

Walks amid wild life: As I lost weight and my joint pain subsided, I wanted to move. My husband has always had a long stride and can move pretty quickly, and now I could finally keep up. We'd find beach trails, farm trails, and just rural mountain roads where we could park and walk for an hour or two, taking in the scenery and fresh air and dreaming big dreams.

Drives with stunning views: If we wanted to explore farther afield, Saturday afternoons morphed into long drives to nowhere in particular. We'd pick a direction or city, and just go—similar to the road trips from my childhood. With good tunes and enough gas, these date drives gave us time to talk for hours or listen to good music or a favorite podcast.

Music sessions: In the last couple of years, we got way encouraged to return to listening to music. Rather than just put on any playlist, we got into the habit of playing our favorite music—from now or way back when—for each other. Inevitably, stories about the music began to pour out of us and we discovered new things about each other—which is totally exhilarating for two folks who've been together for coming up on 20 years.

Podcast co-listening: This is a rather new habit for us that we're still exploring. We both enjoy podcasts but we rarely commute anywhere with each other on a daily basis. Instead, we started playing podcasts aloud in our home. Snug up in front of a fire, listening to a podcast, you begin to feel a little hokey, like it's the 1950s, but then you sort of love that nostalgic feeling too.

FIVE BITS OF ADVICE FOR TRANSFORMING IN A COUPLE

I know many couples who embark on health upgrades, quite successfully, together. Bravo to them. For me, the path was less clear. If you've tried to get actively well with your partner and haven't achieved your desired results, I'd encourage you to take a step back, examine why it may not have worked, and consider some of the following bits that came up along my journey.

1. *Respect your separate wellness paths.* Try as you may, partners and spouses do not consistently transform together. It is not realistic to expect that my wellness transformation will work in the same way for someone else, including my partner. Two individuals could go on elimination diets and have radically different experiences. Be okay with keeping your paths separate and respect your individual journeys.

2. *Plan your joint meals together.* Just because my husband and I ate in unique ways some of the time, doesn't mean that we wouldn't include each other in meal planning. In fact, it's even more critical to do some upfront planning when one of you is embracing a new way of eating. It can be as simple as one person proposing dishes and the other offering up feedback, but draw up something to make sure everyone knows what to expect and can be involved in the meals.

3. *Don't skip date nights.* If the two of you don't continue to find ways to have fun together while one of you is on a transformative path, you run the risk of feeling disconnected. Date nights or day dates, whether at your favorite restaurant, the local beach, or squarely in front of your stove, are an important part of any coupling and shouldn't suffer because one of you, say, eats a little differently. Schedule those dates in a calendar, if that helps you keep having them.

4. *No partner left behind.* There may be times during your transformation when you feel lonely or distant from your partner or spouse. Perhaps you're both just having off days or perhaps your new way of eating is leaving your partner feeling a little left out. Share how it feels to be eating differently and listen to your partner's feelings, too. Listening builds understanding and gives you a chance to dispel any potential jealousy or resentment.

5. *Rediscover all the reasons you love each other.* Since food and body size were such a focus for us, reducing and revising our food connection felt uncomfortable at first. But our relationship is about way more than food. Once the excess food stopped, we reclaimed all the other reasons we were together and that kept us more in sync (and more in love). Cultivate new ways to spend your time together and try all those things you've wanted to try in the past.

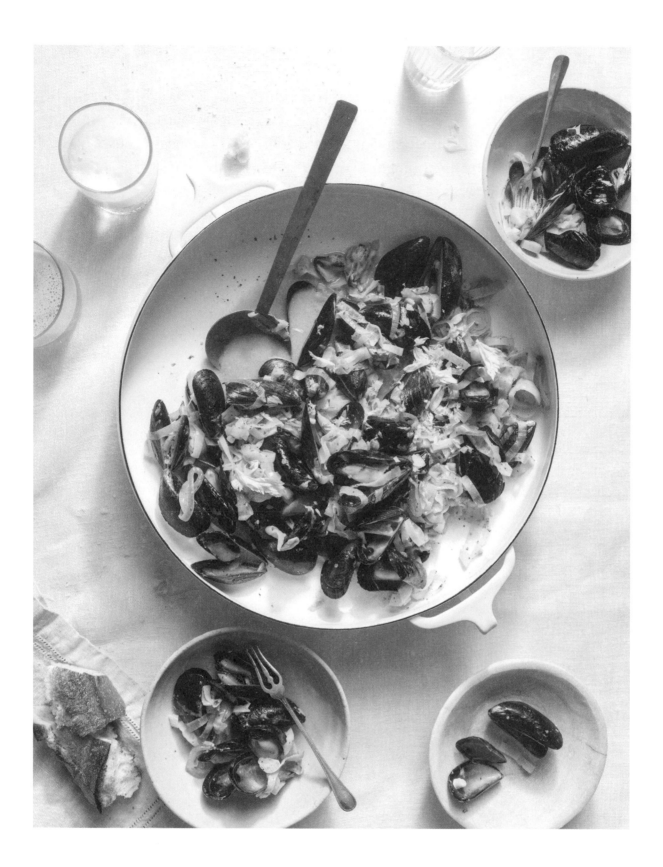

Braised LEEK AND BEER MUSSELS

This dish is like French-style braised leeks met a heap of mussels and fell in love. It's the sort of dish you place between two (or four) people who know each other very, very well. Share it with the sort who don't mind twirling leeks like makeshift pasta, so they revel in braised liquids that dribble down the side of your mouth. Make sure they're the type who are totally cool with picking mussels from shells with bare hands if forks take too long, which they often do. You'll want to dredge big, not small, hunks of baguette through the bowl, so avoid diners who may give you a weird look about that. This is a dish best shared with partners, lovers, and the very closest of friends.

Serves 2 to 4

FREQUENCY: *A couple times per month*

FOOD PREFERENCES: *DF, GF, NF, RSF*

HANDS-ON TIME: *20 minutes*

TOTAL TIME: *35 minutes*

---

2 tablespoons refined coconut oil

1 large shallot, thinly sliced

¾ pound (12 oz; 340 g) leeks, white and light green parts, thinly sliced and soaked/drained

3 tablespoons coarse-ground Dijon-style mustard

One 12-ounce (355 ml) can pilsner-style beer

1 teaspoon sea salt, divided

1 tablespoon capers, drained, rinsed, and coarsely chopped

2 pounds (904 g) mussels, cleaned and beards removed

3 tablespoons finely diced celery leaves (from a bunch of celery)

Baguette, for serving

1. Heat the oil in a large pot with a lid over medium-high heat. Once warm, add the shallot and sauté until it begins to wilt, 4 to 5 minutes. Add the leeks and mustard and stir until the mustard is dispersed. Sauté until the leeks are fully wilted, 5 to 7 minutes. Stir in the beer, ½ teaspoon of the salt, and the capers, and then let the mixture come to a boil. Lower the heat to simmer for 10 minutes to help develop the flavor.

2. Raise the heat back to medium high and bring the mixture back to a boil. Add the mussels, cover the pot, shake it a few times over the heat, and let it steam just until the mussels open, 3 to 4 minutes. Remove the cover and toss to ensure the leeks are all over the mussels.

3. Pour the entire contents of the pot into a large, deep bowl. Sprinkle with the remaining ½ teaspoon salt and garnish with the celery leaves. Serve immediately with an extra bowl for shells, forks for twirling up the leeks into your mouth, and a baguette for dipping in the broth.

ROASTED VEGETABLE DIP
with Olive and Oregano Crackers

This is fine fare for a night when you have a little extra time in the kitchen. Instead of traditional store-bought dips and chips, I roast whatever veg is in my fridge or larder—making sure to include some nice mushrooms like shiitakes for the flavor pop—and toss them in a powerful blender with a few pantry ingredients. You can certainly eat the dip as a sandwich spread or just with a spoon and some yogurt; however, I encourage you to take the time to make the crackers. With olives and oregano pressed into the dough, these crackers are kind of exciting and salty in a way a cracker should be.

*Makes about 2 cups of dip and
32 to 40 crackers*

FREQUENCY: *A couple times per month*

FOOD PREFERENCES: *DF, NF, RSF, V*

HANDS-ON TIME: *40 minutes*

TOTAL TIME: *2 hours*

. . . .

FOR THE ROASTED VEGETABLE DIP

4 ounces (115 g) wild mushrooms
   (such as shiitakes) with stems
   cleaned, trimmed, and halved

1 medium parsnip or carrot, cleaned
   and roughly chopped

1 small red onion, peeled and cut
   into six pieces

3 small garlic cloves, peeled

3 tablespoons plus ½ cup (120 ml)
   extra-virgin olive oil, divided, plus
   more for garnish

1 teaspoon sea salt, divided

12 twists freshly ground black pepper

¼ teaspoon red pepper flakes

One 15-ounce (425 g) can white beans,
   drained and rinsed

1 teaspoon sherry vinegar

2 tablespoons water

MAKE THE ROASTED VEGETABLE DIP

1. Preheat the oven to 350°F (177°C).

2. Place the mushrooms, parsnip, onion, and garlic cloves on a large baking sheet, separated into their own sections. Drizzle 3 tablespoons of the oil between them all, tossing them about until well coated. Sprinkle ½ teaspoon of the salt across the veg. Roast for 20 minutes. Remove from the oven and cool for 10 minutes.

3. Add the roasted veg to a powerful blender or food processor along with the remaining ½ cup olive oil, remaining ½ teaspoon salt, ground pepper, pepper flakes, beans, vinegar, and water. Whiz until smooth-ish but still chunky. Taste and add more salt or pepper. Serve in a clean bowl with an extra drizzle of olive oil, a sprinkle of flaky sea salt, and mushroom powder, if desired, alongside the crackers. Store the dip an airtight container in the fridge for up to 2 days.

MAKE THE OLIVE AND OREGANO CRACKERS

1. Add the flours, salt, and oregano to a large mixing bowl. Add the oil and mix it in with a fork until well distributed. Add the water and stir until a wet dough comes together.

2. Turn the mixture out until a floured work surface. Knead the dough until it's smooth, adding a smidge more water (if too dry) or flour (if too wet), as needed. The dough shouldn't be sticky.

3. Dust your work surface with flour once again and roll the dough out into a ¼-inch-thick rectangle. Sprinkle the diced olives evenly over the dough. Fold the dough over a few times and knead the olives into the dough to distribute them well. Add more flour to the surface if the olive liquid drips out onto it. Form the dough into a small ball. Cover with a damp kitchen towel and rest for 10 minutes.

continued

Flaky sea salt, to garnish

Mushroom Powder (page 54),
to garnish (optional)

FOR THE OLIVE
AND OREGANO CRACKERS

⅔ cup (2¾ oz; 80 g) all-purpose flour,
plus extra for dusting

⅔ cup (2⅔ oz; 75 g) whole wheat flour

1 teaspoon fine sea salt

4 tablespoons dried oregano leaves

4 tablespoons extra-virgin olive oil

½ cup (120 ml) water

½ cup cured black olives, pitted,
patted dry, and finely diced

Flaky sea salt, for sprinkling

4. Arrange two racks in the center of your oven. Preheat the oven to 400°F (204°C).

5. Line your work surface with parchment paper. Divide the dough in half and work with one half at a time, keeping the other under the kitchen towel. Dust the parchment with flour and roll out the dough on it as thinly as possible—the general shape is up to you. Gently slip the parchment with the dough onto a baking sheet. Use a sharp knife or pizza cutter to create long 2-inch-wide cracker shapes, and then slice them in half. Sprinkle the dough with flaky sea salt. Repeat this process with the other half of dough.

6. Bake the crackers for 10 to 12 minutes or until golden brown. If you rolled them thicker, cook them a few minutes longer but watch them closely so they don't get too brown. Remove from the oven and cool to room temperature. Break the crackers apart into long crackers or smaller shapes, as you like. The crackers keep well stored in an airtight container for a few days.

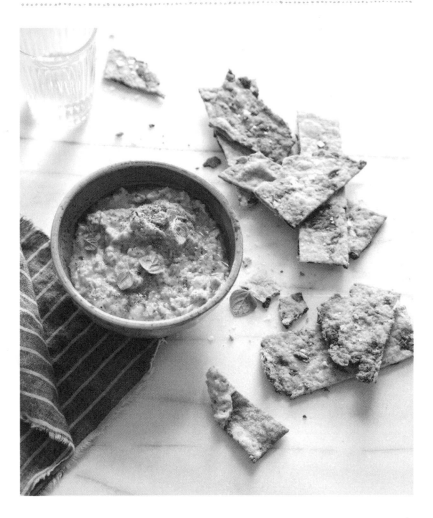

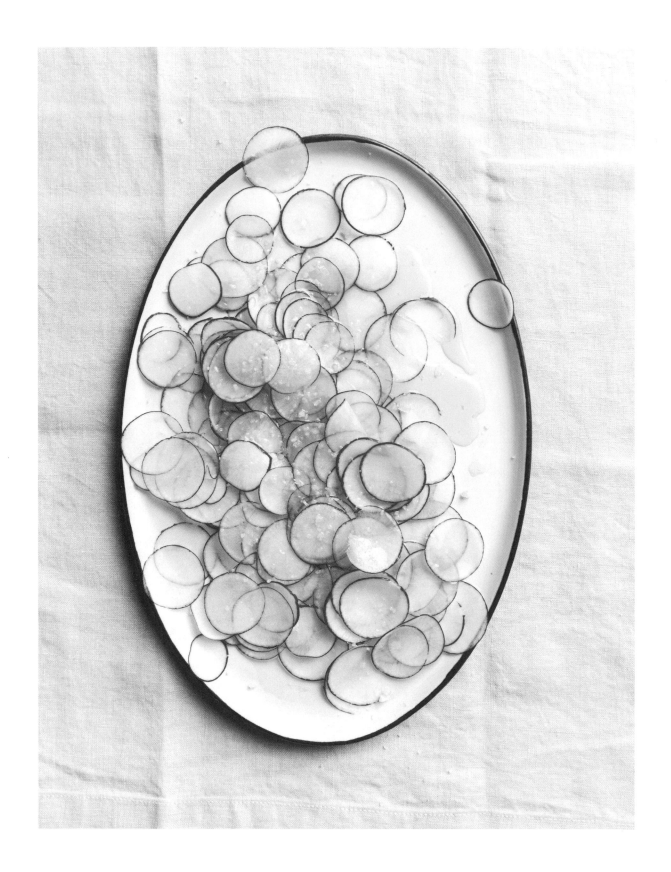

RADISH CARPACCIO *Snack Plate*

One Friday night, my husband and I were part of an impromptu cocktail party on a friend's rooftop deck in Montreal. Our host, Chloe, in a laid-back Quebecois way, thinly sliced a bunch of old radishes from the back of her fridge. With a few flourishes, she turned those tired, tiny globes into an elegant apéro hour snack that was equally sharp and sweet alongside our whiskeys and wine.

It's important to get whatever veg you use—radishes, turnips, cucumbers, and carrots are all fine—into a very thin sliver and I use a mandoline to make this happen. They're super affordable online—just be ultra-careful that you use the finger guard and keep your fingers far away from the blade.

It's equally paramount that you allow the veg to rest once you drizzle the oil and salt. In those 5 minutes, the salt draws out the pure veg flavor, making a radish taste even more like a radish, and the oil adds a rich sweetness. Please choose a high-quality and flavorful olive oil, as there's nothing to hide a lower-quality oil here. Present the platter with small forks and little plates so folks can pull as many as they'd like to nibble from the platter.

Serves 2

FREQUENCY: *A couple times per month*

FOOD PREFERENCES: *DF, GF, NF, RSF, V*

HANDS-ON TIME: *5 minutes*

TOTAL TIME: *10 minutes*

1 bunch radishes (about 8 small radishes), leaves reserved for another use

1 tablespoon extra-virgin olive oil

½ teaspoon flaky sea salt

1. Slice the radishes as thin as you can get them with a mandoline (make sure to use the finger guard). Scatter the slices on a serving plate.

2. Drizzle the oil and sprinkle the salt across the radishes, trying to ensure that each radish slice grabs a drop or two of oil and a few salt flakes. Let rest for 5 minutes and serve.

NICOISE PASTA SALAD *with Basil Dressing*

This is a quickish dish that I turn to quite frequently when I've made no advance dinner plans but know I have some lingering vegetables in the fridge. I prefer to use a mild lettuce or even torn Swiss chard leaves alongside a variety of mixed vegetables like tiny cooked potatoes, green beans, cucumbers, radishes, garden peppers, onions, tomatoes, and celery. Choose what you like to eat and blanch anything that you want to take the raw flavor off of, like green beans or maybe garden peppers.

The point, here, is that there's more veg than pasta but a little pasta helps make this even more filling. Choose a pasta shape—something small and bite size—that matches the sizes of your veg. My favorite pasta to use in this dish is casarecce because it's similar in size to green beans, but other shapes like orecchiette, penne, and cavatelle work well. I prefer to use tuna in olive oil. It has a few more calories than the water-packed kind but retains more flavor, which means it tastes good and I feel satisfied. Satisfaction is an important part of feeding yourself. Plus, the oil used is typically unsaturated and heart-healthy—a good-for-you bonus.

This recipe makes about 1 cup of dairy-free pesto dressing, so you may have a little left over. It works on so many foods beyond pasta salad, such as eggs, tacos, and potatoes.

Serves 4

FREQUENCY: *A couple times per month*

FOOD PREFERENCES: *DF, GF, RSF*

HANDS-ON TIME: *10 minutes*

TOTAL TIME: *30 minutes*

· ·

8 ounces (226 g) dried bite-size, gluten-free pasta

1 tablespoon plus ½ teaspoon sea salt, divided

1 teaspoon plus ½ cup (120 ml) extra-virgin olive oil, divided

1 small bunch basil (about 10 sprigs), stems cut and discarded

ingredients continued

1. Fill a large pot with 1 quart of water and set it on the stove to come to a boil. When it boils, stir in 1 tablespoon of the salt and the dried pasta. Cook, stirring occasionally, until the pasta is cooked al dente to your package directions. Drain in a colander, toss with 1 teaspoon of the oil, and set aside to cool.

2. To make the dressing, add the basil, nuts, remaining ½ cup oil, water, lemon juice, remaining ½ teaspoon salt, and pepper to a powerful blender. Blend until smooth.

3. Combine the pasta, greens, veg, and olives in a very large bowl. Set aside.

4. Pour half the dressing on the pasta salad. Toss to combine until there's dressing on every bite. Fork the tuna across the top of the pasta salad. Serve with remaining dressing, on the side, for folks to add as they like.

⅓ cup pine nuts

¼ cup (60 ml) water

2 tablespoons lemon juice (from about
  1 medium lemon)

10 twists freshly ground black pepper

3 cups mixed greens, like butter lettuce,
  romaine, and radicchio

1 cup fresh vegetable of your choice,
  cut into bite-size pieces

½ cup pitted olives, nicoise or kalamata,
  halved

Two 5-ounce (142 g) tins solid pack
  light tuna in olive oil

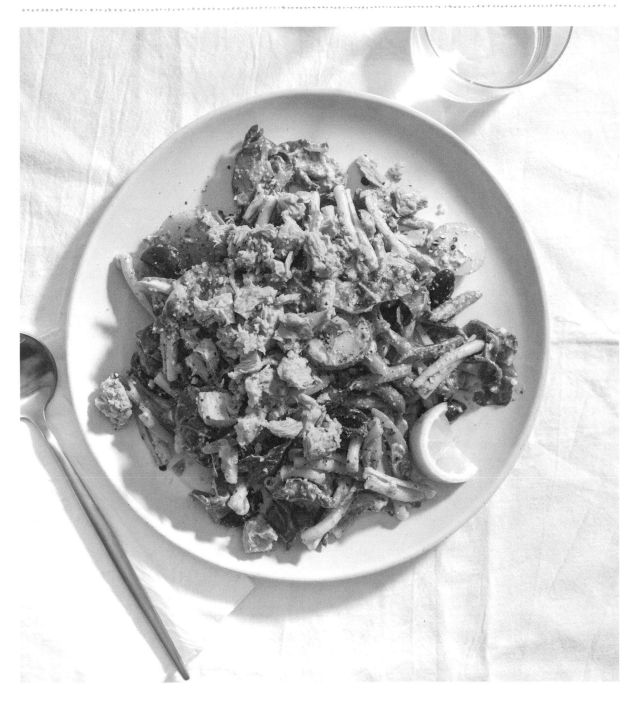

Veggie FRIED RICE

This fried rice isn't perfect. In fact, it's quite the opposite. I created the recipe to use up the remaining few carrots, half onion, and whatever else I had lingering before a grocery trip. I've made it a hundred different ways and have swapped in everything from peas, collards, tiny bits of corn, scallions, cauliflower, and broccoli crowns. Choose a variety of vegetables that lend vibrant colors and nourishment. You may also opt to add shrimp, scallops, or scrambled eggs but then the dish is not vegan, obviously.

If you prefer to ignore my measurements altogether, go for it. A little extra of this or less of that won't ruin the dish; it will just make it your special recipe. But let's be clear: this dish is meant to be more vegetables than rice. It's a hefty dose of your daily vegetables mixed in with filling brown rice. The flavors and textures will remind you of a more wholesome version of Chinese takeout with lots of green.

Use a high-quality sesame oil and soy sauce because these two ingredients really flavor the dish. And if possible, choose a chili paste that's not loaded with sugar. I use a homespun variety from the remains after fermenting a pot of Fermented Hot Sauce (page 49) from summer peppers. Alternatively, you can buy the bottled stuff from your region's Asian market.

I love to start the weekend with this big, pretty bowl of fried rice. It's a little ritual that I've been able to keep up while still leading an everyday wholesome kind of life. And, sometimes, I even use cauliflower rice.

Serves 4

FREQUENCY: *Once per week*

FOOD PREFERENCES: *DF, GF, NF, RSF, V*

HANDS-ON TIME: *20 minutes*

TOTAL TIME: *20 minutes*

3 tablespoons coconut oil

1 tablespoon chili paste

1 medium red onion, peeled and thinly sliced

6 large garlic cloves, peeled and finely diced

3 medium carrots, cleaned and finely chopped

ingredients continued

1. Heat the oil in a wide non-stick pan set over medium-high heat. Stir in the chili paste, onion, garlic, and carrots, and cook until the onions are translucent, 3 to 4 minutes. Add the cabbage and chard stems (not the chard leaves, yet). Toss with other ingredients and cook until slightly limp, 3 to 4 minutes. Add the chard leaves. Toss and cook until incorporated, 1 to 2 minutes. Add the rice and sprouts. Toss with the other ingredients and cook until well incorporated, 3 to 4 minutes. Add the soy sauce and fold into the other ingredients until they're well coated. Cook for 1 to 2 minutes and then turn off the heat.

2. Stir in the sesame oil. Sprinkle with chopped cilantro and serve with lime wedges on the side.

¼ head cabbage, thinly sliced

3 Swiss chard or kale stalks, thinly sliced; chop and reserve stems separately

4 cups cooked rice

1 cup bean sprouts

3 tablespoons gluten-free soy sauce, or to taste

3 tablespoons toasted sesame oil

½ cup finely chopped cilantro leaves

Lime wedges, for serving

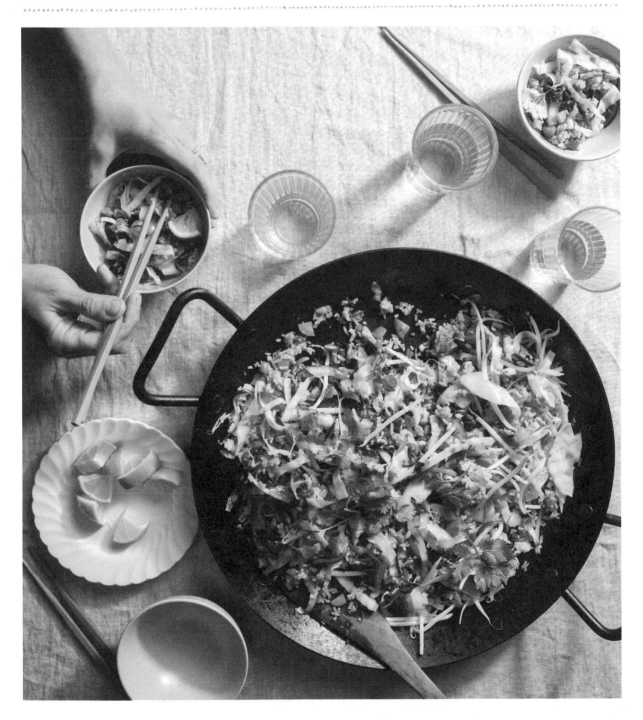

A Better BOLOGNESE

A simmering pot of Bolognese reminds me of Sunday dinners at my Italian grandmother's house. You could smell the meaty red sauce as soon as you pulled into the driveway. Piled high on endless bowls of fresh pasta, Bolognese always hugged me from the inside in a way that only a grandmother's cooking could. When that flavor craving hits me now, I make a healthier version that feeds the food memory in, I hope, a very respectful way.

Instead of ground meat, I use plant-based protein crumbles and typically choose a pea protein variety that's soy-free. To create a deeper flavor, I continue to use red wine (the alcohol burns off leaving just a taste of it in the pot). I also add in a secret flavor bomb: mushroom powder. My recipe takes mere minutes to make so whiz up a big batch for your spice shelf—you can use it in everything that asks to be a bit more savory. Instead of milk or cream, I add a stunning richness to the pot with homemade crème fraîche (soak the cashews and make it in advance, so it's at the ready in the fridge). And please do not omit the nutmeg. It won't make it taste like a cookie; it simply adds a warming spice that's original and critical to the dish.

This Bolognese is a lot more wholesome than the big pot of simmered ground meat and milk from my youth and, though it takes a few steps, I hope you'll give it a shot when only a big bowl of warmth will satisfy you on a frigid night.

Makes about 6 cups

FREQUENCY: *A couple times per month*
FOOD PREFERENCES: *DF, GF, RSF, V*
HANDS-ON TIME: *25 minutes*
TOTAL TIME: *1 hour 25 minutes*

. . . .

4 tablespoons extra-virgin olive oil, divided, plus more for seasoning/serving

1 large purple eggplant, sliced in half lengthwise

3 shallots, finely diced

3 large garlic cloves, peeled and finely diced

8 ounces (230 g) wild mushrooms, diced to the size of the protein crumbles

¼ cup Mushroom Powder (page 54)

½ teaspoon red pepper flakes

1 teaspoon sea salt, plus more for serving

ingredients continued

1. Preheat the oven to 350°F (177°C). Drizzle 2 tablespoons of the oil on the eggplant (1 tablespoon per cut side). Place the eggplant cut side down on a rimmed baking sheet. Roast for 30 minutes or until very soft and a dark golden brown. Allow to cool before scraping the meat from the skin and chopping it up. Set the eggplant flesh aside and discard the skin.

2. Heat the remaining 2 tablespoons oil in a Dutch oven set over medium heat. Add the shallots and garlic, and sauté until translucent with just a touch of golden color, about 2 minutes. Add the mushrooms and sauté until wilted, about 3 minutes. Add the mushroom powder, pepper flakes, salt, and black pepper. Stir until the mushrooms are well coated with the spices and cook until your kitchen begins to fill with those aromatics, 3 to 4 minutes.

3. Add the wine and let it cook off its alcohol and reduce over 4 minutes, making sure to stir up all the flavor bits stuck to the bottom of the pan. Stir in the reserved eggplant, protein crumbles, tomatoes, stock, and crème fraîche. Grate in the nutmeg. Let the sauce come to just a boil. Reduce the heat to low, cover partially letting a bit of the pot peek through, and simmer for 20 to 25 minutes to mesh all the flavors. Stir occasionally to scrape up any pieces sticking to the bottom of the pot.

4. Shut off the heat and add salt and black pepper to taste, along with a small swig of olive oil. Stir in the fresh herbs. Serve over pasta, roasted potatoes, or on good toasted bread.

12 twists freshly ground black pepper,
   plus more for serving

¾ cup (180 ml) dry red wine

11 ounces (312 g) plant-based protein
   crumbles

2½ cups canned whole tomatoes,
   crushed by hand, or crushed/
   diced tomatoes

1 cup (240 ml) vegetable stock

½ cup (120 ml) Crème Fraîche (page 43)

⅛ teaspoon freshly grated nutmeg
   (from a whole nutmeg)

8 sprigs basil, finely diced

2 sprigs oregano, finely diced

Roasted potatoes, pasta,
   or toasted bread, to serve

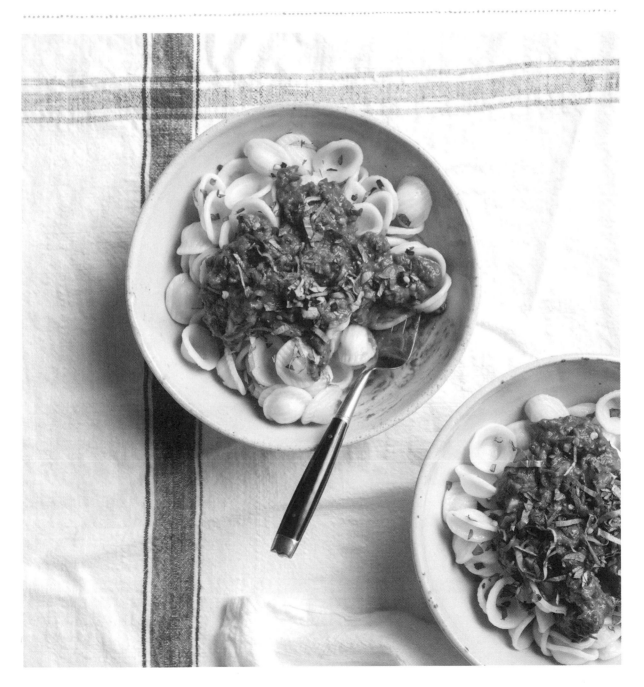

PASTA *with Cauliflower and Capers*

This is another comforting dish that comes together in under 30 minutes, making it perfect Friday night food. My partner chooses and makes the pasta to perfection, meaning just before al dente, and opens a bottle of wine. I bring the sauce together with pantry ingredients and fresh cauliflower.

Since a Friday night fridge can be pretty bare, leave out the celery if you've run out; the sauce will be just as nice with only onions and garlic. No white wine? Use red wine. I always have homemade tomato sauce in my pantry, since I make quarts of Spicy Tomato Sauce during late summer. If all you have is a tin of tomato sauce, use that. If all you have is a tin of diced tomatoes, use that thinned with a bit of water. No capers? Try chopped olives. The yogurt isn't necessary but adds a nice richness. You can use unsweetened almond milk in a pinch. Don't skip the green on top but celery leaves or basil work well, too.

Serves 2 to 3

FREQUENCY: *A couple times per month*

FOOD PREFERENCES: *DF, GF, NF, RSF, V*

HANDS-ON TIME: *15 minutes*

TOTAL TIME: *30 minutes*

· ·

8 ounces (227 g) semolina or gluten-free pasta (like caserecce, trofie, or strozzapreti)

2 tablespoons extra-virgin olive oil

½ medium white onion, peeled and chopped

1 large garlic clove, peeled and thinly sliced

ingredients continued

1. Heat 4 quarts of water in a large pot over medium-high heat. Once it comes to a boil, add in a big handful of sea salt (at least 3 tablespoons). Add the pasta and cook according to your pasta package directions. Cook the pasta about 1 minute less than recommended, as it will finish cooking in the sauce. Drain the pasta, reserving ½ cup pasta water.

2. Heat the oil in a separate shallow, wide pan over medium heat. Add the onion, garlic, and celery. Sauté until everything begins to wilt and soften, 5 to 6 minutes. Add the tomato paste and cook for 1 to 2 minutes. Add the wine and cook for 1 to 2 minutes. Add the cauliflower, salt, and pepper, and toss around until well coated. Stir in the tomato sauce and capers. Let the mixture come to a simmer and cook until the cauliflower is fork tender, about 10 minutes, stirring frequently. Turn off the heat and stir in the yogurt.

3. Add the pasta and a couple tablespoons of pasta water to the pan and toss together gently. Add a little more pasta water, if needed, to get the sauce to coat the pasta with silkiness. Sprinkle with parsley and a bit more salt, to taste. Serve immediately.

2 large celery stalks, thinly sliced

1 tablespoon tomato paste

½ cup (120 ml) dry white wine

1 medium cauliflower, diced into
    ½-inch pieces

½ teaspoon sea salt, plus more for
    the pasta water and seasoning

12 twists freshly ground black pepper

2 cups Spicy Tomato Sauce (page 35)
    or one 14.5-ounce (411 g) can
    tomato sauce

2 tablespoons capers, drained
    and chopped

2 tablespoons unsweetened,
    plain plant-based yogurt

3 tablespoons finely diced parsley

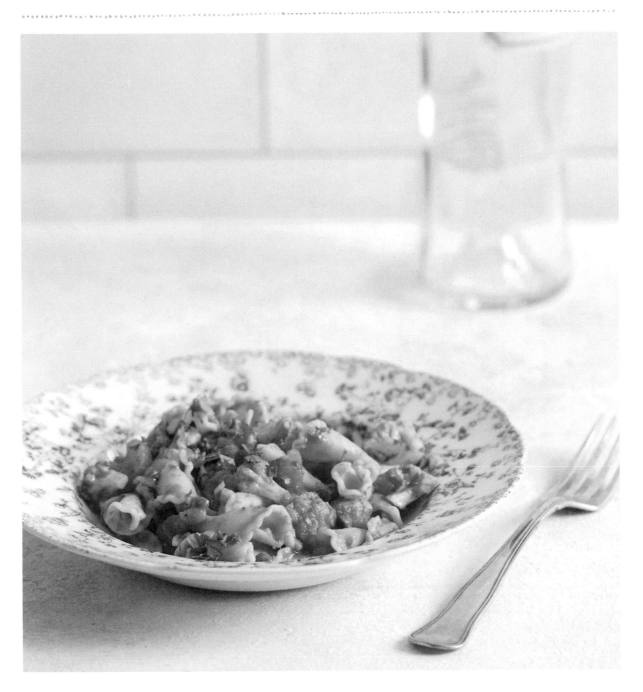

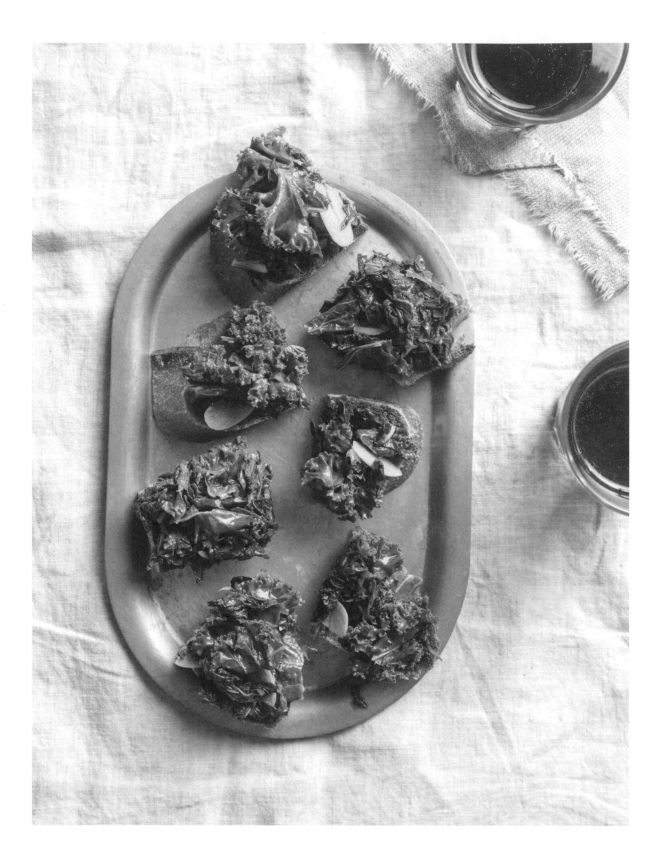

Garlicky-Green TOASTS

If you are looking for nifty ways to incorporate more greens into your meals, this recipe is for you. It's easy, accessible, lip-smacking, and savory. It's also versatile. An egg on top of a single slice of toast makes this equally interesting and more filling for some.

I recommend that you drift into the weekend with greens on toast. It also makes a lovely nibble when friends drop by, especially with a hearty cocktail or a glass of deep red wine.

Make sure to use a solid green that will still retain some shape on your toast. I'm more likely to use Lacinato or curly kale versus something flimsy like baby kale or young spinach, but all of them will taste great. Cook the thinner greens for a minute or two less.

Serves 4 (as snack) or 2 (as meal)

FREQUENCY: *A couple times per month*

FOOD PREFERENCES: *DF, NF, RSF, V*

HANDS-ON TIME: *15 minutes*

TOTAL TIME: *15 minutes*

. . . .

1 large bunch curly kale (about 8 stalks) washed and dried

2 tablespoons extra-virgin olive oil

1 large garlic clove, peeled and thinly sliced

¼ teaspoon sea salt, plus more for seasoning

¼ cup (60 ml) water

1 teaspoon balsamic vinegar

6 twists freshly ground black pepper

4 small slices sourdough bread, toasted

1. Remove the stems from each kale leaf, gathering the long leaves into a wide stack, reserving the stems for a future pot of stock. Slice across the width of the kale stack into 1-inch strips. Turn the cutting board or the kale and slice again into a ½-inch dice. Take your knife through the kale again, dicing as you go, to ensure it's as close to bite-sized pieces as possible. You'll have a big pile of well-diced kale.

2. Warm the oil in a frying pan set over medium heat. Add the kale, garlic, and salt. Toss and fry until the kale has wilted slightly, about 1 minute. Add the water and cover the pan for 3 minutes. Remove the cover, stir in the vinegar and black pepper, and cook for 1 minute more. Turn the heat off. Taste and add more salt, if you like.

3. Divide the kale evenly on top of the four toast slices. Slice each toast into three pieces to create smaller segments. You'll have about 12 toasts in total. Serve immediately while it's still warm.

My Kind of NACHOS

Nachos are iconic fast food that have become a yellow cheese flavor bomb. They were first made in Mexico with fried tortillas, a little shredded cheese, and sliced jalapeños and served as an appetizer. They've turned into a highly caloric pile of everything typically served as a main course that's loaded with fat. While there's nothing wrong with that once in a while, nachos are tough territory for those who don't eat dairy.

For me, nachos are less about the cheese and more about the varied textures and toppings. I want each chip to have a little bit of everything, including a mix of warm toppings and cool toppings. And if I'm going to enjoy a highly caloric pile of fried tortilla chips, I certainly want them to be nutritious on top of extremely satisfying—one may say, I want to get my money's worth.

My nachos have layers of punchy flavors and include smooth, garlicky bean spread; spicy, crispy, chorizo-like tofu; meaty, wild mushrooms; bright, pickled salad turnips; avocado triangles; and a zippy lime crème fraîche. I don't even try to re-create a dairy-free cheese sauce because (1) anything I'd create would not appeal to traditional nacho eaters and (2) there are other ways to craft that creaminess that a good chip deserves. And just so we're clear, the right tortilla chips are crucial. Pick up a bag that contains the fewest ingredients; the best versions are made from non-GMO white corn, sunflower oil, salt, and lime. Even my husband has no idea how he went from eating cheap commodity tortilla chips to the higher-priced, well-crafted tortilla chips available on some shelves today—but he wouldn't go back. (Me: "Need anything at the market?" Him: "Just the expensive tortilla chips.")

The Tofu Chorizo is adapted from a recipe by Mark Bittman that appeared in the *New York Times*. Mark has written many wonderful books, including *How to Cook Everything Vegetarian* and *VB6: Eat Vegan Before 6:00 to Lose Weight and Restore Your Health . . . for Good*. He's got an inspiring way with vegetables and I credit him for some of my early interest in vegetable-forward meals.

Don't feel like you need to create all the layers in the recipe. It's all simple work but multiple steps, so leave anything out that feels extraneous for you. If you do make all the layers, you may have leftovers so use them to liven up your dishes the rest of the week. You can certainly layer everything in a nice oven-proof dish but I make and eat these nachos right off a parchment-lined tray. This meal paired with a drink as the sun sets will comfort (and nourish!) you after a hard week, promise.

Serves 2

FREQUENCY: *A couple times per month*
FOOD PREFERENCES: *DF, GF, RSF, V*
HANDS-ON TIME: *1 hour*
TOTAL TIME: *1 hour 15 minutes*

MAKE THE MY KIND OF NACHOS

1. Heat 1 tablespoon of the oil in a frying pan over medium-high heat. Add the garlic cloves and fry in the oil, tossing a few times, until golden brown on all sides. Transfer the garlic to a powerful blender. Lower the heat and carefully pour the pinto beans and their liquid into the pan. Raise the heat back to medium and cook until it simmers, about 3 to 4 minutes. Turn the heat off and cool for 5 minutes. Add the contents of the pan to the blender with the garlic and add the salt. Blend until smooth and silky. Set aside for the moment.

continued

FOR THE MY KIND OF NACHOS

2 tablespoons extra-virgin olive oil,
    divided

3 small garlic cloves, peeled

One 15-ounce (425 g) can pinto beans,
    beans and liquid

½ teaspoon sea salt, plus more
    for seasoning

Tofu Chorizo (recipe follows)

4 ounces (115 g) maitake or hen of
    the wood mushrooms, cleaned
    and sliced

⅓ bag white corn tortilla chips

Quick Pickled Turnips (page 56)
    or some other pickle

1 avocado, pitted, peeled, and sliced
    into tiny rectangles

Lime Crème Fraîche (page 43)

1 small bunch cilantro (about 10 sprigs),
    stems cut and discarded

FOR THE TOFU CHORIZO

One 14-ounce (397 g) block extra-firm
    tofu

2 tablespoons extra-virgin olive oil

1 small white onion, peeled and chopped

3 small garlic cloves, peeled and
    finely diced

1 tablespoon chili powder

1 tablespoon cumin

¼ teaspoon cinnamon

½ teaspoon sea salt, plus more to taste

1½ tablespoons apple cider vinegar
    or coconut vinegar

2. Make the Tofu Chorizo now, following the instructions below.

3. Preheat the oven to 375°F (191°C). Line a rimmed baking sheet with parchment paper.

4. Heat the remaining 1 tablespoon oil in the frying pan over medium-high heat. Add the mushrooms and sauté until they wilt and release some of their water, about 5 minutes. Sprinkle with salt if desired and set aside for the moment.

5. Arrange a single layer of tortilla chips on the parchment-lined baking sheet. Place a dollop of pinto bean spread on each chip. Scatter the mushrooms across the chips, aiming to get one slice on most chips. Sprinkle the tofu chorizo across the chips. Bake for 8 to 12 minutes, until everything is warmed through, including the chips, to your liking.

6. When the nachos emerge from the oven, top with the turnips, avocado, and crème fraîche. Sprinkle with cilantro leaves and extra salt. Serve immediately.

MAKE THE TOFU CHORIZO

1. Drain the tofu and pat it dry with a paper towel or kitchen towel. Let the tofu sit in the towel for about 15 minutes so that some extra water is extracted.

2. Heat the oil in a frying pan over medium-high heat. Add the onion and garlic, and sauté until they wilt a bit, about 5 minutes. With clean hands, break up the tofu into small crumbles and add them to the pan. Cook, stirring and scraping up the pan frequently, for at least 10 minutes until the tofu begins to get crispy and golden.

3. Lower the heat to medium. Sprinkle the chili powder, cumin, cinnamon, and salt on top. Cook another 10 minutes, stirring frequently, until the tofu gets fully crispy and golden and is well covered with spices. The fragrance should fill the air around you. Stir in the vinegar and more salt to taste. Set aside for the moment.

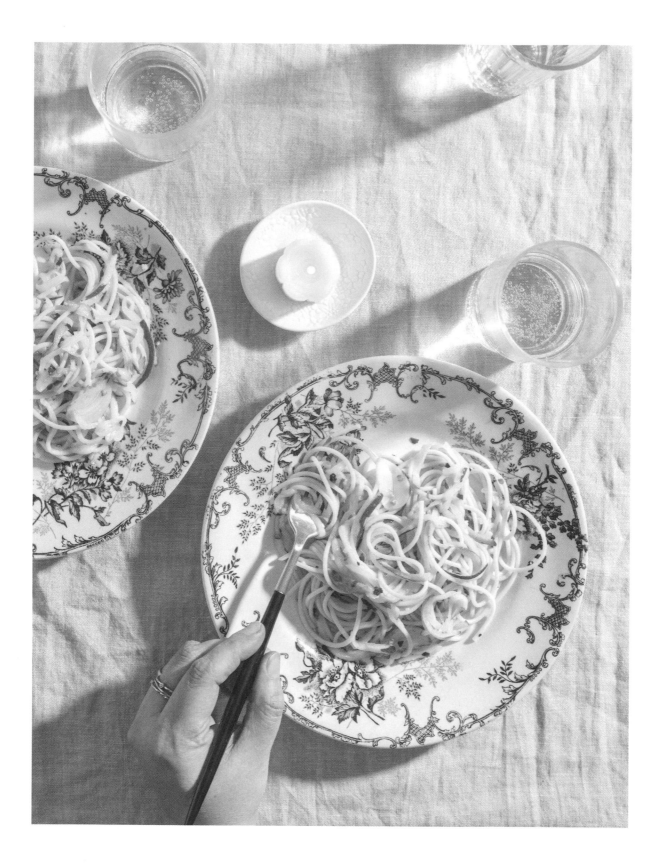

Spicy ZUCCHINI SPAGHETTI

This is a quick pasta dish that easily qualifies as comfort food but is also filled with silky shredded vegetables, which is the real bonus. There's more veg than pasta, purposefully, because the veg does wilt down considerably.

Shred the zucchini on a box grater and zen out to the repetitive movement or use the shredder attachment on a food processor to speed up the process. In the fall, I shred small piles of zucchini explicitly to make this dish in the winter. Overall, it is much better with freshly shredded zucchini in season but when you're overloaded with a harvest, you can freeze it up knowing you'll still get a solid dish off-season. (If you have the time, thaw and drain the frozen veg in advance.)

As written, the recipe is only mildly warm from the red pepper flakes. Oftentimes, I'll double the amount of pepper to make it even more picante. This dish is gluten-free if you use gluten-free pasta, which I do often and it's wonderful.

Serves 2 to 3

FREQUENCY: *A couple times per month*

FOOD PREFERENCES: *DF, GF, NF, RSF, V*

HANDS-ON TIME: *20 minutes*

TOTAL TIME: *20 minutes*

¼ teaspoon sea salt, plus more for pasta water and seasoning

8 ounces (227 g) semolina-flour or gluten-free spaghetti

2 tablespoons extra-virgin olive oil

3 medium garlic cloves, peeled

¼ teaspoon red pepper flakes

2 small zucchini, shredded

1. Heat 4 quarts of water in a large pot set over medium-high heat. Once it comes to a boil, add in a big handful of salt (at least 3 tablespoons). Add the pasta and cook according to your pasta package directions. Cook the pasta about 1 minute less than recommended, as it will finish cooking in the sauce. Drain the pasta, reserving ½ cup of pasta water. Don't begin making the sauce until the pasta is well on its way to done.

2. Heat the oil in a shallow wide pan over medium heat. Add the garlic cloves and sauté until the garlic is golden (but not burned) on all sides, 5 to 6 minutes. Remove from the pan and let cool. Add the pepper flakes and cook for 1 to 2 minutes. Add the shredded zucchini and salt, and toss around in the oil until slightly wilted. Add the pasta and 2 tablespoons of pasta water, or more, if needed, to bring a whisper of a sauce together that just coats the pasta with silkiness. Thinly slice the garlic and toss it into the pasta. Sprinkle with a bit more salt, to taste, and serve immediately.

PINEAPPLE, LIME, CHILI

When I make dessert on a Friday night, it's usually something like this easy-peasy dish. There isn't much to it but its simplicity makes the flavor punch so exciting. Quite frankly, it tastes like a very good-for-you version of a fruity cereal from my childhood (and maybe yours).

In addition to dessert, this dish makes a stunning side dish on a summer's day, perhaps served with something just off the grill and a massaged kale salad. It's easy to double, triple, or even quadruple for a party.

Serves 2

FREQUENCY: *Once per week*

FOOD PREFERENCES: *DF, GF, NF, RSF, V*

HANDS-ON TIME: *10 minutes*

TOTAL TIME: *10 minutes*

One quarter large pineapple, cleaned and sliced into ¼-inch-wide pieces

⅛ teaspoon chili powder

½ teaspoon lime zest (from about 1 medium lime)

Spread the pineapple on a plate. Dust with the chili powder and lime zest. Serve immediately or store in the fridge, for no more than an hour, uncovered, until ready to serve.

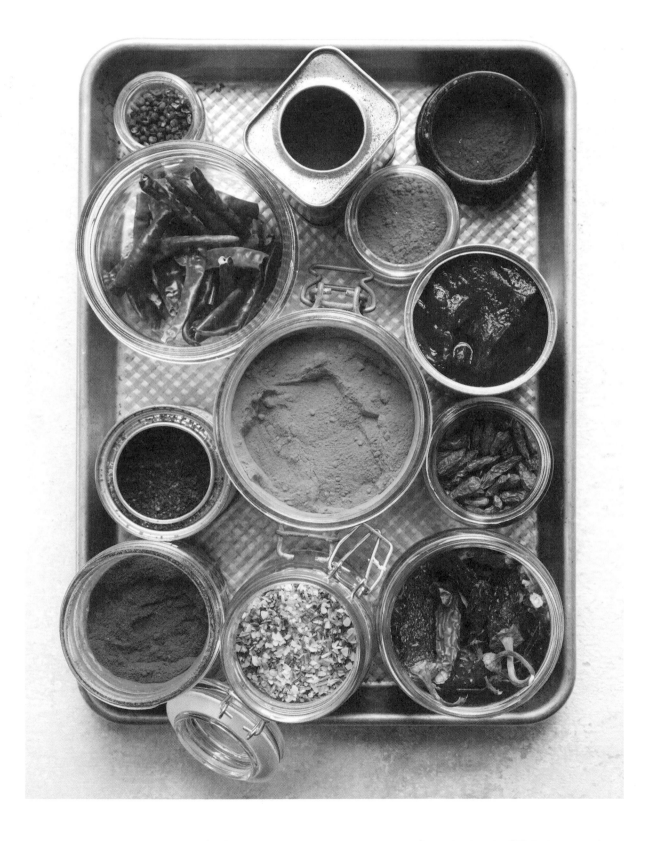

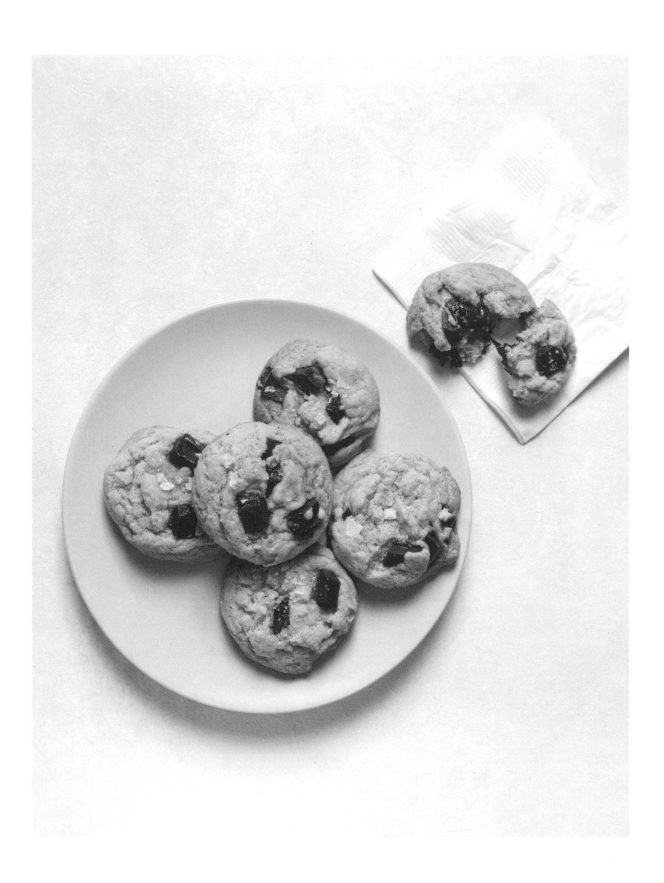

Vegan CHOCOLATE CHIP COOKIES

I'll make this cookie dough early on a Friday morning (or even late Thursday night) to bake off just in time to serve hot from the oven on Friday night. The batter needs to rest anyway—to help it hydrate—and that rest makes me look like a champ, the sort of champ who pulls fresh cookie dough from the fridge and presents hot cookies in 10 minutes flat.

I adapted this recipe from the one created by Erin Patinkin and Agatha Kulaga, the two women who own and operate Ovenly Bakery in Brooklyn, New York. They make a chocolate chip cookie that you'd never know is vegan and I replaced the refined sugar with sugars that are a little bit lower on the glycemic index. Remember, these cookies still contain sugar—you'll taste the sweetness in the first bite—but you'll also taste a caramel-like flavor that comes to life when you cook coconut palm sugar.

I do promise you this, few people will be able to notice these cookies are vegan and refined-sugar free. Yes, they taste that good.

Makes 20 cookies

FREQUENCY: *A couple times per month*

FOOD PREFERENCES: *DF, NF, RSF, V*

HANDS-ON TIME: *30 minutes*

TOTAL TIME: *12 hours 30 minutes*

. . . .

2 cups (8½ oz; 240 g) all-purpose flour

1 teaspoon baking powder

¾ teaspoon baking soda

½ teaspoon fine sea salt

1 cup (5¾ oz; 160 g) dairy-free
   dark chocolate chips (no higher
   than 60 to 70 percent cocoa content)

½ cup (3¼ oz; 95 g) maple sugar

½ cup (3½ oz; 100 g) coconut palm
   sugar

½ cup plus 1 tablespoon (95 ml)
   safflower oil

¼ cup plus 1 tablespoon (75 ml) water

½ teaspoon vanilla extract

Flaky sea salt (such as Maldon),
   for garnish

1. Whisk together the flour, baking powder, baking soda, and fine sea salt in a large bowl. Add the chocolate chips to the flour mixture and toss to coat.

2. Combine the sugars with the oil, water, and vanilla extract in a separate large bowl and whisk briskly until smooth and incorporated, about 2 minutes. If there are sugar clumps, break them up with the back of a spoon or your hand before whisking.

3. Add the dry mixture to the wet mixture. Stir with a wooden spoon or a rubber spatula until just combined and with no flour visible. Do not over-mix.

4. Cover with plastic wrap. Refrigerate the dough for 6 to 12 hours. Do not skip this step.

5. Preheat the oven to 350°F (177°C). Line two rimmed sheet pans with parchment paper. Remove the dough from the refrigerator and let sit for 10 minutes. With an ice cream scoop or a spoon, portion the dough into 1 tablespoon (2-inch) mounds. Sprinkle the balls of dough with flaky sea salt. Bake for 10 to 12 minutes, until the edges are just golden, turning the rack once to ensure even cooking. Do not over-bake.

6. Cool the cookies for 5 minutes, and then move them to a wire rack to cool completely before serving.

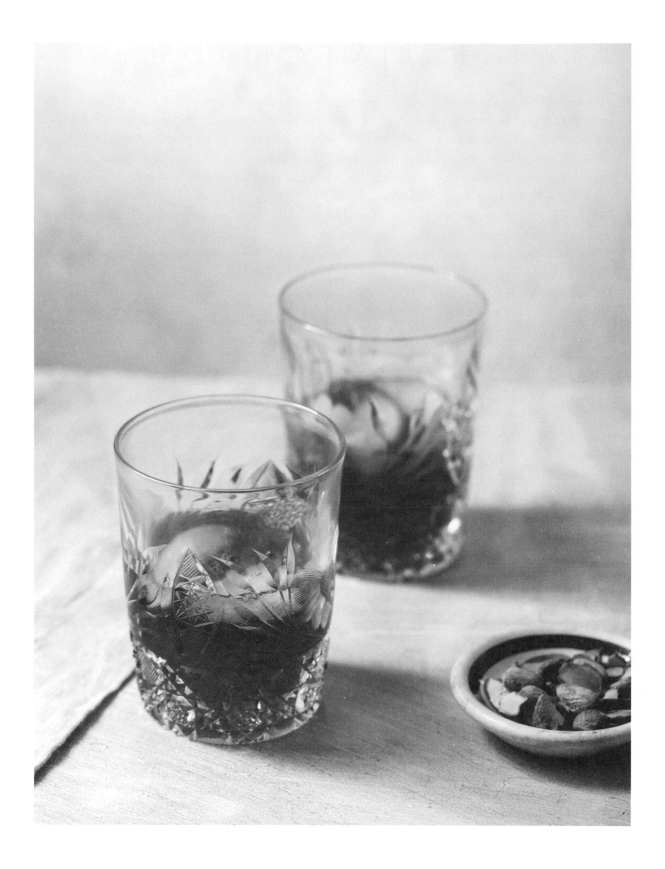

SBAGLIATOS *for Two*

During active wellness mode, I avoid the sugar in cocktails. However, during everyday wellness mode, I add in a single cocktail on a weekend night, as long as some of the ingredients are homemade and the overall cocktail offers other nutritional benefits, like with this Sbagliato.

This cocktail is a worthwhile option for a few reasons. First, it only has three ingredients: Campari, sweet vermouth, and sparkling wine. Campari is a bitter aperitif infused with herbs, oranges, and rhubarb that supposedly aids digestion. I can only confirm for myself that a few drops of Campari in soda water have helped me forget an indulgent meal on several occasions. The sweet vermouth in this drink is homemade, infused with a huge pile of bitter elements, herbs, and spices, and with far less sugar than the store-bought sort. And sparkling wine is wine, something that I do drink on the regular. Altogether, they make a famous Italian drink that came to life when a busy bartender used sparkling wine instead of gin in a Negroni. The Sbagliato, meaning "mistaken" or "wrong" in Italian, was born and it's my go-to cocktail.

The classic recipe is 1 part Campari to 1 part vermouth to 1 part sparkling wine. I've been known to prefer an even lighter Sbagliato by doubling the pour of sparkling wine. In this way, you can use a half-ounce each Campari and vermouth with a full ounce of sparkling wine. It's a lighter drink but a drink nonetheless. You do what works for you.

Makes 2 drinks

FREQUENCY: *A couple times per month*

FOOD PREFERENCES: *DF, GF, NF*

HANDS-ON TIME: *5 minutes*

TOTAL TIME: *5 minutes*

. . . .

2 ounces (60 ml) Campari

2 ounces (60 ml) Vermouth, homemade
    (page 62) or store-bought

Ice, for serving

Two 3-inch orange rinds,
    for garnish

2 ounces (60 ml) sparkling wine
    or prosecco

1. In a glass cocktail tumbler, stir together the Campari and sweet vermouth. Divide equally between two lowball or rocks glasses, over a couple ice cubes.

2. Twist an orange rind over the ice and add to each glass. Gently pour 1 ounce of sparkling wine over the ice in each glass. Serve immediately.

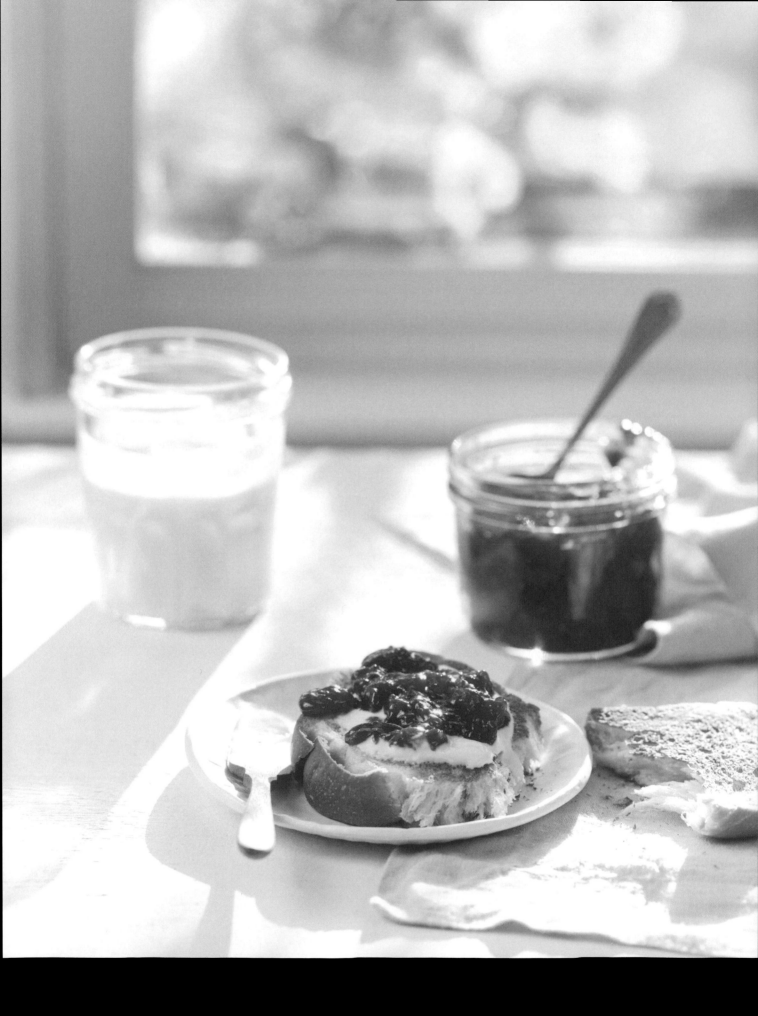

7

EMBRACE A NEW YOU
Recipes for Revitalizing Spring Foods

A wellness journey is just that—a journey. Along the way you're sure to encounter moments of uncertainty, anxiety, and fear. But I know you have the strength to do this. As you work every day to focus on your good health, a new sense of self will arise. You'll be stronger, happier, and way more comfortable in your skin. The parts of your life that may have seemed impossible previously may, in fact, become just a little less complicated.

This chapter includes recipes inspired by my own new sense of self. I finally love all the lighter spring ingredients and what that fresh food does for my body.

The Rebirth in Spring

I FIND SPRING TO BE THE MOST CHALLENGING season (and the most dreaded). It's a time when the world shouts at us about transforming our bodies and ourselves for the summer months ahead—swimsuits and peekaboo bikinis parading up and down every balmy beach and sunny backyard. Judgment from others feels omnipresent and it's really hard, for me anyway, to stay emotionally strong.

Traditionally, spring emerged as the antidote to the cold weather holidays, a time when I often indulged in everything. In the past, during the holiday season, I practiced the art of overspending on gifts and celebrations; I allowed myself to eat every single thing in sight; and I made daily holiday drinks a thing because I needed them just to get through the over-consumerism, overeating, and all the guilt.

However, once the first buds pop, hinting that transformation time is here, society wants to forget the heaviness of winter and, goodness, so do I. But sadly, the media leads the charge. In fact, January's "new year, new you" message turns toward a full calling for a March metamorphosis. In every magazine and marketing campaign, we're informed that it's now time to really take getting healthy seriously by eating far less and shedding a little or a lot of weight.

Instead of the cozy coats of winter, which covered every inch of our bodies, we're now advised to shed those weighty clothes, show way more skin, and, if we want to really embrace the shift toward lightness, change out our entire wardrobe immediately. Instead of well-worn boots, slip into short skirts that bare legs—and spend a small fortune on proper leg tanning. Hurry up, quickly, because swimsuit season—a moment when every body part will need proper tanning—is just a few months away.

If you're not doing all of these things, then, let's be real, you're not a legitimate woman. Of course that's not true, but it's how I felt every single spring since I realized just how big the world thought I was. I've harbored so much guilt for not doing my "proper duty" as a lady, the sort who should get to eating less, exercising more, wardrobe overhauling, and prettifying every body bit as soon as possible. Frankly, if you're not transforming, you're not with the program. And I was definitely not with the program.

For most of my life, I wore baggy clothes to hide all my puffy parts. Forget prettifying myself; more than anything, I wanted to cover up and hide from the world, never more so than in the warmer months. My clothes stayed loose fitting; no short-shorts and mini-skirts for me. Even if I made the effort to update some piece, any piece, of my wardrobe, at the local mall, the fat girl options were limited, unless, of course, I wanted to wear one of those large muumuus made famous by Mrs. Roper in the eighties sitcom *Three's Company*. The elegant actress Audra Lindley rocked those frocks but they really weren't prime fashion for a teen or twenty-something hoping to feel fresh, young, and new. Even if all I wanted was a new pair of jeans and couple cool t-shirts, I'd have to shop in stores geared more toward fifty-somethings.

Spring fashion has simply never been for me or for thousands of other big girls. I wore jackets and sweaters for as long as possible. Boots and sneakers have always provided way more padding for all-day city walking so I shunned open-toed flat shoes as they provided zero comfort and super-strained muscles. And most shops didn't cater to my size anyway, so shopping became such a tedious act that I avoided it at all costs. And let's not even begin to discuss shopping for swimsuits.

Since a seasonal wardrobe shift wasn't available to me, I stayed in my same tired, baggy clothing year-round. To cope, I'd simply eat the same tired, indulgent food, which didn't help me fit into the most transformative of all seasons.

THE FOOD OF SPRING

Spring eating was never really fun for me. As a reaction to the overly generous winter foods, the types that are meant to pad us up and provide a bit of warmth, spring food is the exact opposite. Seasonal eating means consuming light dishes using fresh spring produce just dug from a local farm. And, hello, you'd better eat a salad at every meal or something was gravely wrong with you. *Sheesh*, everything was wrong for me.

Instead of jumping on the trendy mixed greens and balsamic dressing train of the nineties, I was firmly planted on the other side of the tracks. Sitting amid my salad-eating college girlfriends, I'd shovel away at my pile of hearty animal protein, mashed potatoes, and gravy. Forget those leafy greens, I much preferred to comfort myself with (and perhaps wallow in) a cheeseburger and a pile of cheese-laden French fries. Even at breakfast, when fellow classmates were spooning dainty piles of yogurt and fruit onto their plates, I'd top my bowl of strawberry yogurt with seventeen handfuls of sugary granola—always to some girlfriend's dismay. My food choices garnered unanimous looks of pity from friends and non-friends, and left me feeling pretty bad on most days.

Once in a while, a girlfriend would implore me to grab a tossed salad instead of something more filling or replace potatoes with broccoli. On those days, probably the most confusing of all my food days, I'd receive equally inflated looks but not of pity. Instead, the looks were more of concern or disbelief.

You see, there's this sort of damned-if-you-do and damned-if-you-don't thing that happens when others judge what fat girls eat, and spring was prime time for food shaming. If I ate anything I wanted unreservedly in public, whether in a college cafeteria or a regular restaurant, I'd receive unfriendly stares or eye rolls that suggested, "oh, yet another fat girl who doesn't take care of herself." The looks were disdainful and mean.

However, if I chose that more reasonable tossed salad or a simple plate of vegetables, I'd get curious and insulting inquiries. Someone would always undoubtedly say, "Are you sure that salad is going to be enough for you?" At first, I'd legitimatize the question with an answer, but soon I learned it was healthier to just disengage. Even if the question came from a concerned girlfriend, it felt like a backhanded insult. On all my not-prettified, unpolished fingers and toes, I could count the dozens and dozens of times others judged me based on the food in front of me. This was a regular thing, people.

Ultimately, the new produce of spring—dark leafy greens, rhubarb, peas, strawberries, and all those tiny (not oppressively large) new potatoes—is not to blame for the food shaming. These wonderful little bits of nature didn't make me feel bad. I made me feel bad. I let those looks of judgment, many from total strangers, influence how I thought of myself. I already felt uncomfortable eating indulgent food in front of people. Very soon into young adulthood, I began to feel uncomfortable eating all the good spring foods, too. Eventually, I decided to eat privately in my apartment or bedroom, to simply avoid the bad feelings and to basically avoid the world's gaze.

EMERGING WITH A STRONGER SENSE OF SELF

Spring is so different since I started to really love myself. It's so hard to put these new feelings into words, and not because the feelings are hard to describe. It's hard to talk about because I feel a lot of shame for believing all the hype created by the media (and, in turn, my brain) for so long. It's hard to stop letting the world judge you and feel self-possessed and strong at the core.

I'm ashamed that I bought into the metamorphosis nonsense every single year. I suppose, as a young uncertain thing, I didn't know much better. But as a strong and powerful adult woman, I feel regret for letting the media shape what I thought of myself. I know who I am now. I know how I want to spend my spring days. I know what I want to eat, how I want to dress, where I want to go, all that I want to do. Most notably, I know what I believe. You see, once you start to love yourself, you begin to discover your authenticity; you begin to understand and accept your imperfections; and you begin to appreciate every part of your truth, the frailties, the excellence, and the potential.

Spring has now replaced fall as my favorite season. After eating lots of good food through the winter months—the sort of dishes that are filled with more veg and a lot less not-so-great stuff—I crave the ingredients of spring. My body has finally sent a memo to my brain to say, "Let's officially eat all you want of that just-dug produce right this second." It tastes so great, feels so good in my body, and it gives me the sort of alert energy I need to tackle whatever is before me.

I still want super comforting food—for better and for worse, food will always provide comfort to the big-little girl inside me. I minimize and manage the cravings, and really love that big-little girl the best I can, but instead of wanting to stick with the same old filling winter foods, I want to give her all the crisp, gleaming produce of spring because she deserves all the very good foods. I promise that you do, too.

All that said, I do not go through a huge rebirth experience every spring. Each day of the year is a new day full of immense possibilities and I don't wait for the media's March metamorphosis plea. In fact, forget the media. I don't have to believe them. I have to believe me.

Instead of gorging on the wrong foods, I now eat the easygoing foods of spring, with my own special comfort food twists. Instead of buying an entirely new wardrobe, I have my own kind of fashion. And rather than hide myself away, I now strut into each new day. I imagine it's how my mother must have strutted back in her days, albeit in a different sort of uniform but one that makes me feel just as fierce. I embrace the warmer weather and I'm ready for all the new adventures.

MY NEW KIND OF FASHION

As I began to eat differently and feel more in control of my body, I also developed a keener sense of self. I suppose tracking your food and listening to your body will give you deeper insight into what works for you and what needs to be tossed altogether. As I got smarter on the topic of me, I began to appreciate every inch of my body, however wobbly or thick.

Simultaneously, I also started to stand up straighter. Instead of slouching, I stood alertly, ready for whatever was coming my way. My stomach pulled in a little and my stride, never very distinct in the past, got more purposeful; I walked everywhere with a newfound intent that was totally foreign to me. In fact, it felt so great to walk that I wanted to do it quite frequently; my body had suddenly told my brain that it was time for me to move.

As I moved more and stood more thoughtfully, my clothes became even looser. I couldn't wear some of the duds in my closet any longer and, gosh, I didn't really want to. Most were cut in such a way to cover up my gut or generous bottom. Just like I had cleaned out my kitchen pantry, I applied the same purpose to my closet and piled it all into large black garbage bags. Garments that were now too large were cleaned, folded, and donated. Instead of holding on to all those bigger-sized pieces, just in case I'd need them again down the line, I determinedly bid farewell to the attire that had gotten me this far and set out to find my new kind of fashion.

Slowly, as if testing myself to see what felt good, I added a few new pieces to my wardrobe. Rather than source loose plus-size pieces, I scoured the Internet for modern fashion pieces that felt more like the young person inside me. Remember, when I was in my twenties, the only plus-size clothing available was made for fifty-somethings; the fashion industry really just didn't prioritize plus-size younger women and if they did have a large size here or there, those bigger pieces were reserved for women of a certain age with a certain income who would spend big bucks for a size 20 dress.

By the time I felt better in my body, the fashion industry was starting to catch up—frankly, they are mostly still in catch-up mode—and I locked down a pair of dark skinny jeans that were tight, fit my bum snugly, and comfortable to both walk and sit in. I got a jean skirt too—not because I'm big into jean skirts but because I never got to wear them when they were the "it" fashion in the eighties. Now that a few brands made a jean skirt that finally fit the nearly 70 percent of women in America who are plus size, I snatched it up and wore it with pride.

After those two new pieces, I added in black leggings, smart flannel shirts, pop-culture t-shirts, and boots. All of the aforementioned were figure fitting, rather than loose, because that's what finally felt good on me. Remember, I'm not skinny but I have a shape that deserves respect and I didn't want to hide my body any longer. I loved myself and if that meant the jeans would fit snugly or the t-shirt would accentuate my ample bosom, then bring it on.

Eventually, I determined my uniform, the sort of fashion I want to be in all the time, regardless of my work or my age. Just like loving comfort food, I love comfort clothing. I like how it feels to wear tighter jeans. I prefer trimmed down basics like straight-up t-shirts and button-up shirts. And, get this; I love skirts and dresses. They make it easy for me to just get on with life rather than hem and haw at my closet, like I'd done for decades. I'm still experimenting with clothes but my kind of fashion is both comfortable and fun and, definitely, ever-changing.

Through my boosted sense of self and garment upgrade, I've learned that fashion is just a tool. It's just a way to keep your naked parts covered. Fashion enhances my identity but it isn't my identity. I've unlocked my fashion voice and found clothes that make me feel good but my message matters way more than any piece of clothing I wear. I define who I am and I define what I wear and—thank goodness—there are so many more options for us these days. My clothes are tighter, there's far less material, and my closet has a trimmed-down set of garments that get me through the day with my sort of style.

FIVE MANTRAS THAT MAY HELP

If you want to embrace a new way of eating or new way of thinking about yourself, then you should do that in whatever way makes sense to you. But no matter what anyone tells you—including the media or your family and friends in their sometimes flawed ways—you are enough just as you are.

Either way, focus on the positive. I did a lot of mental work to understand my past, appreciate my present, and be enthusiastic for my future. Through it all, I have become more positive and optimistic. I've shifted away from the fat girl mindset and toward a mindset that sees my beautiful body and all its beautiful potential.

Sometimes, I've recited mantras—either out loud or silently—to acknowledge and push through rough moments or momentous mindset shifts. Perhaps repeating these to yourself, either during a quiet moment in a proper bath or just before you get out of bed in the morning, will help you, too. It feels silly for a moment but, eventually, it feels great.

1. *I am grateful.* There is so much goodness around you, even when it doesn't always feel that way. I repeat this mantra when I need to remind myself that I have so much that is good. Just chanting these words gets me to recall all the good stuff and instantly pulls me from a sad or tough moment.

2. *I am awake.* Reciting these words is my way to ensure I'm living in the present with purpose. Some say these words during a yoga practice, to experience each moment on the mat, but I use the words in my everyday life as well, to keep me aware. I sometimes say these words or, an alternative; "I am here," to myself on airplanes, just before takeoff.

3. *I am okay.* I often use this mantra when I don't quite feel okay or when I need that little push to feel all right. I also use it when I discover something new about my past, something that may stress me out, because it is indeed the past. And, in the present, I'm okay.

4. *I am perfect.* I believe I was made the way I am purposefully. I repeat this mantra not because I think I'm perfect in the traditional sense of the word. I do so to remind myself that even with my flaws and imperfections and wobbly bits, I am enough just the way I am.

5. *I am love.* I am unique and I may have bad days when I don't say the right things or make a multitude of mistakes daily but I am also full of love. Sometimes it takes me a series of mistakes to learn the best lessons but, still, I am full of love. Love for others and love for myself.

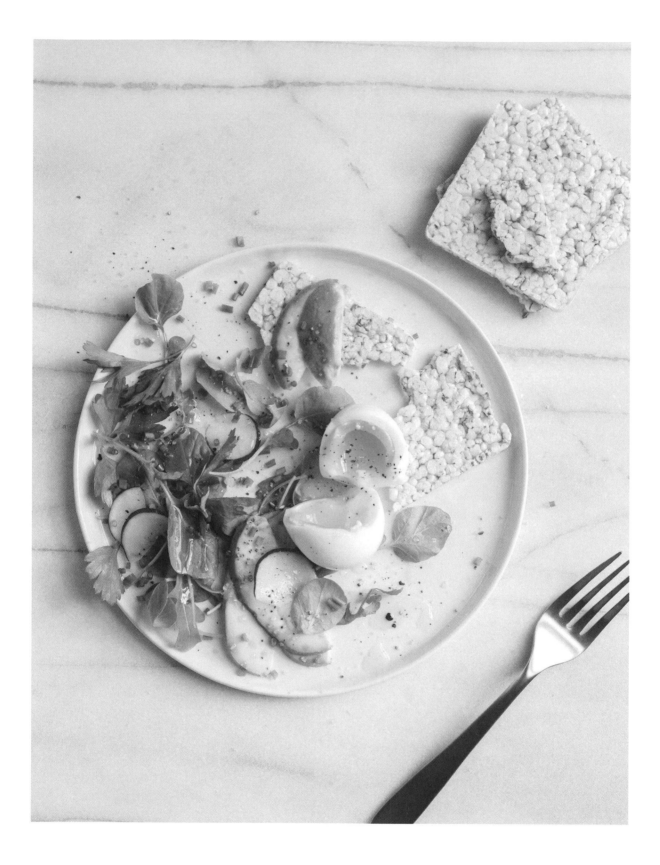

AVOCADO, SOFT-BOILED EGGS, THIN RICE CAKES

On the mornings when I'm not sipping a smoothie, I'm typically eating creamy oats or this. Especially in the spring, when farm eggs fill the markets. I get a lot of satisfaction from the protein-filled egg (the whites and the yolk); the fresh avocado is fatty and rich; and the thin rice cakes provide a bit of something filling to chew on. Don't get too stressed about whether you eat one or two eggs; do what your body needs. I make a bunch of boiled eggs and start with one, grabbing a second, if I feel like it, or perhaps save it for the road. Store the rest in the fridge for the next few days.

In the time it takes to boil the eggs, I cut, peel, and slice my avocado. Assemble it all on a plate, as you like, and slide a few leftover veg slices into the mix, as you'll likely have something green in your fridge. If you have pickled veg in there, even better.

Serves 1

FREQUENCY: *Almost everyday*

FOOD PREFERENCES: *DF, GF, NF, RSF, Veg*

HANDS-ON TIME: *10 minutes*

TOTAL TIME: *10 minutes*

. . . .

1 or 2 eggs

½ ripe avocado, pitted, peeled, and thinly sliced

2 thin, square rice cakes

⅛ teaspoon sea salt

1. Bring a medium pot of water to a boil over medium-high heat. Once it boils, add the egg(s) to the water and reduce the heat to a simmer. Let the eggs simmer in the water for 6½ minutes. Drain them and rinse with cold water or submerge in an ice water bath to stop the cooking. Peel and slice in half—the yolk should be a bit runny and almost jam-like. If they're fresh eggs or difficult to peel, let them sit in the cold water for 10 to 15 minutes to firm up a bit.

2. Arrange the egg halves on a plate with the avocado slices and rice cakes. Sprinkle the salt over the avocado and eggs. Slide some avocado slices onto a rice cake and alternate bites of the rice cake with the soft-boiled eggs.

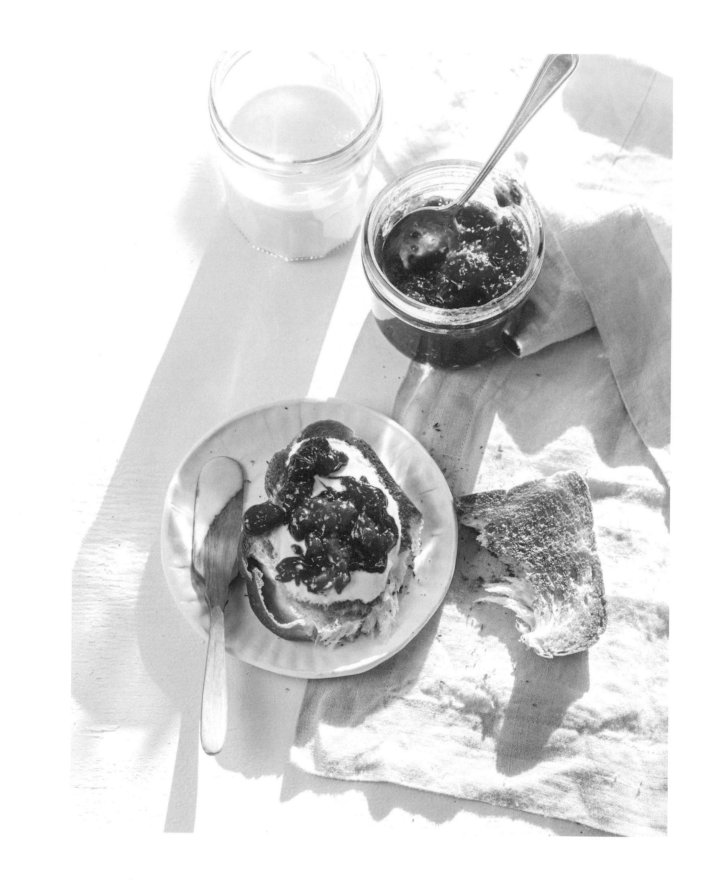

SMOKY STRAWBERRY JAM *and Yogurt Toast*

Toast is my preferred vehicle for jam—together, they are the truest of duos, making each other even better. And spread on top of a high-quality slice of bread with cashew yogurt, this smoky jam really tells the right sort of story: I'm a little bit sweet, a little bit savory, and, altogether, the kind of treat you want in your life. The Roasted Stone Fruit Rhubarb Jam (page 60) would be wonderful in this recipe, too.

I did not give up preserving in this new way to food. In fact, it's hard for a preserver to stop preserving. It's forever a part of me and I had to figure out a new way to enjoy preserves now and again. Instead of using cane sugar, I turn to honey or maple sugar. I also use a lot less sweetener because fruit doesn't really need that much if you still want to taste the fruit, not just the sweet.

West Coast strawberries are available year-round, but the tiny round East Coast ones that start tart and end sweet are an even more precious treasure that work wonderfully here.

Serves 1

FREQUENCY: *Once per week*

FOOD PREFERENCES: *DF, GF, RSF, Veg*

HANDS-ON TIME: *5 minutes*

TOTAL TIME: *5 minutes*

. . . .

FOR THE SMOKY STRAWBERRY JAM (MAKES ABOUT 3 HALF-PINT JARS)

2 pounds (904 g) fresh strawberries, cleaned and hulled

⅔ cup (160 ml) water

1 cup plus 1 tablespoon (12.75 oz; 361 g) light honey, divided

¼ teaspoon smoked paprika

1 tablespoon powdered fruit pectin

FOR THE SMOKY STRAWBERRY JAM AND YOGURT TOAST

1 tablespoon Cashew Yogurt (page 42) or other unsweetened, plain plant-based yogurt

1 slice Sandwich Bread (page 34) or your favorite bread, toasted

1 tablespoon Smoky Strawberry Jam

TO MAKE THE SMOKY STRAWBERRY JAM

1. Put two small plates in your freezer. (I keep a few small plates in there at all times during jam season.)

2. Dice the strawberries into about ½-inch pieces. Add the strawberries, water, and 1 cup of the honey to a shallow wide pan. Bring to a boil and cook over medium-high heat for 20 minutes, until some of the fruit has broken down and some of the liquid has evaporated.

3. Stir together the remaining 1 tablespoon honey, smoked paprika, and fruit pectin in separate small bowl. Add 1 tablespoon of the jam mixture and stir until a slurry or paste forms. Stir into the strawberries on the stove.

4. Cook the jam for 10 to 15 minutes longer to remove even more water and until the mixture gets darker and a bit shinier. It may also begin to stick to the bottom of the pan. Stir frequently to prevent any scalding of the fruit. The jam is ready when a dab added to one of your frozen plates stiffens a bit and doesn't run as you rock the plate back and forth. After 15 minutes, pull the jam regardless because it will set up a bit when in the jar. Allow to cool for 3 minutes.

5. Clean your jars in hot, soapy water. Sterilize the jars by running them through a dishwasher at the hottest setting or boiling them in a pot on the stove for 10 minutes. Allow to air dry.

6. Carefully ladle the jam into your jars. Allow to cool completely and then store in the fridge for up to 3 weeks.

TO MAKE THE TOAST

Spread the yogurt on the toasted bread. Spread the jam on top of the yogurt. Serve immediately.

CRISP VEGETABLES *with Green Yogurt Sauce*

On some nights, dinner is just this and a glass of wine. I always feel downright righteous as I munch on veg slices between sips of wine, as if the wine is my just reward for eating so very well. But more often, I make this recipe for guests; as a starter it serves six to eight people.

The vegetables listed are merely a guide; you should choose the freshest in-season veg that you get excited to eat raw. I include some stalwarts of typical crudité platters like carrots, green beans, cucumbers, tomatoes, and mix in some special finds like salad turnips, beets, asparagus, or even not-too-juicy figs, sliced. Just make sure to quickly blanch any veg that you'd prefer less raw, like perhaps green beans or asparagus.

The sauce is distinctly herby and bright green, thanks to the avocado. Since it's already loaded with capers, don't salt the dip until you give it a taste. If it's not bright and briny enough, add a bit of salt. Eat this dip immediately after making; it's not at its best when in the fridge for days on end.

Serves 2 to 6

FREQUENCY: *Almost every day*

FOOD PREFERENCES: *DF, GF, RSF, V*

HANDS-ON TIME: *15 minutes*

TOTAL TIME: *15 minutes*

1 small bunch radishes (about
    8 radishes), cleaned and sliced
    lengthwise

1 small head radicchio, leaves
    pulled apart

1 medium cucumber, cleaned and
    sliced thin on the diagonal

1 pound (454 g) small carrots, cleaned
    and sliced in half lengthwise

ingredients continued

1. Place a small bowl that will hold about 2 cups of dip in the center of a platter. Prep all of your vegetables and arrange them on the platter around the bowl.

2. Add the basil, chives, avocado, capers, vinegar, yogurt, oil, and water to a powerful blender. Blend until thick and smooth. Add an extra tablespoon of water, if needed, to loosen it up. Taste the sauce and add salt, if desired. Serve immediately.

12 cherry tomatoes, cleaned

¾ cup green beans or snap peas, cleaned and quickly blanched

1 small bunch basil (about 10 sprigs), stems cut and discarded

1 small bunch chives (about 20 sprigs), any dry tips removed

½ small avocado, peeled

2 tablespoons capers, liquid removed

1 tablespoon coconut vinegar or apple cider vinegar

¾ cup (180 ml) Cashew Yogurt (page 42) or other unsweetened, plain plant-based yogurt

½ cup (120 ml) extra-virgin olive oil

1 tablespoon water, or more as needed

¼ teaspoon sea salt (optional)

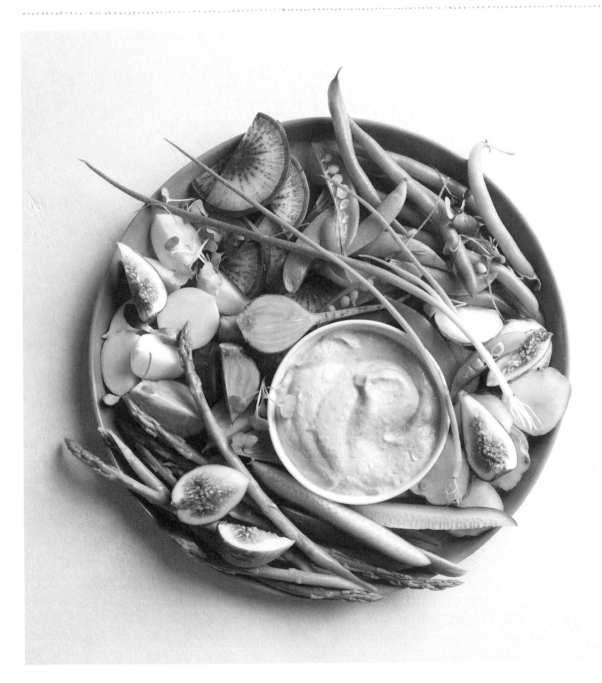

SALMON AND FENNEL *Spring Dinner Salad*

Don't let the light nature of this dish fool you. This spring dinner salad is hearty and filling. The salmon offers a satisfying richness; the couscous adds heft; and the creamy dressed vegetables feel indulgent but aren't in the least. If you are using a very thin piece of salmon, check it early and often so it doesn't overcook. As a little surprise, I tuck strawberries between each of these elements to add a sweet, tangy pop.

This recipe does have multiple steps so make sure you have the time to bring the final dish to life. But once made by your hand, tossed and tucked together, this salad will serve four as a cool dinner and even more when placed on a brunch buffet or added to a multi-course lunch.

Serves 4 to 6

FREQUENCY: *Once per week*

FOOD PREFERENCES: *DF, NF, RSF*

HANDS-ON TIME: *30 minutes*

TOTAL TIME: *55 minutes*

. . . .

FOR THE SALMON AND FENNEL DINNER SALAD

1 pound (454 g) salmon filet (about 1-inch thick), pin bones removed

1 teaspoon sea salt, divided, plus more for serving

12 twists freshly ground black pepper, plus more for serving

2 teaspoons extra-virgin olive oil

2 limes, halved

1 cup pearl couscous

1¼ cup (300 ml) water

⅓ small head Napa cabbage, thinly sliced

1 large fennel bulb, core and fronds removed, thinly sliced (reserve a few fennel fronds for garnish)

2 cups strawberries, washed and quartered

Herby Yogurt Dressing (recipe follows)

1. Preheat the oven to 350°F (177°C). Line a rimmed baking sheet with parchment paper. Place the salmon, skin side down, on the parchment. Sprinkle with ½ teaspoon of the salt and the black pepper. Drizzle the oil over the salmon. Roast in the preheated oven for 12 to 18 minutes (longer for thicker salmon), until a meat thermometer inserted in the thickest part of the fish registers about 115°F to 120°F (46–49°C). I check for doneness at 12 minutes and every few minutes thereafter. Remove the fish from the oven and tent a piece of foil over the salmon until ready to serve, giving it at least 5 minutes to come to medium rare or 125°F (52°C).

2. While the salmon roasts, toast the couscous until it browns on most sides in a medium pot set over medium high heat. Stir or swirl the pot frequently to ensure even browning. This should take 6 to 7 minutes, but watch carefully so it doesn't burn. Once golden brown, pull the pot off the heat and carefully add the water and the remaining ½ teaspoon salt—be careful, it may splash up a little. Stir until combined and return to medium-high heat. Bring to a boil and then lower the heat to medium low. Cover and allow to cook until all the water has been absorbed and the couscous is light and fluffy and just a touch al dente, about 7 minutes. Check it once or twice to make sure it doesn't stick to the bottom of the pan. Remove the pan from the heat and let the couscous cool before handling. My faster cooling method is to spread it on a large plate or baking sheet, with a touch of olive oil to prevent clumping, and let it rest away from the stove.

3. Make the dressing. Add the yogurt, oil, lime juice, honey, salt, and pepper to a medium-size bowl. Whisk together until fully emulsified. Stir in the chives. Chill until ready to use.

continued

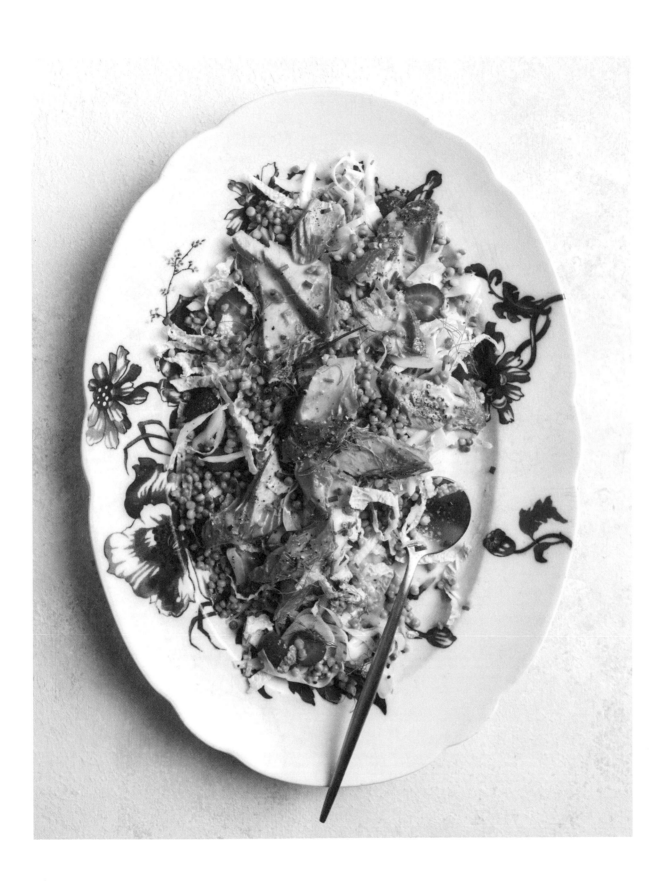

FOR THE HERBY YOGURT DRESSING

½ cup (4½ oz; 125 g) unsweetened, plain plant-based yogurt

½ cup (120 ml) extra-virgin olive oil

4 tablespoons lime juice (from about 2 limes)

4 teaspoons light honey, like clover

½ teaspoon sea salt

24 twists freshly ground black pepper

1 small bunch chives (about 20 sprigs), any dry tips removed, finely diced

4. On a large platter, toss together the cooled couscous, cabbage, and fennel with two-thirds of the dressing until everything is well coated. Add the strawberries to the salad and gently (with your hands) tuck them in and around the veg to get touched with the dressing—be gentle, as they may get mushy or moist if handled too roughly. Break up the salmon with a fork or your fingers and place small 2-inch chunks across the veg. Drizzle with the remaining dressing. Sprinkle with extra salt and pepper. Garnish with fennel fronds and serve.

TUNA SALAD *Lettuce Wraps*

This is one of those I-don't-have-time-to-cook-a-single-thing meals that does the trick for lunch, dinner, or in-between. If 5 ounces of tuna is more than you want, just fork out half and save the rest in a new airtight container for the next day or a snack later in the day. If your tinned tuna has added salt, omit the sea salt in the recipe.

Serves 1

FREQUENCY: *Once per week*

FOOD PREFERENCES: *DF, GF, NF, RSF*

HANDS-ON TIME: *10 minutes*

TOTAL TIME: *10 minutes*

One 5-ounce (142 g) tin solid pack light tuna in olive oil

½ small shallot, finely diced

2 teaspoons vegan mayonnaise

2 teaspoons lemon juice (from about ½ medium lemon)

1 tablespoon finely chopped cilantro

¼ teaspoon sea salt (optional)

2 large butter lettuce leaves, cleaned and dried

1. Fork the tuna from the can into a medium bowl. Add the shallot, mayonnaise, lemon juice, cilantro, and salt (only if your tuna has no salt added). Stir to ensure everything is well distributed.

2. Fill a lettuce leaf with half the tuna. Repeat with the other leaf and remaining tuna. Eat immediately over your plate or over the sink in your kitchen.

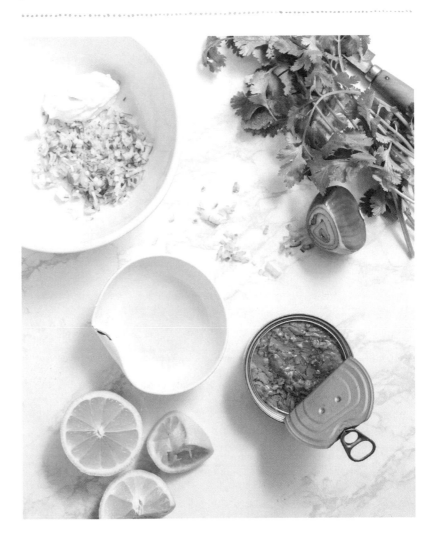

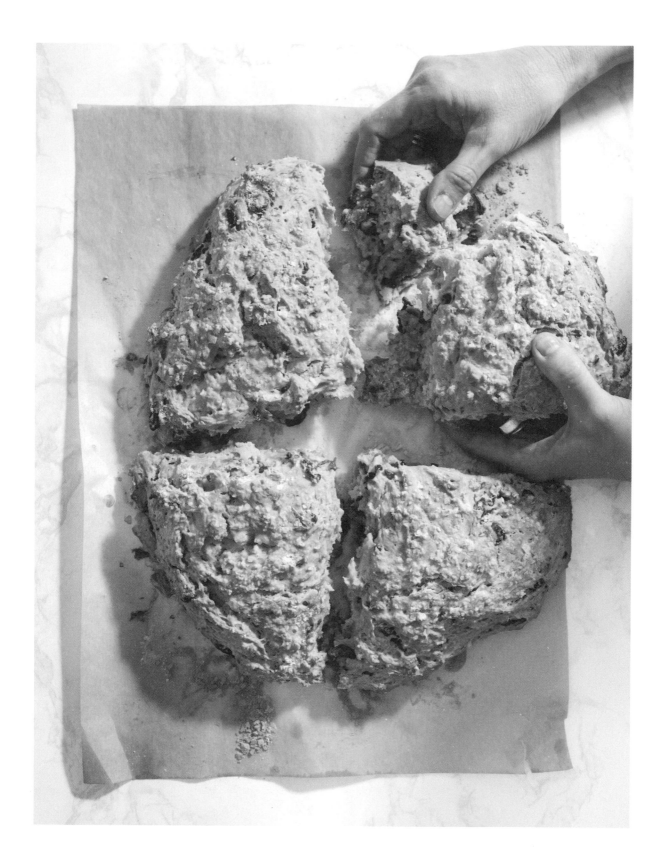

Shallot Thyme SODA BREAD

Early on in my wellness journey, I made a trip of a lifetime to Ireland. Eating wholesome while traveling can be difficult so I packed lemons (for lemon water), tea bags, and snack bars to make sure I always had a little something nourishing in the middle of nowhere. To my delight, the food in Ireland was remarkably good, especially all the from-scratch carbohydrates I'd watch my fellow travelers devour at breakfast.

When I returned home, I set about creating a savory soda bread recipe I could enjoy but that also checked all the texture and flavor boxes. This recipe is vegan as written; however, if you need to swap in animal dairy for any part, it will turn out just fine, too.

Makes one 8-inch (20 cm) loaf

FREQUENCY: *Once per week*

FOOD PREFERENCES: *DF, NF, RSF, V*

HANDS-ON TIME: *40 minutes*

TOTAL TIME: *1 hour 20 minutes*

. . . .

2 tablespoons coconut oil

6 medium shallots, sliced into thin rounds

6 cups (1 lb 9.5 oz; 720 g) all-purpose flour, plus more for sprinkling

1 teaspoon baking soda

1½ teaspoons fine sea salt

4 tablespoons fresh thyme leaves, finely diced

2 cups (480 ml) plus 2 tablespoons unsweetened, plain plant milk, divided

4 tablespoons unsweetened, plain plant-based yogurt

½ teaspoon flaky sea salt

1. Preheat the oven to 425°F (218°C). Line a baking sheet with parchment paper and a heavy sprinkle of flour.

2. Warm the coconut oil in a skillet over medium heat and add the shallots. Sauté and caramelize until the shallots become translucent and golden brown, about 10 minutes. Remove from the heat to cool.

3. Sift the flour, baking soda, and fine sea salt into a large mixing bowl. Add the thyme and cooled shallots, tossing to distribute both well.

4. In a smaller bowl, whisk together 2 cups of the milk and the yogurt until blended. Make a well in the middle of the dry ingredients. With a clean hand, stir the wet ingredients into the dry ingredients until there are no dry patches and the dough is well-combined but still a little rough and tacky; do not over-mix. Don't forget to mix in the extra flour underneath the dough. Wash and dry your hands.

5. With a floured rubber spatula, push the dough out of the bowl and onto the lined and floured baking sheet. Form it into an 8-inch round. With a floured knife, cut an X about 2 inches deep into the dough making sure not to go all the way to the baking sheet. Brush the remaining 2 tablespoons of milk all over the top and sides of the dough to encourage the browning. Sprinkle with flaky sea salt.

6. Bake for 30 to 40 minutes, until the top is golden in color and the loaf sounds hollow when tapped on the underside. The bread's internal temperature should be at least 190°F (88°C). Cool before breaking into quarters, slicing, and serving.

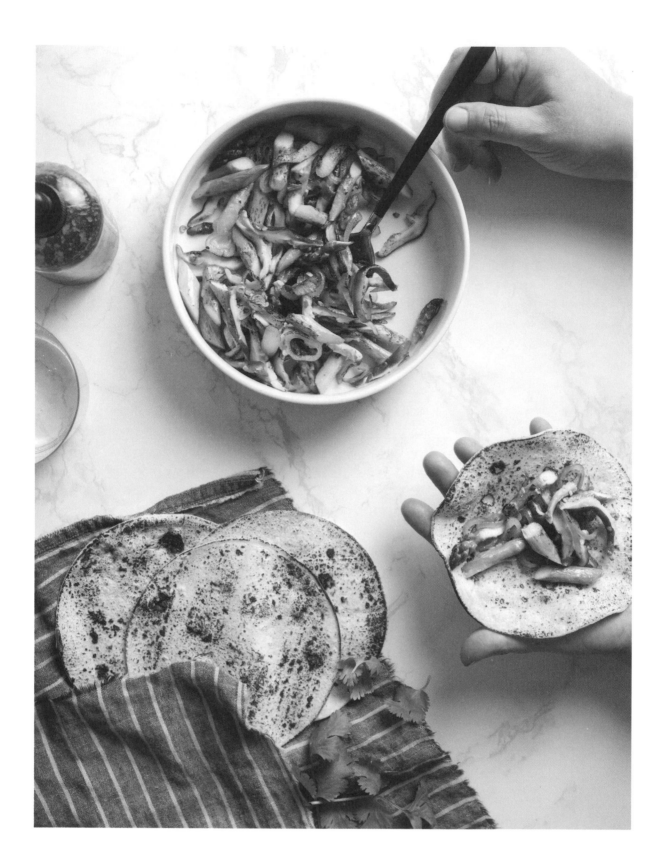

SPRING VEGETABLE *Stir Fry, Tortillas, Hot Sauce*

Growing up in a Latin household practically obligates you to put everything, anything, in a tortilla. In my life, I've been known to stuff all of the following into a tortilla to make an instant meal or snack: fried or soft-boiled eggs, tofu wedges, melted butter, melted cheese, any bean, all varieties of rice, sliced and salted tomatoes, fish and seafood, fresh soft herbs (with melted cheese), pickled veg, hot cherry peppers, tomato-dressed pasta, salad, bacon, boiled potatoes, corn off the cob—you get the idea.

With all that in mind, I like to stuff the best of every season into a tortilla, too. You choose any vegetables you like or whatever's hanging around in your fridge. I particularly like to sauté the season's first everything—like peas, asparagus, mushrooms, ramps, and greens—for a wholesome, satisfying dose of spring that motivates me to make more good spring dishes. Garnishes are optional but highly encouraged.

Serves 1 (as a meal)

FREQUENCY: *Almost everyday*

FOOD PREFERENCES: *DF, GF, NF, RSF, V*

HANDS-ON TIME: *15 minutes*

TOTAL TIME: *15 minutes*

2 tablespoons extra-virgin olive oil

5 medium asparagus spears, cleaned, stemmed, and sliced in 1-inch pieces

½ small white onion, peeled and thinly sliced

5 large shiitake mushrooms, cleaned, stemmed, and sliced

2 scallions, garlic scapes, or ramps, trimmed and thinly sliced

¼ teaspoon red pepper flakes

1 tablespoon apple cider vinegar or coconut vinegar

½ teaspoon sea salt, plus more for seasoning

2 Tortillas, homemade (page 36) or any natural, sugar-free corn tortillas

Fermented Hot Sauce (page 49) or store-bought hot sauce, for serving

Cilantro leaves, for garnish

1. Add the oil to a wide pan set over medium-high heat and sauté the asparagus, onion, mushrooms, and scallions until slightly wilted, 5 to 7 minutes. When nearly done, sprinkle the pepper flakes and vinegar over the vegetables and cook for 1 to 2 minutes longer. Season with salt and set aside.

2. In a separate pan set over medium-high heat, cook each tortilla for 30 seconds to 1 minute on each side. Split the vegetables between the tortillas. Serve with extra salt (as needed), hot sauce, and cilantro leaves.

Rhubarb SNACKING CAKE

This cake is yet another way for me to honor my favorite spring produce: rhubarb. The recipe is adapted from the cookbook *Chickpea Flour Does It All*, written by the incredibly talented Lindsey S. Love. Her cookbook is revelatory—yes, you really can do anything with chickpea flour—and the recipes are inventive and delicious. I cook with it quite frequently, as her recipes are gluten-free, dairy-free, and vegetarian. I say, "cook *with* it" because the joy of new cookbooks is finding inspiration from them to create your own dishes to please your palate or that of your family.

Since I'm known for my sweet tooth, I wanted a simple cake recipe that I could adapt for any fruit at any time of year. Lindsey's recipe uses more lemon while I added almond and vanilla extract to make my version nuttier. Using unsweetened plant yogurt creates an incredibly moist crumb, which is something I quite enjoy. You can use fresh or frozen rhubarb. Fresh rhubarb will float to the top and remain visible after the bake; frozen rhubarb will sink to the bottom of the cake (try tossing frozen rhubarb in flour to keep it from falling). Either way, it's cake and it's good. A little loose coconut cream, whipped from both the thick cream and loose water in a can of coconut milk, with vanilla bean seeds and maple syrup, makes for a nice topping along with toasted sliced almonds.

Makes one 8- by 8-inch
(20 by 20 cm) cake
FREQUENCY: *Only on a special occasion*
FOOD PREFERENCES: *DF, GF, RSF, Veg*
HANDS-ON TIME: *15 minutes*
TOTAL TIME: *1 hour*

⸱⸱⸱⸱⸱⸱⸱⸱⸱⸱⸱⸱⸱⸱⸱⸱⸱⸱⸱⸱⸱⸱⸱⸱⸱⸱⸱

Coconut oil, for greasing

½ cup (1½ oz; 43 g) chickpea flour

3 tablespoons finely ground
    almond flour

2 tablespoons arrowroot powder

1 teaspoon baking powder

½ teaspoon baking soda

ingredients continued

1. Preheat the oven to 350°F (177°C) and grease an 8- by 8-inch (20 by 20 cm) pan with coconut oil.

2. Add the chickpea and almond flours, arrowroot powder, baking powder, baking soda, and salt to a medium bowl. Whisk until well combined.

3. Whisk the sugar and egg together in a large bowl until the sugar dissolves into the egg. Add the oil, yogurt, and almond and vanilla extracts. Whisk those together until well combined.

4. Fold in the dry ingredients, bit by bit, until no dry steaks remain. Then, fold in 1 cup of the rhubarb. Pour the batter into your greased pan. Sprinkle the remaining ¼ cup rhubarb across the top of the cake. Bake for 30 to 35 minutes, until a wooden skewer comes out clean when pressed into the center of the cake. Cool before slicing off a square; I typically slice this cake into nine pieces about 2½ inches (6.4 cm) square, but you do whatever you need.

⅛ teaspoon sea salt

¾ cup (4 oz; 120 g) lightly packed
   maple sugar

1 egg

¼ cup (60 ml) safflower oil, plus more
   for greasing

½ cup (4½ oz; 125 g) unsweetened,
   plain plant-based yogurt

½ teaspoon almond extract

½ teaspoon vanilla extract

2 fresh rhubarb stalks, cut into
   ½-inch pieces, or frozen (1¼ cups)

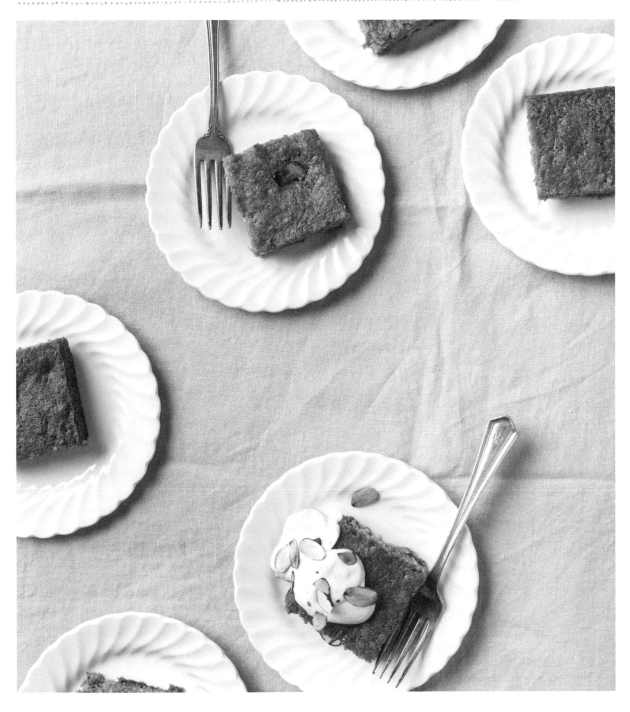

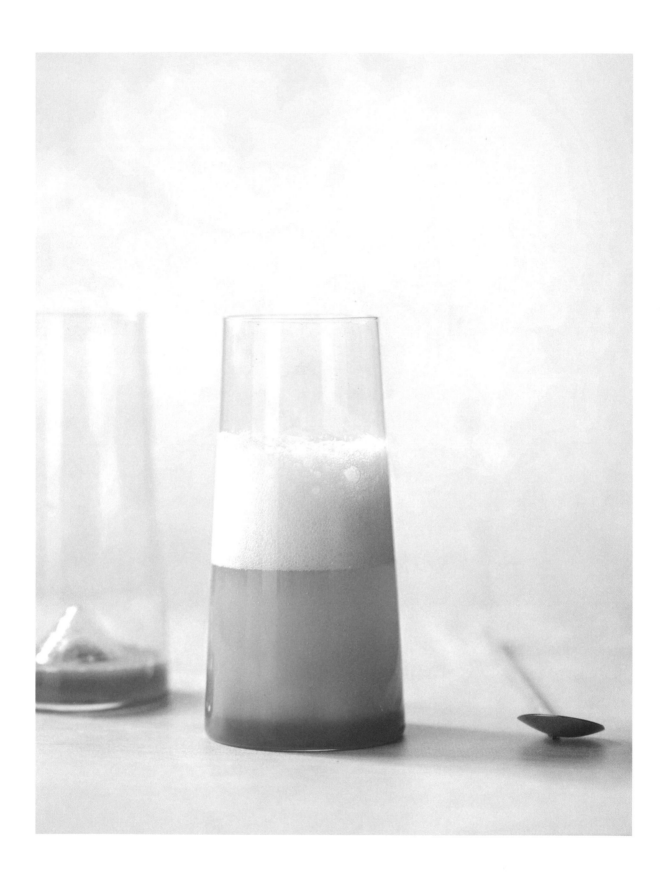

Rhubarb Honey SHRUB SODAS

When I say I love rhubarb, I mean there are six pounds diced into two sizes and frozen in my freezer right now. With all that rhubarb handy, I couldn't resist adding a rhubarb drink recipe to this spring-focused chapter.

Instead of simple syrup, I offer a shrub recipe. It's another way to get apple cider vinegar into your body. Apple cider vinegar is a natural preserver (it's frequently used to preserve fruit and pickle veg) but has also been thought to kill off certain types of bacteria, clear up your skin, lower blood sugar responses, increase that feeling of fullness (which may lead to weight loss), reduce risks of heart disease, lower cholesterol, and slow the growth of cancer cells.

To be fair, much of this hasn't been verified with human studies but it does me no harm to make apple cider vinegar a part of my food life. I frequently use it in place of other vinegars, especially in salad dressings. I drink a shot in water during the colder months to fend off viruses and during the season changes to aid my allergies. I sprinkle it on sautéed vegetables at the end of cooking for a little brightness. And, I drink it in shrub form.

Makes about 1½ cups of shrub (enough for 12 drinks)

FREQUENCY: *Only on a special occasion*

FOOD PREFERENCES: *DF, GF, NF, RSF, Veg*

HANDS-ON TIME: *10 minutes*

TOTAL TIME: *40 minutes*

. . . .

4 thick rhubarb stalks, chopped into 1-inch pieces

¾ cup (9 oz; 255 g) light honey

1¼ cups (300 ml) apple cider vinegar, divided

1 cup (240 ml) cold sparkling water (carbonated) per drink

1. Add the rhubarb, honey, and 1 cup of the vinegar to a pot over medium heat. Bring to a simmer and cook until the rhubarb breaks down into shreds, about 10 minutes. Remove from the heat and let it sit for 20 minutes.

2. Strain the mixture through a sieve or a strainer lined with cheesecloth into a bowl or jar. Do not press the mixture, just toss it about a little to encourage straining.

3. Stir in the remaining ¼ cup vinegar and store it in the fridge in an airtight container until ready to use or up to 2 weeks.

4. To make an individual soda, add 2 tablespoons of shrub mix to a glass with 1 cup of cold sparkling water. Serve immediately.

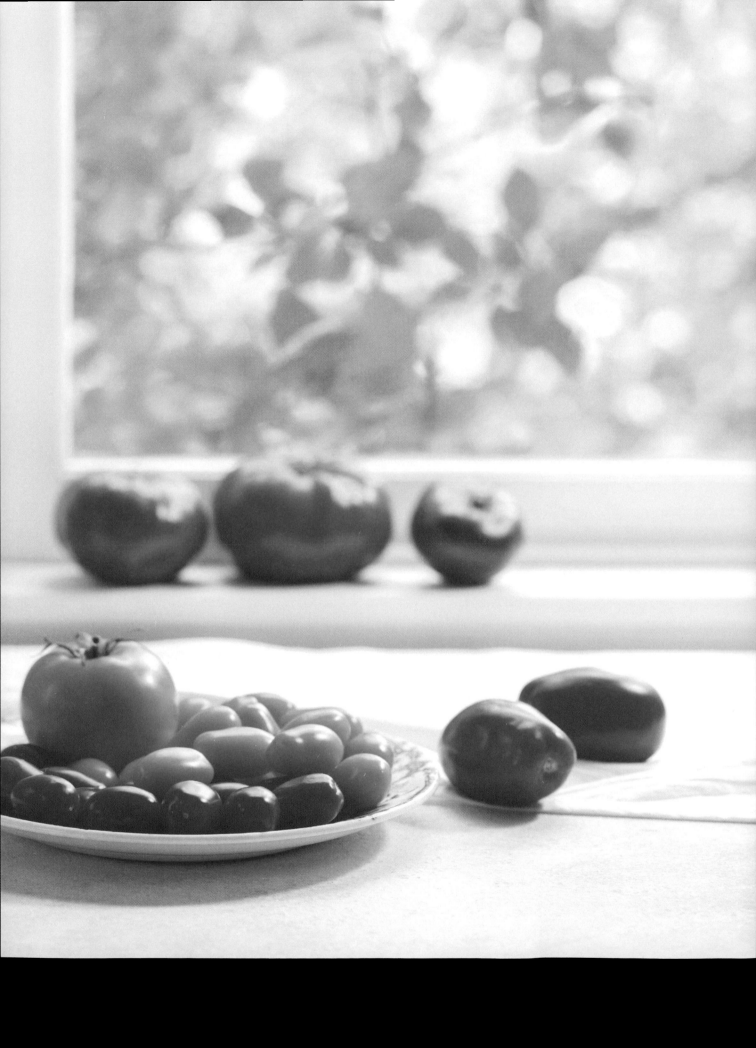

8

CELEBRATE LIFE

Recipes for Everyday Wellness Mode

After taking control of your body and your good health, you will feel ready to take on the world. It's time to finally shed everything that's been holding you back. It's time to live out your wildest dreams. It's time to live life to its fullest and make that self-love stick for life.

This chapter was inspired by my big adventures and learning to incorporate good-for-you indulgences into every single day. You'll find recipes for easy breakfasts, grilled dishes, and even homemade pizza. Several dessert and cocktail recipes are also scattered throughout to provide some inspiration for enjoying food to the max.

Restriction Doesn't Work

AFTER YEARS OF LIVING A LIFE OF RESTRICTION in a body that swelled rather than slimmed, I've learned firsthand the mental devastation of letting yourself down again and again. Each time, I felt like that idealized version of me was moving further and further away. If I couldn't do something as simple as keep off a few or a ton of pounds, then I certainly couldn't do all the other things I wanted to do in life.

It's devastating to feel like you may never be able to fulfill your life's calling and make good work due to your size. It's distressing to feel like you can't enjoy the best parts of life—real adult love, moments of peace, travel for joy—because your body is so unfixable. It's shattering to feel like some of your dreams—which, for me, included living like a local in other places—may never come to life because you have no control over your own body.

After decades of these screwed-up beliefs, I'm so over it. I'm tired of letting myself down. I've tired of hating every inch of me. Since getting well on all the good foods that come from plants *slowly* rather than quickly and taking the time to appreciate every inch of me *inside and out*, I've finally broken the make-believe connection between being skinny and being perfect.

I've finally learned that there is no perfect version of me and putting my life on hold until she appears is useless. Not only am I enough just as I am each and every day, but living my best life and putting my dreams into action is what leads me to real wellness. Just like you have to love yourself even when you don't yet really love yourself, you also have to take the tiny steps to live your best life in order to create your best life. Waiting until the right moment—until you have a beefy bank account, until you're the perfect size—is explicitly putting a hold on living your best life. Doing all this hard work to learn to love me has made it clear that there is no perfect anything, there's only you and me doing the very best we can to be happy as soon as possible.

Nowadays, I make tiny changes that stick and I strive to make myself happy in a healthy-ish way. I care so much for the big-little girl inside of me who experienced more than just food restrictions. She felt sad and demotivated all the time—and was frequently made to feel less-than—and it's time she enjoy every part of life.

Today, I savor life. I take care of myself, eat well, and charge toward adventure. And I certainly don't pause my dreams, waiting for some prehistoric diet to cure me before I try this or do that. Instead, I put my dreams into full-on go mode all the time, take my chances, and hope for happy-ish results.

One of my long-wished dreams was to run away to some beautiful place with my partner. After years of the daily nine-to-nine grind (because that's the Internet life, truth), I craved something different, a new way to live. For the last few years, we've finally changed how we live some of the year. We run away together for a spell each year and our lives, including the food, are so much better for it.

MOONLIGHT IN VERMONT

When we stepped through the back door of the school-house, we were certain it would let us down in every possible way. Local friends, neighbors, and the actual owner had told us it was *very rustic*, using the words repeatedly and emphasizing the *very*—enough to make us worry. "It's *very rustic*," the owner said. "You should see it before you decide to rent it."

After a two-hour drive through mountainous roads, we arrived to take a look at the place up close. We stepped in, cautiously, only to find a huge vaulted ceiling that made a loft of the entire first floor of the property. As the town's original schoolhouse, built back in the early 1800s, we were sure we'd find odd rooms and random walls, but stepping into a light-filled loft was a happy surprise.

Tiptoeing through the rest of property as if we'd surely stumble upon something scary, we found a large living space with enough room for family to lounge about; a dining room table that could fit ten; a separate nook for four to enjoy the green mountain views; a pretty banged-up bathroom, wallpaper peeling throughout; and a kitchen that was the size of my kitchen island back in Boston.

It was clear that an army of mice had taken up residence in every kitchen cabinet and on every surface, but the bones of the room weren't so bad and the small appliances were serviceable. And once I took in the kitchen views—of century-old, bursting with green, maple trees, a breathtaking hill, and a mountain farther afield—I knew I could cook anything in here just fine.

We popped the stuck screen door open and stepped onto a fading deck that was covered in moss, boards rickety from years of snow and no protective care. The sound, though, was mesmerizing. A brook trickled by the road across the street, echoing the tune of rushing water up to the house. With the windows open, it seemed that peaceful tone might lull us to a fairly restful sleep.

After five days of cleaning the place from top to bottom, we fully moved in and did, indeed, sleep undisturbed, well, until the birds took over with their sweet tune very early in the morning. But we had a hard time staying mad at them for too long.

We rented that old falling-apart place to experiment with living between two places, because everyone wishes for a life in some vacation spot but we knew it wasn't as simple as hot coffee on chilly, dewy mornings and barbecues on the back deck most nights. Very few people talk about the more-money-more-problems nature of taking care of another structure, let alone a dilapidated one that needed thousands of dollars invested to just bring it up to date. We wanted to see what that felt like, at some low barrier to entry where we didn't own the actual property and could forget about it when we drove away each week.

But probably more important than that, we wanted to have the summer both of us had witnessed others experience over the years, one of pure fun. We worked so hard, always prioritizing our responsibilities and de-prioritizing our personal joy waiting for the perfect moment, a larger savings account, or (for me) a perfect summer body. This was the summer to do all the pleasing things we had missed out on: we'd four-wheel drive on heavily wooded roads; take long walks across neighboring farms; dine outside under the stars every single night; and just sit still, listening to the chatty brook across the road and the siren song of the crickets that made it impossibly hard to leave every Sunday evening.

Unlike some of our friends and neighbors with slightly deeper pockets, we had a monthly budget we struggled to keep to each month and we vowed that this Vermont life could not increase that budget; among other things, we had to split our food budget between both houses and eat like paupers in order to make all this jive. In order to feel the fun, we didn't want to feel any pain.

Instead of filling two unique pantries with two of everything, we split every ingredient between our city home and our country home, including all the condiments and spices which got parsed out into old jars and little baggies. We traveled back and forth with a cooler in the trunk at all times—and carted all the ingredients we needed for a few days' worth of meals. We purchased most everything in our regular city grocery store and brought it north because food prices inflate during the summer in Vermont. We had to economize if we were going to stick to our budgets.

The only exception to the grocery rule was for certain produce and farm-raised meats. Since we were in our Vermont place on the weekends, we visited a regular farmers market every Saturday and searched out deals on vegetables and fruits. Produce that is both local and organic happens to be a bit harder to find in the city— many big-box grocery stores cart in a lot of produce from farther away—so we valued whatever was grown or raised not far from our schoolhouse. Often, we'd just go directly to the Vermont grower, however far away, pick the produce ourselves, and cart it back in our cooler (which really was a permanent fixture in the Jeep).

Learning to navigate a smaller kitchen was odd at first but, eventually, quite liberating. In our snug kitchen, we had everything we needed—ingredients, plates, cookware, glasses, utensils—and nothing more. I discovered that we didn't need much more than that to make a great meal. The produce was so good that a powerful blender or certain whisk was an unnecessary luxury that really didn't fit in such a rustic home and the tiniest of kitchens. The oven worked well, so many of the recipes in this chapter, dishes that came to life during our summers of fun, were made in an old but simple four-range, gas stove with only a sheet pan, cast iron pan, and a casserole dish. Unless they were made on the deck, of course.

There was a nice grill out back, one that hadn't seen much use nor much love over the years, but after a few hours of cleaning, it was ready to fire up. In fact, we tried to cook outside as much as possible but alternated between the stove inside and the grill depending on the dish. Over very low fires in the grill, I'd simmer Eggs in Tomato Sauce (page 215) and cook large pans of Smoky Paella with Fennel (page 262). On higher heat, I'd roast whole potatoes and grill everything from vegetables and stone fruit to the occasional bit of animal protein.

Ultimately, we ate so well during our summers away and not because we spent liberally. In fact, though we work in the city most of the week and eat out occasionally, our Vermont weekends felt like three months of vacation where we ate far better than any restaurant meal. With all that beautiful produce, we made some of the best meals of our lives. And most of the good dishes came to life on Saturday nights, when we turned up the volume on the music and the food.

SATURDAY NIGHTS

Since we worked office-style gigs that kept us in the city during the week, we visited Vermont on the weekends and during extended vacation time. We relished every brief moment away so when we got there, we generally stayed around the schoolhouse. Once we unlocked that door, we truly never wanted to leave, unless it was for a walk down the road past the local sugar house (a maple syrup maker) or for a drive up Mount Hunger to take in our favorite view from the steep mountain road—the locals joke that their favorite view of New Hampshire is from Vermont (*ba-dum ching*).

As well, instead of venturing out for meals, we cooked most everything. This kept us on budget and allowed me to make dishes that both appealed to that vacation-kinda-life and kept me balanced. On short vacations of my past, I'd give myself full-on permission to eat anything I wanted, without regard to its effect on my body. But on this new style of vacation, the type where we got to feel relaxed every single week, I really didn't want to alter my way of eating nor eat a lot more than I ate normally back home. There was genuinely no need to; the real indulgence was finally living a more adventurous life.

Without Friday night picnics (see page 144), since we were often on the road north then, we wanted to create a healthy-ish environment for enjoying really good food and long talks with each other and our visiting friends. Saturday nights became our dining-in nights—they incorporated everyday pantry ingredients and organic produce from the local farmers market, but were amped up a little by a few new rituals.

In the early morning post-breakfast, we'd venture to a large market of thirty-some farmers, food and drink makers, foragers, and crafters who lugged their harvest or goods to sell over the course of four hours. Fueled on coffee (him) and tea (me), we'd explore the stands, say hello to the vendors we came to know well, and pick out what looked good to us. I spent a lot of time with the mushroom forager—as mushrooms provide a variety of nutrients and distinctly rich flavors to dishes—and quite liberally grabbed produce for the evening meal. Don built a budding friendship with the farmer who raised grass-fed cows a few towns away, and filled our freezer and the evening meal with some well-raised beef. I typically avoided beef but this beef, eaten in the right proportions and only occasionally, made me feel so good. Everything went into a cooler while we took the long way home.

After a day of reading or whatever suited us, like napping, cocktails started early. Before planting our bodies into deck chairs, he'd mix up a cocktail and I'd typically grab a glass of wine or small sipper of excellent tequila—some studies show that tequila can lower blood sugar and cholesterol—usually with a little citrus-spiked sparkling water on the side. I often had sparkling water on hand, as it provided a little pause between drinks, often two drinks max, but still felt like I was a part of the party. On extra special nights, I'd make some homemade infusions (specifically, orgeat syrup) during the day and he'd whiz up a drink, like a Mai Tai for two.

With drink in hand, we'd proceed with making our meal. And on some Saturday nights, a steak dinner is practically a ceremony for us. One of us may ready the grill, feeding it wood until it reaches a scorchingly high heat. The other makes a simple rub of coarse salt and freshly pounded black pepper. The steak rests on a plate at room temperature to ensure it will cook more evenly and then it's liberally dusted with the rub. Potatoes are roasted first, directly over the flame to create light char marks, and then placed almost rotisserie-style on a high rack at the top of the grill to finish cooking slowly, far from the embers. Once the potatoes are well on their way, the steak goes on the grate, close enough to the fire to cook but far enough from the flame to avoid too much blackening—a little creates a nice texture, a lot makes everything taste burnt.

Eager and ready to do something more with my hands (besides hold a glass of wine), I'll always make a chimichurri sauce—a very green, raw sauce composed of whatever soft herbs have not yet wilted or a fresh find from the Saturday farmers market, garlic, red pepper flakes, enough oil to thin it out, and enough vinegar to brighten even the starchiest of potatoes. While the steak rests, we set a table and light short candles.

The season may determine the choice cooking method or even the quintessential recipe, but the ritual plays out the same. It's all very romantic and an experience I may curb a bit here or there, but I don't think I could relinquish it indefinitely. I tell you this story as I bet there are powerful rituals in your life so closely tied to food, perhaps indulgent or even very bad-for-you food. I believe it's okay, even compulsory, to retain a few easygoing food rituals that are meaningful to you and whoever you love. Love is so very long and life is so very short.

On summer evenings when we were sure to have guests and perhaps even little kids over, I might instead make some pizza dough from scratch, kneading it by hand on the rickety counter instead of using a fancy mixer. After rising over a few hours and then 20 minutes in a very hot oven, the pizza would emerge—sometimes with cheese, often without—and I'd instantly spread a just-tossed green salad on top, making sure the salad's dressing was bright enough to pop against the fried dough.

Whatever the dish, we made it all in a leisurely way and ate it slowly, savoring only what we needed to feel full enough because there was also Blueberry Plum Crisp Pie (page 228). Seriously though, to eat mindfully is something I still struggle with every day but it's a skill I work hard to practice anytime I pass food through my lips. My eating typically involves some long pauses, talking between bites, and gently reminding myself to delight in every morsel and moment. It's often a bit easier for me to remember this in Vermont, where I feel the space to appreciate every piece of produce, each ethically raised animal part, and all those green hills from where it all came.

FIVE BITS OF ADVICE TO DO WHAT YOU LOVE NOW

My summers are the best of my life and—thankfully—I have maintained my weight loss and stayed super balanced. I live every day to its fullest, no longer waiting for some amorphous future to arrive or my perfect body to materialize. I grab on to all the good experiences right now. I say yes to anything that seems exciting. I do what I love in the moment and enact plans to live out my dreams in the present. Each time I choose to do something that I love, I show myself love. Those individual acts of love form an everlasting pattern that keeps me loving me. The greater the love, the more I stay balanced and well.

Don't wait for the right moment, for a bulking bank account, or for the perfect body to live your best life. Start as soon as possible. To help you get going and perhaps have the <insert season here> of your life, consider these bits of advice:

1. *Believe that your dreams are possible today.* You can do anything you want to do, regardless of body size, budget, time, and responsibilities. Don't wait for the perfect moment because there is no perfect moment. Certainly, there are a few exceptions—like if you want to climb a mountain, you may want to be somewhat strong enough to make the climb. But the only way to climb that mountain is to take a first step and then a second and then a third now (not next year). (My yoga teacher explains that to go far, you must start near. And that nearest step, the first one, is the most important.)

2. *Choose experiences that make your life worth living.* Dreams aren't only career-, money-, or love-based. To be fully balanced, don't forget to follow the dreams that make you excited to wake up in the morning. I absolutely have very vivid professional ambitions that I work to achieve daily. I also have dreams that are about pure joy. Pursuing a holistic set of dreams keeps me fulfilled, happy, and balanced.

3. *Learn to live with much less.* I know firsthand how challenging it is to pursue any given dream without ample time, life flexibility, or money. I, however, choose to make my dreams happen within the means that are possible at the moment, which may involve altering budgets and reshaping expectations. Perhaps my bank account and commitments won't permit a summer in France but I found Vermont's green mountains to be just as beautiful and, in some ways, even more vibrant. I live with a little less in my city life to enjoy my dreamy country life.

4. *Savor and appreciate the seasons.* Whatever you dream and do, enjoy every single moment because they are, inevitably, fleeting. Take in the change of seasons and incorporate any takeaways into your everyday life. I preserve food but you may choose to preserve images of the changing leaves in fall, soar down all the slopes in winter, or simply admire a late spring shower from your perch. Sometimes, taking a few moments to write down any thoughts in a journal helps remember and relish the experience and all its gifts.

5. *Living your dreams supports self-love.* Living your best life is not an exercise in indulgence or recklessness. Done within whatever means works for you, these achievements feed your soul and foster even more dreams. You are taking care of you and that's the ultimate in self-preservation and real self-love.

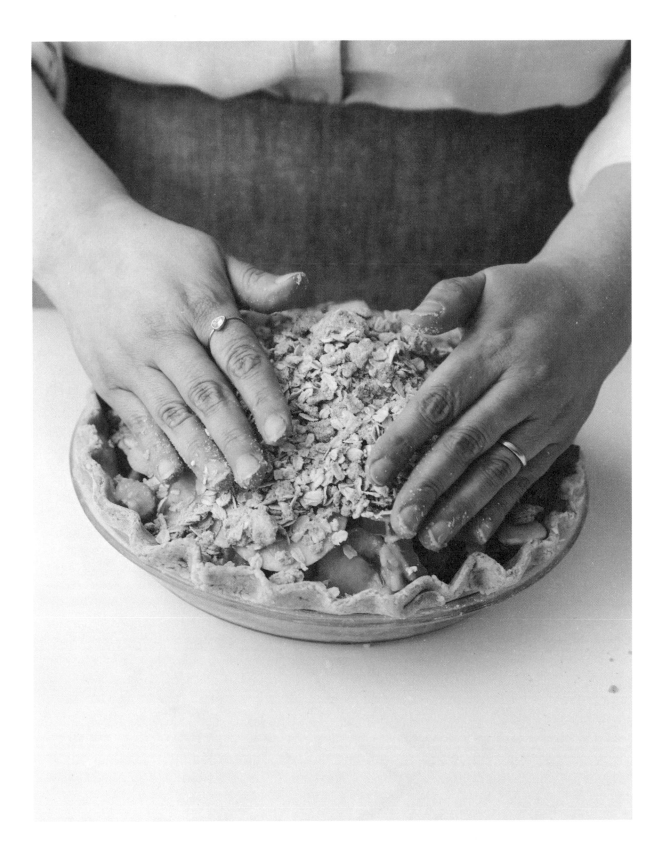

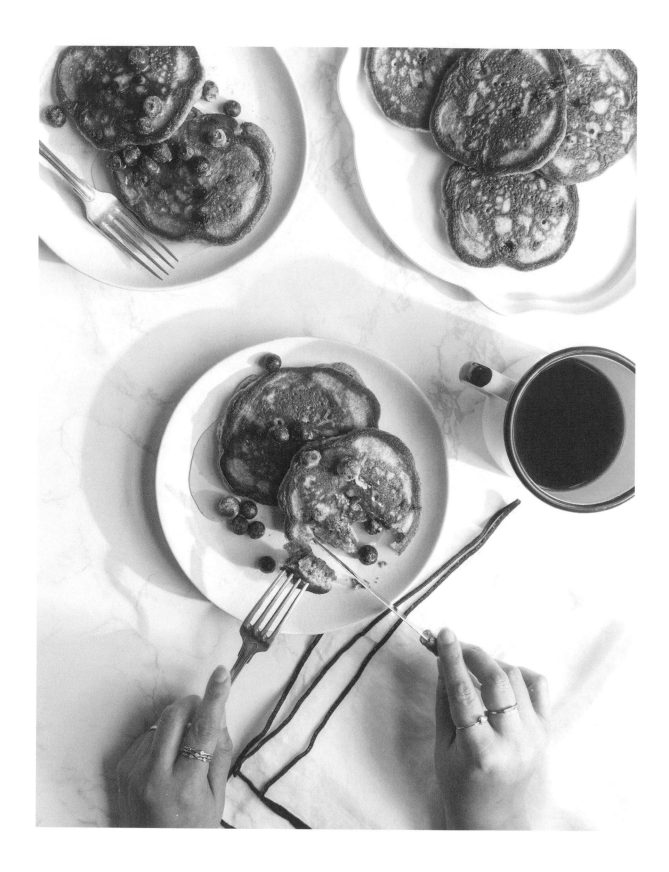

Blueberry BUCKWHEAT PANCAKES

These pancakes have changed my life and, most definitely, my summer life. They make Saturday morning baking super fun and remind me of summertime pancakes at the various camp-style programs from childhood. Their joy comes from how easy it is to bring together a comforting dish that's healthy-ish and satisfying. Just mix the dry ingredients together, mix the wet ingredients together, mix them together, and fold in your fruit.

Blueberries are always in my freezer so they're a top choice but strawberry slices, raspberries, banana slices, and dark chocolate chips all work well. There's a little bit of honey in the batter, which makes them slightly crunchy on the edges in a very good way. I like to add a bit of maple syrup to a small stack but many friends have eaten them just as they are with two hands.

Makes about a dozen 4-inch
(10 cm) pancakes

FREQUENCY: *A couple times per month*

FOOD PREFERENCES: *DF, NF, RSF, Veg*

HANDS-ON TIME: *45 minutes*

TOTAL TIME: *45 minutes*

· ·

1 cup (4¼ oz; 120 g) all-purpose flour

⅓ cup (1½ oz; 40 g) buckwheat flour

4 teaspoons baking powder

½ teaspoon fine sea salt

2 eggs, beaten

2 tablespoons light honey

5 tablespoons vegan butter or coconut oil, melted and cooled, plus more for cooking

1 cup (240 ml) unsweetened Cashew Milk (page 41) or other unsweetened plant milk

1 tablespoon lemon juice (from about ½ medium lemon)

1 cup fresh or frozen blueberries, plus more for serving

Maple syrup, for serving

1. Whisk the flours, baking powder, and salt together in a large bowl. Set aside.

2. Whisk the eggs and honey together in a medium bowl. Add the butter, milk, and lemon juice, and whisk until well blended.

3. Mix the liquid ingredients into the dry ingredients until no flour streaks remain. Don't overmix; the batter may be a little lumpy. During the final stir, fold in the blueberries until coated. Let the batter rest for 10 minutes.

4. Add a teaspoon of vegan butter to a preheated skillet set over medium-high heat. Pour ¼ cup of batter into the pan; it should spread to about 4 inches so you can fill your pan up with 2 or 3 pancakes. Cook for about 4 minutes and flip just after tiny bubbles form around the outside edges of the pancakes. Cook for 2 to 3 minutes longer. Repeat until you've used all the batter. Serve immediately with extra blueberries and maple syrup.

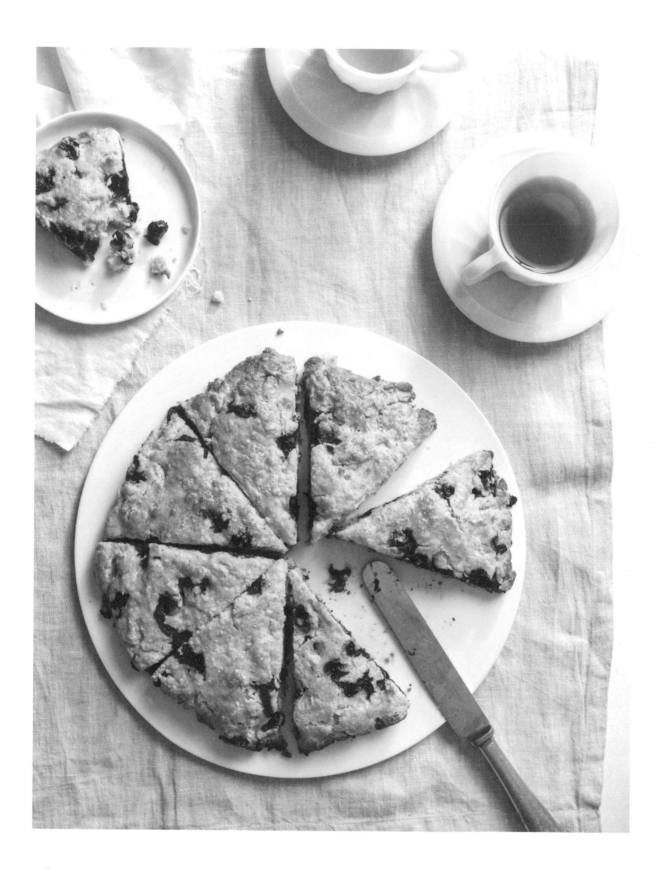

Blueberry SCONES

These are my summer house scones. If people have house wine, I can have summer house scones. The batter comes together in a flash and can be modified to create dozens of variations (see the Sweet Potato Cranberry Scones, page 244, for example). Feel free to switch up the blueberries, increase the maple sugar (if you like a sweet scone), or use a different extract. I'm particularly fond of substituting in orange juice for half the milk and fiori di sicilia extract during the winter holidays.

Makes 8 scones

FREQUENCY: *A couple times per month*

FOOD PREFERENCES: *DF, NF, RSF*

HANDS-ON TIME: *15 minutes*

TOTAL TIME: *30 minutes*

* *

6 tablespoons coconut oil (in solid form), plus more for greasing the pan

2½ cups (10⅔ oz; 300 g) all-purpose flour

2 teaspoons baking powder

½ teaspoon sea salt

¼ cup (1⅜ oz; 40 g) lightly packed maple sugar, plus more for sprinkling

2 eggs, separated

1 cup fresh or frozen blueberries

⅔ cup (160 ml) unsweetened, plain plant milk

½ teaspoon vanilla extract

1. Preheat the oven to 375°F (191°C). Line a baking sheet with parchment paper and grease it with the extra coconut oil.

2. Combine the flour, baking powder, salt, and sugar in a large bowl.

3. Cut the coconut oil into small pieces and blend it quickly and lightly into the flour mix, using your fingertips. Don't let it melt on your fingertips.

4. With a fork, stir in the egg yolks lightly. The yolks will leave tiny yellow clumps throughout the bowl.

5. With a large spoon or rubber spatula, stir in the blueberries.

6. Add the milk and vanilla, mixing just until the dough holds together without crumbling. Add additional milk to the dry spots in the bowl, if needed.

7. Pour the dough onto the center of the parchment and, using the parchment paper or oiled hands, form it into a round, about 9 inches (23 cm) across and 1 inch (2.5 cm) deep. Slice the round into eight large uniform pie-shaped pieces, pulling them away from each other slightly with the knife. Brush the tops with the egg white and sprinkle with extra maple sugar, if you like.

8. Bake the scones for 18 to 22 minutes, until lightly browned. Let cool briefly before serving.

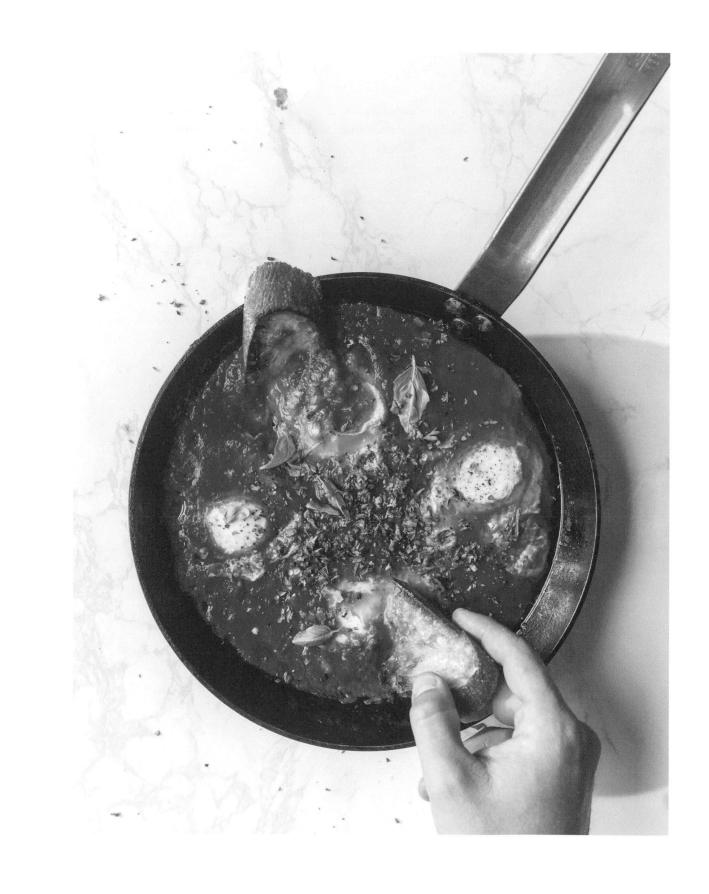

EGGS *in Tomato Sauce*

I make this classic dish quite frequently when I want a solid meal in less than 15 minutes at any time of day. When I'm living in Vermont, I always have organic, cage-free eggs in my fridge and a jar of my Spicy Tomato Sauce in the pantry. Simmer it together and sprinkle on a few fresh herbs. This dish dazzles in its simplicity and the way it nourishes, in any season really.

Serves 2 (as a main dish)

FREQUENCY: *Once per week*

FOOD PREFERENCES: *DF, NF, RSF*

HANDS-ON TIME: *10 minutes*

TOTAL TIME: *15 minutes*

. . . .

1 tablespoon extra-virgin olive oil

1 large garlic clove, peeled and thinly sliced

2 cups (480 ml) Spicy Tomato Sauce (page 35) or your favorite tomato sauce

4 eggs

4 small slices sourdough or Italian bread

Sea salt

Freshly ground black pepper

4 to 6 basil leaves, thinly sliced, for garnish

1 tablespoon minced parsley, for garnish

1. Heat the oil over medium heat in a large skillet with a lid. Swirl the pan to ensure it's well covered in oil. Add the garlic slices and sauté for just a minute to remove some raw flavor. Stir in the tomato sauce and cook until slightly bubbling, 1 to 2 minutes. With a spoon, make four divots in the sauce for the eggs.

2. Break each egg into one of the divots. Cook for a minute uncovered so the whites begin to set. Cover the pan and cook the eggs until the whites are set but the yolks are soft underneath, about 3 minutes.

3. While the eggs cook, lightly toast your bread slices in a toaster, in the oven, or in a separate pan.

4. Remove the lid from the pan and sprinkle the eggs with salt and pepper, to taste. Bring to the table in the skillet. Garnish with basil and parsley. Serve immediately with the toasted bread.

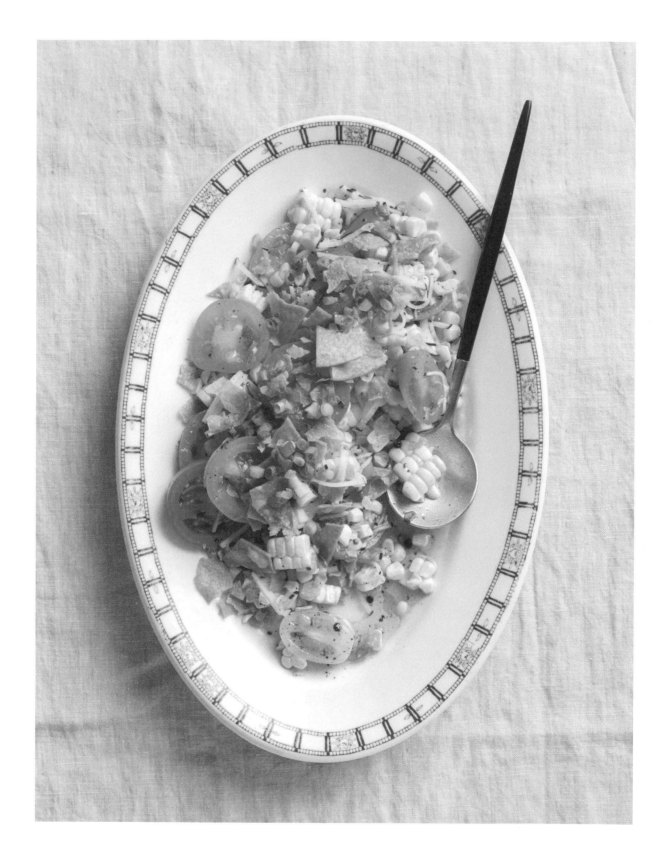

CORN, RADISH, TOMATO,
and Tortilla Chip Salad

This is a fork and knife kind of salad, as it has all sizes of vegetables that need cutting or scooping up into your mouth. It's a summer salad, no doubt, but one that's hefty enough to be a lunch-time main when made with large in-season tomatoes. That said, I actually developed this on a summer morning when traditional eggs or pancakes just sounded so heavy. I chopped and stirred the ingredients together and hand-crushed tortilla chips on top. It satisfied beautifully alongside an iced coffee.

Add a whole lot more tortilla chips, if that's your thing. Or remove the chips altogether and serve the salad on top of garlic rubbed toast. As for the cobs, I reserve them and simmer a big batch of corn stock for the freezer because it makes all sorts of chowders incredibly flavorful.

Serves 4 to 6

FREQUENCY: *Once per week*

FOOD PREFERENCES: *DF, GF, NF, RSF, V*

HANDS-ON TIME: *25 minutes*

TOTAL TIME: *25 minutes*

4 scallions, trimmed and thinly sliced

1 pound (454 g) large ripe heirloom
tomatoes

½ teaspoon sea salt, plus more
for seasoning

2 tablespoons coconut vinegar or
apple cider vinegar

2 tablespoons extra-virgin olive oil

10 twists freshly ground black pepper,
plus more for seasoning

2 cups fresh corn (sliced from about
4 ears)

2 small radish bunches (about
16 radishes), cleaned and julienned

About 10 salted tortilla chips, crushed

1. Soak the scallions in cold water for 20 minutes to crisp them up. Drain and pat dry with a paper towel.

2. Slice the tomatoes into medium-size wedges. Dust them will a heavy pinch of salt and let them sit for 10 minutes to further bring out their flavor.

3. In a medium bowl, mix together the salt, vinegar, oil, and black pepper. Add the tomatoes, corn, radishes, and half the scallions, and toss gently with clean hands to coat each veg well. Taste and season to taste with more salt and pepper, but don't add too much salt as the tortilla chips are also salty.

4. Gently arrange the veg on a large platter to create a pretty presentation. Sprinkle the tortilla chips and remaining scallions atop the dish and serve immediately.

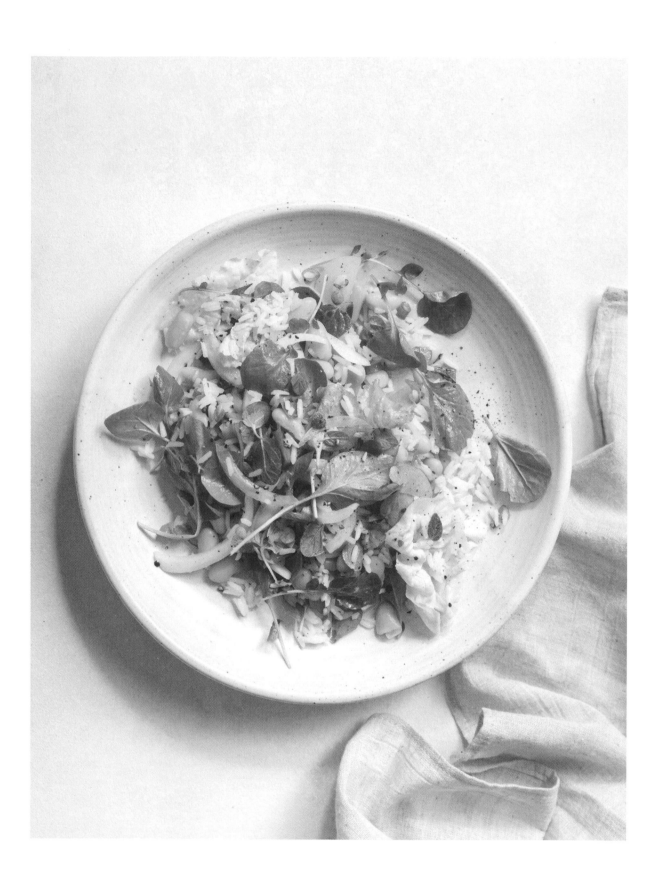

Italian-Style LEFTOVER RICE SALAD

It may seem strange to suggest adding Spanish rice to an Italian-style rice salad but it feels natural to me as my family was a mix of both of these cultures. There was plenty of rice in my childhood as we ate it for practically every meal and always managed to have half a pot leftover that lingered into the next few days. As long as you have leftover rice lingering in your fridge, you can toss this dish together within 15 minutes and it will satisfy immensely—something to do with all those greens, the creamy white beans, and the starchy rice. In the summertime, I mix this together for a quick al fresco lunch and often add in a little tinned tuna.

Serves 2

FREQUENCY: *Once per week*

FOOD PREFERENCES: *DF, GF, NF, RSF, V*

HANDS-ON TIME: *15 minutes*

TOTAL TIME: *15 minutes*

. . . .

2 tablespoons extra-virgin olive oil, divided

1 cup leftover rice or Spanish Turmeric Rice (page 127)

2 tablespoons lemon juice (from about 1 medium lemon) or red wine vinegar

2 handfuls mixed young salad greens

2 scallions, trimmed and finely diced

½ medium sweet white onion, peeled and thinly sliced

1 cup (9¼ oz; 262 g) cooked cannellini beans

4 sprigs fresh oregano, leaves removed, stems discarded

Sea salt

Freshly ground black pepper

1. Add 1 tablespoon of the oil to a shallow frying pan set over medium heat, and sauté the rice until it's just warmed through. Remove from the pan and set aside for a moment.

2. Drizzle the remaining 1 tablespoon oil and the lemon juice along the inside of a large salad bowl. Add the greens, scallions, onion, beans, and oregano leaves. Add the rice, and salt and pepper to taste. With clean hands or a fork and a spoon, gently toss everything together, coating it with the lemon juice and oil that's inside the bowl. Taste and add more salt and pepper, if needed. Enjoy immediately.

Ahh-Maizing TOMATO PIZZA

Homemade pizza (versus the takeout pie from the local pizza joint) is less likely to cause me to have a bloated stomach or to gain weight. I don't eat seventeen slices, just one or two, tops. But every time I make and eat homemade pizza in moderation, it satisfies my pizza craving so I can carry on in everyday wellness mode without any worry, stress, or guilt. I feel great when I eat this Sicilian-style pizza and make it for family and friends quite often.

The dough is based on a recipe by the brilliant J. Kenji Lopez-Alt, author of the bestselling cookbook *The Food Lab* and a chef who focuses on the science of cooking. His recipe is bonkers-good and stunning every time. I made a few tweaks for the more wholesome home cook and even created a dairy-free pie that delivers on richness without the cheese. This pie is covered with corn cream and sliced tomatoes, and then sprinkled with fresh arugula a moment before serving. Make sure your dough has a warm place to rise in the kitchen and that your oven goes as high as 450°F (232°C). And always use the very best extra-virgin olive oil—you'll taste it in every bite.

Serves 6 to 8

FREQUENCY: *A couple times per month*

FOOD PREFERENCES: *DF, NF, RSF, V*

HANDS-ON TIME: *30 minutes*

TOTAL TIME: *3 hours*

. . . .

FOR THE SICILIAN-STYLE PIZZA DOUGH

3½ cups (14⅞ oz; 420 g) bread flour

2 teaspoons sea salt

1 teaspoon active dry yeast

½ cup (120 ml) extra-virgin olive oil

1½ cups (360 ml) room temperature water (98–105°F/37–41°C)

MAKE THE SICILIAN-STYLE PIZZA DOUGH

1. Whisk together the flour, salt, yeast, and 2 tablespoons of the olive oil in a large bowl. Add the water and mix together with a wooden spoon until a shaggy dough comes together. The dough will be sticky. Dump the mixture onto a floured surface and knead for 5 minutes until soft and smooth, adding extra flour here or there to make a less sticky dough. Let the dough rest for 5 minutes under a clean, damp dish towel. Return to kneading for 5 minutes longer until a soft and smooth dough comes to life, adding only a little extra flour as needed—the dough shouldn't need too much flour during the second knead.

2. Pour the remaining 6 tablespoons of oil onto a rimmed 13- by 18-inch (33 by 46 cm) baking sheet and spread it over the entire inner surface with your hands. Transfer the dough to the baking sheet, turning it in the oil a few times until well coated. Then, gently press the dough into a large square or rectangle. You will not be able to stretch the dough to the entire size of the baking sheet, but push and stretch as far as you can. Pick up the dough, stretch it by hand, and let the olive oil run underneath. Cover the baking sheet with plastic wrap and let the dough rise at room temperature for 1 hour. Gently pull the dough to the corners of the pan with your fingers, lifting it to allow the olive oil to run underneath. Re-cover it with the plastic wrap and let it rest at room temperature for 1 to 1½ hours more, until it has spread very close to the rim of the pan and risen up to the rim. You can now proceed with making your pizza.

continued

FOR THE AHH-MAIZING
TOMATO PIZZA

2 tablespoons extra-virgin olive oil

2 oregano sprigs, leaves removed,
    stems discarded

2 cups fresh corn (sliced from about
    2 ears)

½ teaspoon sea salt, plus more to taste

½ cup (60 ml) vegetable stock or water

1 pint (9¾ oz; 275 g) cherry tomatoes,
    halved

2 cups arugula, cleaned and dried

MAKE THE AHH-MAIZING TOMATO PIZZA

1. Heat 1 tablespoon of the oil in a frying pan set over medium heat. Add the oregano leaves and sauté for just a minute or two. Add the corn and the salt. Sauté, stirring frequently, just until it's cooked through, 3 to 4 minutes. Remove the oregano and discard. Carefully scoop the corn into a powerful blender along with the stock. Puree for at least 30 seconds until creamy and smooth. Chill the corn cream until ready to use.

2. Preheat your oven to 450°F (232°C). Carefully remove the plastic wrap from the pizza dough. Spread the corn cream across the surface of the dough, leaving about a 1-inch margin for the crust. Dot the corn cream with cherry tomato halves, cut side up, ensuring even coverage. Sprinkle with more salt and drizzle with the remaining 1 tablespoon oil. Bake the pizza for 20 to 25 minutes, until the bottom is crisp and brown, and the top is just beginning to get golden brown, too. Allow to cool for 5 minutes before cutting and serving. Sprinkle with the arugula just before serving.

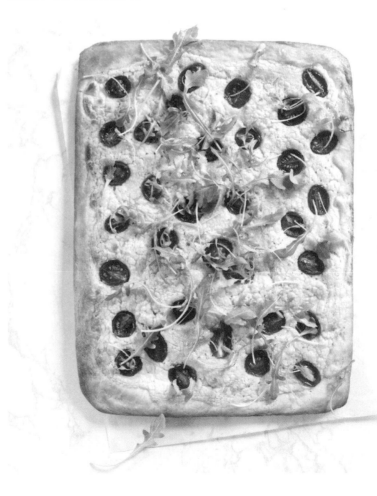

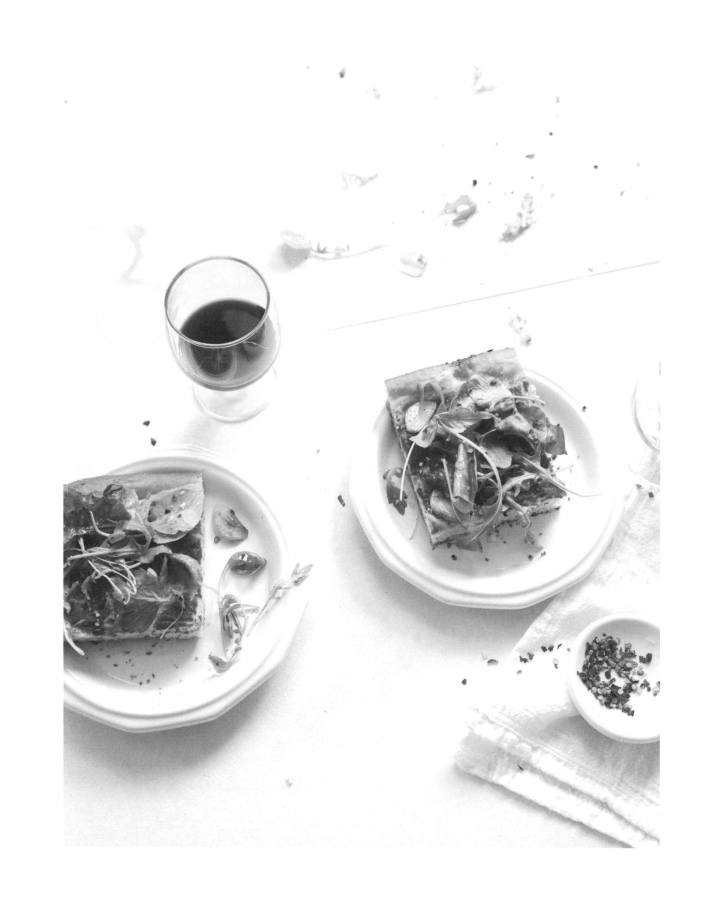

Garlicky-Green PIZZA

This is another version of a Sicilian-style pizza that's very garlicky and exceptionally green because it's topped with a lightly dressed salad. It's made in the style of a true marinara-style pizza, but without cheese. Instead, the toppings include Spicy Tomato Sauce, slivers of fresh garlic, and a simple garden-style salad gently tossed with red wine vinegar.

If you're a fan of the sweet and spicy flavor mash-up, try a drizzle of Hot Honey on this pizza. It makes this already-satisfying meal a little extra special.

Serves 6 to 8

FREQUENCY: *A couple times per month*
FOOD PREFERENCES: *DF, NF, RSF, V*
HANDS-ON TIME: *30 minutes*
TOTAL TIME: *3 hours*

. . . .

5 tablespoons extra-virgin olive oil,
  divided

8 large garlic cloves, peeled

1 Sicilian-Style Pizza Dough (page 220)

1 cup (240 ml) Spicy Tomato Sauce
  (page 35) or your favorite
  homemade sauce

Sea salt

3 cups chopped fresh greens,
  such as spinach or arugula

1 tablespoon red wine vinegar

12 twists freshly ground black pepper

Hot Honey (page 57), for serving
  (optional)

1. Warm 2 tablespoons of the oil in a shallow frying pan over medium heat. Pan fry the garlic cloves, whole, until they get golden brown on all sides, which should take no more than 5 minutes. Remove to a bowl to cool and let the oil cool as well. Once cooled, slice the garlic cloves into thin slices. Save the garlic oil for seasoning your pizza. Set aside.

2. Preheat your oven to 450°F (232°C).

3. Carefully remove the plastic wrap from the pizza dough. Spread the tomato sauce across the surface of the dough, leaving about a 1-inch margin for the crust. Dot the tomato sauce with garlic slices, ensuring even coverage. Sprinkle with salt and drizzle with 1 tablespoon of the olive oil. Bake the pizza for 20 to 25 minutes, until the bottom is crisp and brown. Allow to cool for 5 minutes.

4. While the pizza is baking, toss the greens with the remaining 2 tablespoons olive oil, vinegar, and salt and pepper to taste. When the pizza has cooled and just before serving, sprinkle the salad across the pizza. Cut and serve with the reserved garlic oil or the hot honey if desired, on the side for drizzling.

THE PERFECT RIB-EYE STEAK
with Whole Grilled Potatoes and Chimichurri Sauce

After achieving my active wellness mode goals, I added a little organic, grass-fed steak back into my way of eating. I did it less so for the sake of eating meat again. The flavor is certainly incomparable but it's not essential to my palate. I make a steak now and again more so to honor a past food ritual and share a hearty dining experience with someone I love.

When choosing a steak, especially a rib-eye, look for a highly marbled piece, with white veins running throughout, as that fat will create a lot of flavor once it melts over the high heat. A less marbled piece of meat may become tough after a cook. I source my organic grass-fed beef from a Vermont farmer but, sometimes, I pop into old-fashioned butcher shops to ask questions and love how they often refer to a rib-eye as a Delmonico steak. The term feels fancy and special, and eating meat should indeed feel significant since, let's be honest, a life was taken to get it to your plate.

Because there's so much delicious fat on a rib-eye, grilling it can sometimes spark a fire so be very alert of any rogue flames. A few years ago, I was introduced to the reverse sear method, so when there's no grill in sight (or even when there is), I take that path. It guarantees a perfectly cooked steak every single time. And I feel quite powerful wielding my tongs, placing and then flipping a perfect slab of red meat in a very hot pan.

This recipe typically serves at least two—four if you're light eaters, one if it's the only steak you'll have all year. I sometimes serve it with a pan of roasted and charred Brussels sprouts or a bright lemony green salad, or both. But if I'm going for quintessential steakhouse style, I'll offer a pile of whole grilled potatoes along with chimichurri sauce. The sauce entwines with the dry potatoes and the drippy steak, creating a sort of enhanced dressing that's been unmatched time and time again.

The potatoes don't have to be grilled; you can simply roast them dry on a baking sheet in the oven. The sauce is well suited to everything—these potatoes, a steak, a whole-roasted fish, and all kinds of vegetables, especially crisp-edged turnips or caramelized cauliflower.

Serves 2

FREQUENCY: *A couple times per month*

FOOD PREFERENCES: *DF, GF, NF, RSF*

HANDS-ON TIME: *15 minutes*

TOTAL TIME: *1 hour 40 minutes*

FOR THE PERFECT RIB-EYE STEAK

½ cup black peppercorns

½ cup coarse (not flaky) sea salt

1 pound (454 g) bone-in rib-eye steak, about 1-inch thick

1 tablespoon grape seed oil or other high-heat cooking oil

MAKE THE PERFECT RIB-EYE STEAK

1. Prepare the salt and pepper rub. Grind the peppercorns into a coarse grind with a mortar and pestle. You can also grind them with a spice or coffee grinder. Just be sure to clean out your grinder by whizzing up uncooked white rice in it just before and after you grind the peppercorns. Toss the ground peppercorns and salt together in a bowl until well-distributed and light gray in color.

2. Preheat the oven to 250°F (121°C) with the rack in the center position. Pat the steak dry thoroughly with a paper towel.

continued

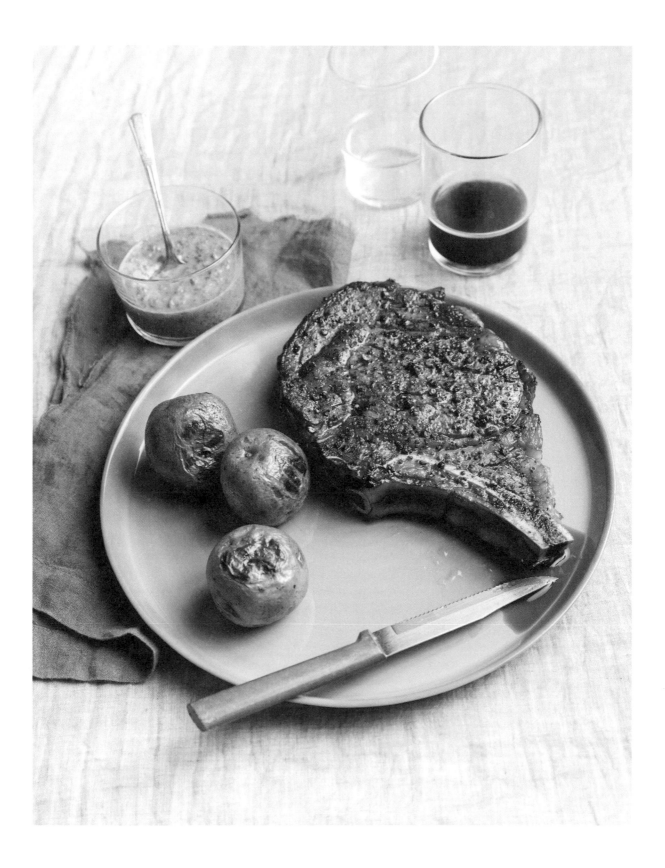

Ten 3-inch, thin-skinned potatoes,
cleaned and dried

Chimichurri Sauce (page 48)

3. Sprinkle and rub the steak on all sides with the salt and pepper rub. Start with a tablespoon of the rub and add more to suit your preference— the more you add, the spicier and saltier the finished steak. Reserve any unused rub in an airtight jar for up to 1 year. Ideally, let the steak stand for 1 hour at room temperature or up to 8 hours in the fridge. But if you only have 10 minutes, that's fine too.

4. Place the steak on a rimmed baking sheet and slide it into the oven. Roast until the internal temperature registers 105°F (41°C) for a rare steak or 115°F (46°C) for a medium-rare steak, about 15 to 20 minutes. The steak will be the juiciest, most tender, and flavorful at these temperatures but feel free to roast it to your preference. Remove from the oven.

5. Heat a cast iron skillet or stainless steel pan over medium-high heat. Add the oil to the pan and swirl until it's well-coated and just begins to smoke. Sear the steak for no more than 30 seconds on both sides and up to 20 seconds on its sides, until you get a nice seared golden color. The final internal temperature of the steak should be 120°F (49°C) for a rare steak or 130°F (54°C) for a medium-rare steak.

6. Transfer the steak to a plate and let rest for 15 minutes before slicing and serving.

MAKE THE WHOLE GRILLED POTATOES AND CHIMICHURRI SAUCE

1. Fire up the grill to between 400°F and 450°F (204–232°C).

2. Place the potatoes directly on the grates (if the potatoes fall through your grates, cook them at 400°F/204°C in your oven) but to the right or left of the main fire. Close the grill lid and cook for 20 to 25 minutes, opening only once to turn them over. (In an oven, this may take closer to 40 minutes.) The potatoes will be ready when they are easily pierced with a fork and have light grill marks all over the skin. Remove them from the grill and cover with foil.

3. Serve the potatoes with the chimichurri sauce and the steak.

STEAK *au Poivre*

I've enjoyed Steak au Poivre on multiple occasions, often made by women my mother's age. It's possible that they learned how to press peppercorns into beef tenderloin from Julia Child's *Mastering the Art of French Cooking*. In fact, I believe Child was one of the first to offer a written recipe for the dish to American cooks. No doubt, my mother-in-law learned it from her and made it for special gatherings when I started dating her son, perhaps first showing off to a new guest and, eventually, showing me that he'd need plenty of quality dishes put before him if we stuck together long-term. I hope I've done her as right as possible.

A few years ago, David Tanis presented a stunningly simple recipe for Steak au Poivre in the *New York Times*. I was initially deterred, as cream is an essential part of the pan sauce that coats the crusted steak, but not for long. I pulled out a jar of my homemade crème fraîche, which is made from cashews, and plotted along to make my version of his dish. I use a lot more peppercorns, and oil instead of butter. I also include bourbon in the pan sauce, because it's the only moment I really get my bourbon fix. I hope this dish gives you a moment to indulge while respecting your dairy-free ways.

Serves 2

FREQUENCY: *A couple times per month*

FOOD PREFERENCES: *DF, RSF*

HANDS-ON TIME: *30 minutes*

TOTAL TIME: *5 hours*

. . . .

Two 12-oz (340 g) boneless rib-eye
   or New York strip steaks, about
   1-inch thick

¼ cup black peppercorns

Fine sea salt

1 tablespoon grape seed oil or other
   high-heat cooking oil

2 medium shallots, finely diced

1½ cups (360 ml) vegetable or beef stock

1 tablespoon bourbon

¼ cup (60 ml) Crème Fraîche
   (page 43)

1. Preheat the oven to 250°F (121°C) with the rack in the center position.

2. Pat the steaks dry thoroughly with a paper towel. Using a mortar and pestle or a spice grinder, grind the peppercorns until coarsely crushed.

3. Sprinkle and rub the steaks on all sides with salt. Divide the crushed black pepper between the two steaks, pressing the pepper into the steak surface with your hands. Let sit for 10 minutes.

4. Place the steaks on a rimmed baking sheet and slide it into the oven. Roast until the meat thermometer registers 105°F (41°C) for a rare steak or 115°F (46°C) for a medium-rare steak, about 15 to 20 minutes. The steaks will be the juiciest, most tender, and flavorful at these temperatures but feel free to roast them to your preference. Remove from the oven.

5. Heat a cast iron skillet or stainless steel pan over medium-high heat. Add the oil to the pan and swirl it until it's well-coated and just begins to smoke. Sear the steaks for no more than 30 seconds on both sides and up to 20 seconds on its sides, until you get a nice seared golden color. The final internal temperature should be 120°F (49°C) for a rare steak or 130°F (54°C) for a medium-rare steak.

6. Transfer the steaks to a plate and let sit while you make the sauce.

7. Add the shallots to the same pan in which you cooked the steaks and sauté until they begin to wilt and brown, 1 to 2 minutes. Add the broth and bring to a simmer. Stir in the bourbon and continue to simmer until the sauce is reduced by half, 2 to 3 minutes. Stir in the crème fraîche and cook until sauce thickens slightly, about 2 minutes.

8. Return the steaks to the pan and cover with sauce, turning once. Transfer to plates and serve immediately.

Blueberry Plum CRISP PIE

What's a Vermont summer without a solid blueberry dessert? The tiny berries—at once tart and sweet—grow everywhere and pick-your-own patches dot many scenic byways. I pick or buy flats upon flats of navy gems, enough to fill my freezer for an entire year's worth of smoothies, scones, pancakes, oatmeal, and, of course, blueberry pie. In recent years, a few daring farmers have planted plum trees. Together, blueberries and plums taste like what dark blue and purple might taste like together—deep, inky, and indulgent.

My mash-up of these two fruits takes the form of a very easy pie. Instead of two pie doughs (top and bottom), this dish has just one. The top comes together from a mix of oats, almond flour, all-purpose flour, cinnamon, and maple sugar, forming a crisp layer that blends into the fruity layer. When those two layers meet, they create a surprising layer that's both fruity and bar-like. A proper and modern New Englander may say, it's pretty awesome.

I use the tiniest of wild blueberries and damson plums and, out of season, you can find both in the freezer section of most grocery stores nowadays. If plums are hard to find, try diced peaches. If seedless Concord grapes are available wherever you are, use those in place of the plums because that combo is equally heavenly.

This pie can be made a day in advance. The pie will set more firmly and the flavor will improve in the extra 24 hours.

Makes one 9-inch (23 cm) pie

FREQUENCY: *Once a season*

FOOD PREFERENCES: *DF, RSF, V*

HANDS-ON TIME: *20 minutes*

TOTAL TIME: *1 hour 15 minutes*

. . . . , ...

1 batch Pie Dough (page 58) or
    1 store-bought vegan pie crust in
    9-inch (23 cm) foil shell

3 heaping cups fresh or frozen
    blueberries

8 small ripe red or purple plums,
    pitted and slivered, or 2 cups seed-
    less concord grapes

¼ cup (1⅜ oz; 40 g) plus 2 tablespoons
    lightly packed maple sugar, divided

¼ teaspoon sea salt, divided

2 tablespoons all-purpose flour

1 tablespoon lemon juice (from about
    ½ medium lemon)

1. Preheat the oven to 350°F (177°C).

2. Place your dough in a 9-inch pie plate or foil shell. Make sure that the dough fits snuggly into all the corners of the plate. Trim off extra dough and crimp the edge as you prefer to create a design and hold the crisp topping in place. Set it in the fridge while you prepare the fruit and crisp. (If you are using a store-bought pie crust, set it in the fridge now.)

3. Add the blueberries, plums, ¼ cup of the maple sugar, ⅛ teaspoon of the salt, the all-purpose flour, and lemon juice to a large bowl. Toss to coat evenly. Set aside.

4. Put the oats, almond flour, cinnamon, the remaining ⅛ teaspoon salt, and the remaining 2 tablespoons maple sugar in a medium bowl and toss until well combined. Divide the coconut oil into teaspoon portions (9 total) and add it 1 teaspoon at a time. With your clean hands, blend everything together until the mixture binds together a bit and looks like coarse breadcrumbs.

continued

1 cup (3½ oz; 100 g) old-fashioned oats

½ cup (1⅔ oz; 48 g) finely ground almond flour

⅛ teaspoon cinnamon

3 tablespoons coconut oil, solid form

1 tablespoon extra-virgin olive oil

5. Remove your pie dough from the fridge. Pile in the fruit mixture, allowing any extra fruit to hump up in the center of the pie. Place your oat mixture on top of the fruit, covering as much of it as you can, and allowing any extra crisp mixture to hump up in the center of the pie. Drizzle the olive oil across the top of the pie.

6. Place your pie on a rimmed baking sheet. Bake for 45 to 60 minutes, until the oat mixture and pie crust are almost golden brown and any fruit that shows through is bubbling. Allow the pie to cool for 20 minutes before serving or place in your fridge to cool completely.

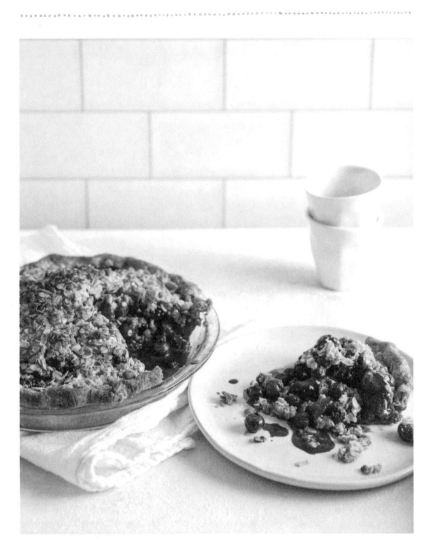

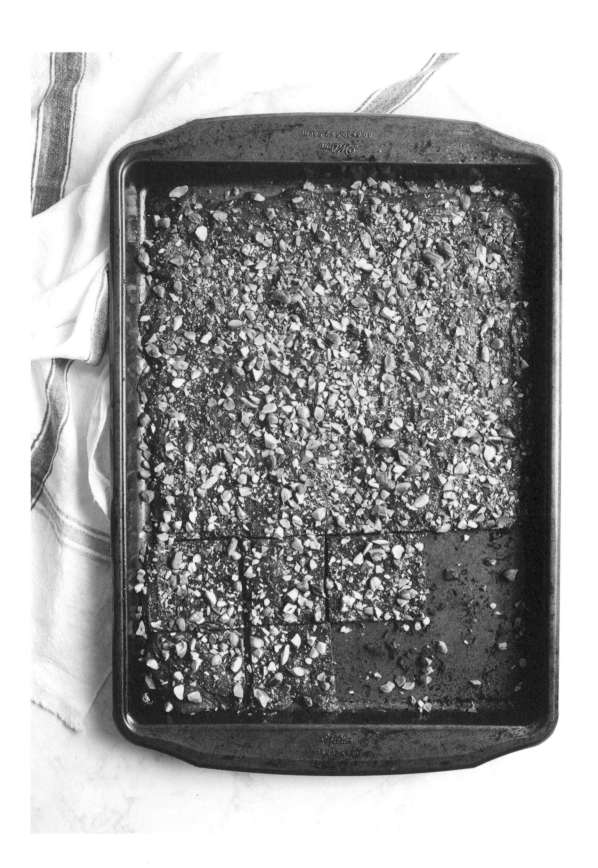

Pistachio Bark BROWNIES

These exceptionally thin brownies look more like bark, but the texture and taste is that of a rich, nutty brownie. The chocolatey flavor comes from raw cacao powder. Cacao is the raw form of chocolate and far less processed than, for example, cocoa powder or chocolate bars. Cacao powder is essentially ground up cacao beans that have not been heated in any way; whereas cocoa powder has been heated and is often sold mixed with sugar. Both cacao powder and cocoa powder are good for you but cacao powder is the purest form and may be the highest source of antioxidants of all the foods on the planet. It's also high in magnesium, monounsaturated fats, cholesterol-free saturated fats, vitamins, minerals, fibers, and protein, making it an excellent way to get a bunch of nutrients. Because it's so pure, raw cacao powder can be expensive. I buy a large bag for the year and use mine to make these brownies and chocolate-flavored pancakes and waffles. I also slip some into my Cacao-Coffee Granola (page 85) and my smoothies on the regular—see my Chocolate Zucchini Smoothie (page 82).

Makes 24 squares

FREQUENCY: *A couple times per month*
FOOD PREFERENCES: *DF, RSF, Veg*
HANDS-ON TIME: *20 minutes*
TOTAL TIME: *45 minutes*

. . . .

½ cup (120 ml) safflower oil, plus
    more for greasing

¾ cup (4 oz; 120 g) lightly packed
    maple sugar

¾ cup (2¾ oz; 80 g) raw cacao powder

¼ teaspoon sea salt

1 teaspoon almond extract

2 eggs

½ cup (1¾ oz; 50 g) spelt flour or
    all-purpose flour

½ cup shelled pistachios, raw and
    unsalted, finely chopped

Flaky sea salt, for sprinkling

1. Preheat the oven to 325°F (163°C) with the rack in the center position. Generously grease a 13- by 18-inch (33 by 46 cm) rimmed baking sheet. Do not line the pan with parchment.

2. Mix together the sugar, cacao powder, and salt in a large bowl. Pour the oil and almond extract over those ingredients and stir until smooth. Add the eggs one at a time, stirring vigorously after each addition, until the batter is thick and shiny. Stir in the flour until no flour streaks remain.

3. Using a rubber spatula or offset spatula, spread the batter into a thin even layer to the edge and into the corners of the prepared baking sheet. (Don't worry if the batter doesn't reach all the way to the corners; do your best.) Sprinkle the pistachios across the batter and press them in slightly with the flat of your hand. Sprinkle some flaky sea salt on top for an extra kick.

4. Bake the brownies for 10 to 15 minutes, until firm to the touch and a tester inserted into the center comes out with moist crumbs and no runny batter attached to it. Let cool for 5 minutes.

5. Cut the brownies into about 3-inch squares with a pizza cutter or sharp knife. Remove from the pan with a spatula and cool completely on a wire rack or piece of parchment paper. Store the brownies in an airtight container at room temperature for up to 5 days.

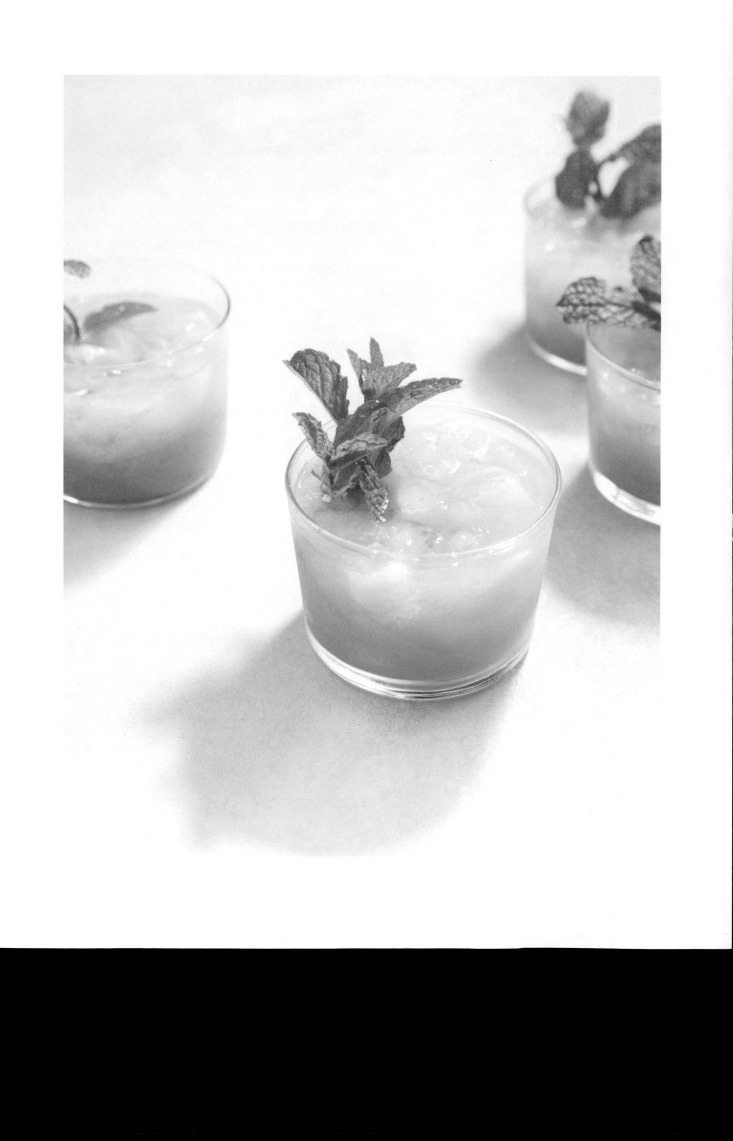

MAI TAI *Cocktails*

Before I started on this path to wellness, I faithfully ate and drank at my favorite Sichuan restaurant weekly. On the surface, this spot is similar to your average Chinese dive but, once you become a regular, you know the experience is far more in tune with some of the best big city dining venues. If you request it, the food can be exceptionally spicy, closer to what you may taste in Sichuan itself. But far surpassing the food, the drinks at The Baldwin Bar are the proverbial bar to which I hold every other cocktail.

During our weekly visits, we fell in with the best bartenders in the world, some of whom have competed and won national championships. They make every sort of drink imaginable, so just rattle off your preferred flavors and a master-piece will find its way to your table. The bar quickly became known for having the region's best Mai Tais, a Polynesian-style cocktail that is said to have been created at a California restaurant in the 1930s or 40s. The recipe varies but it's generally a refreshing mix of rums, Orgeat syrup (almond syrup), lime juice, and other fruit juices.

When I was in active wellness mode, our visits to The Baldwin Bar become less frequent, more like monthly, and my cocktails transformed into white wine or bitter-flavored sodas. Still, when the summer hits and I want to share a fond food memory, I'll make this drink from scratch with slightly more wholesome ingredients, such as maple sugar instead of white sugar in the homemade Orgeat syrup. This recipe makes four drinks served in tiny glasses; it's my way of enjoying the food memory without drinking too much.

Makes 4 small drinks

FREQUENCY: *Once a season*

FOOD PREFERENCES: *DF, GF, V*

HANDS-ON TIME: *10 minutes*

TOTAL TIME: *10 minutes*

. . . .

Ice, crushed

3 ounces (90 ml) dark rum

3 ounces (90 ml) light rum

1½ ounces (45 ml) Orgeat Syrup
(page 59)

1 ounce (30 ml) Cointreau

1 ounce (30 ml) maple syrup

2 ounces (60 ml) lime juice
(from about 2 medium limes)

8 sprigs fresh mint, snipped to fit
your glass

1. Add a handful of ice, both rums, the Orgeat Syrup, Cointreau, maple syrup, and lime juice to a shaker. Close the shaker and shake for 30 seconds. Add fresh crushed ice or a large ice cube to each glass. Strain the cocktail between four small glasses, about 2½ ounces each.

2. Take 2 sprigs of mint and tap them on your hand briskly, almost bruising them, to bring out the mint flavor. Place the bruised mint sprigs in each glass as garnish, repeating for each cocktail. Serve immediately.

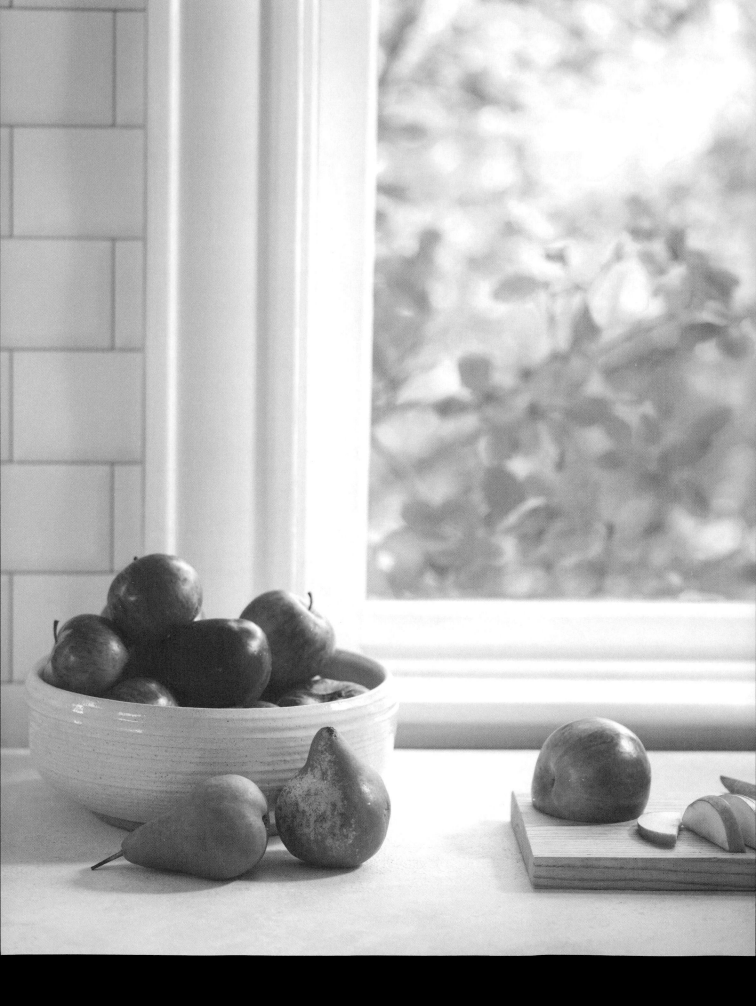

STAY WELL FOREVER

Recipes for Everyday Comfort Foods

It's time to make this change a welcome part of your life for good. When the foods you eat make you feel good, it becomes easier to stay with it. Of course, there are always temptations, and comfort foods can be one of the biggest. Still, rich, flavorful, satisfying food doesn't have to derail all of your good progress.

This chapter includes recipes inspired by all the new comfort foods that now represent the cooler months to me. You'll notice techniques for adding deep flavor in lighter ways and recreations of some of my dearest cold-weather dishes. There's also Sweet Potato Pie (page 278) because I believe there's always room for a slice.

Fall Layers

EVERY YEAR I LOOKED FORWARD TO the closure of summertime. I waited for that first moment when evening sunsets brought a penetrating cold chill instead of a warm, lazy breeze. I was so eager to veer away from fresh fruit and raw vegetables in favor of ample platters of rich pasta, all the cheeses, or long-braised meats and stews. I could finally bid goodbye to barely-there clothing, the sort that made the summer tolerably cool but showed way too much skin. I could, at last, hunker down comfortably in sweater weather.

Fall was my original favorite season precisely because it removed every excuse for a bathing suit and shorts, and forced me to layer on jacket after sweatshirt after long-sleeved top. Instead of baring my legs and arms, I could finally button up all my wobbly flesh where it belonged, under a drab, thick ensemble. Forget polished fingers and toes, I was in thick socks, boots, and mittens way earlier than everyone else because I didn't want to look at my imperfect outer layer any longer than necessary, skin bulging and burned then tanned, freckled, and peeled by the East Coast ocean air.

With more garments on my big-little body, I could finally hide away from everyone's gaze and, quite frankly, avoid the pitied glances at my exposed parts. I still got loaded hugs from my mother, the sort where she sized up how the new season of food fit on my frame, but her adult acquaintances would be less likely to comment on my Popeye-sized arms or well-endowed bosom, both oddly proportioned for such a young, non-athletic girl. I wore scarves every chance I could, to cover up my ample chest from concerned adults and bug-eyed boys.

From my tween years to well into my thirties, my passion for fall followed me every day of my life. If I could just make it from the last day of winter to the first day of fall unscathed, not too banged up from comments or insults, I'd be okay. Much like food, fall and winter provided a comfort blanket to brave back-to-school season or even back-to-work season (after the more casual clothes of summer). By the first day of fall, I'd have all my armor back on and, perhaps, I could at long last feel safe again.

This new way of eating and, ultimately, living has given me a brand new outlook on everything. While spring is my now favorite season, fall holds a very special place in my heart, likely because the big-little girl inside me grabs on to the season like a security blanket. Still, the enlightened adult in me now uses fall as a time for reflection.

ALL THE REFLECTIONS

Ultimately, all the parts of my life have made me pretty strong. I've experienced some tough stuff and the tough stuff has made me braver. I've also experienced some good stuff and the good stuff has made me better. I didn't have a perfect childhood, but gosh, no one does. And to be clear, no one was putting cigarettes out on my arm. There's real pain and suffering in this world, people. We read about it in the news everyday but it's not in the pages of this cookbook. This is fundamentally a happy-ish story.

I do not minimize the sad, humiliating, and somewhat traumatic moments I lived through. I can't forget that all the hard-hitting moments bounded together to form a distorted view of myself. Even with that though, I'm happy, grudge-free, and okay. I *am* okay now.

Forgiveness is a tough topic. Perhaps forgiveness has no place in a cookbook but I am pretty sure it plays an imperative role in the cookbook you're holding right now.

After years of grudges, I've let everyone off the hook for everything they may have done to contribute to my warped view of myself. I really do believe that no one fully understood how candid and qualifying words, delivered ever so casually and even with good intentions, could so resolutely hurt a big-little girl. They had no idea how their words and actions influenced me.

I've forgiven my parents, too. Maybe I didn't wholly forgive them while they were still alive but I have absolutely forgiven them now that they've orphaned me on this planet. I believe my parents had no concept of the potential impact their stinging words or startling actions would have on me. I believe that they did the best they could with whatever they knew at the time.

However, this forgiving feeling didn't surface overnight. After several long talks, many of them quite heated, with my mother, I felt I had adequate time to say my bit, to explain how it felt to receive such charged hugs, and to finally implore her to put those hugs on pause.

As well, I didn't find a way to forgive alone. This forgiveness manifested after a lot of therapy, the sort that taught me the only part of life that was remotely within my control was how I allow myself to feel. I can't control anyone else. I can't control how anyone else feels. I certainly can't control the future. But I can control my reaction to everything that has happened and will happen. And I can choose to forgive, to move on, and be happy enough.

Now, I have not had children but parenting looks like very hard work. My parents did their best and I know you're doing your best, too. I have no business offering up suggestions to parents, even parents to big-little kids. But since I've been that big-little kid—mocked, insulted, and shamed repeatedly for years and years—I want to share what I think I wanted to hear.

I believe that if I had heard the following statements when I was younger, I may have grown up feeling just a little better about myself sooner rather than decades later. Here's what I wished I had heard on repeat, with no caveats inserted—you know, when I wasn't all mischievous or naughty.

> *"You're very smart and very kind."*
> *"You're wonderful, just as you are."*
> *"You can do anything with perseverance and hard work."*

If I had a child, I would not make comments about their appearance at all. I would reserve my guidance and commentary to their performance and quality of character versus how they looked on any given day. I would discourage others from commenting on my kid's appearance. I would encourage my kid to care less about fashion and the money needed to buy it, and more about how they can make the world a better place. I don't know how to do that but I would do my best, like you do. I suppose, ultimately, I would make sure my kid knew that I am on their side all the time.

I am on *my side* all the time now. My feelings for me today are paramount to all the past hurt and damage. I have forgiven myself. I have forgiven myself for hating every part of me; for not believing in me; for feeling like I let myself down; for feeding myself to the point of pain; and for using all sorts of messed-up techniques to comfort the little girl inside me. I forgive myself for using food as comfort and I will continue to forgive myself for that every single day.

Since I have given myself reprieve from all the gristly stuff in my past, I also show myself swift compassion during these colder weather months. I appreciate fall's comfort foods, loaded with heavy ingredients and all sorts of familiar feelings. In fact, comfort food is still my thing but in a new way. If comfort food is your thing, maybe these thoughts and recipes will be of service to you, too.

A NEW THOUGHT ON COMFORT FOOD

Eating more filling foods is a biological inevitability come autumn. It's natural to pack on some insulation—a little more fat keeps us a little bit warmer. In my former life, the calories came in the form of fat-laden animal products, because those rich flavors and greasy mouthfuls both satiated and converted into the kind of fat that made me feel warmer, even if my body temperature didn't necessary go up.

You need fat: it wants to be on your body and becomes a back-up energy source that is stored and used, as needed, to keep you going. Unfortunately, some fats found in animal products contribute to the rise of bad cholesterol in the arteries and are a major risk factor in heart disease. If you eat too much, it could affect your health negatively. Small portions are okay. It becomes riskier when you eat fatty meat or dairy-full dishes morning, noon, and night.

Eating rich comfort foods was crucial to the big-little girl inside me. I put those types of ingredients— beef, pork, cream, butter—in my mouth to ease negative feelings or pain. I ate more than my fair share to give myself a hug from the inside. But no matter how much I ate and how comforted I thought I was, it never eased my bigger issues. I had a lot of mental reckoning to survive before I could understand why I stuffed my face, especially come fall when I finally felt suited up and safe again. I've worked through many of these issues, but I still crave comfort foods.

Today, however, I eat different kinds of fall ingredients because I don't believe you need piles of animal products to make dishes that fulfill on the tenets of comfort food: to provide consolation, a feeling of well-being, and even memories associated with childhood. I focus on making and eating dishes with deeper flavors versus classic cheesiness. I still use animal products, especially seafood, in some of my cold-weather cooking—mainly because I've learned to portion control for myself and I get a lot of satisfaction from feeding other people who crave them—but wholesome vegetables, beans, nuts, seeds, and super-filling fats have become the star of the show. Most of my comfort dishes are now filled with long-simmered beans, sliced orange squash, roasted pumpkin, vinegar-splashed savory greens, and sweet potatoes. I also incorporate considerable but healthy-ish portions of whole grains, semolina and alternative-flour pastas, corn polenta, and dumplings.

Plant-based ingredients provide a different kind of comfort now: They fill me up and I feel good knowing that the vegetables fuel me rather than potentially hurt me. Giving yourself all the vegetables is like giving yourself a big dose of vitamins and nutrients that will provide its own sort of unending comfort as the season progresses. These recipes make me super happy and I hope they fill you up, too.

EIGHT WAYS TO MAKE A TRANSFORMATION A FOREVER THING

I feel pretty strongly that this new way of eating is for life. I'll experience hits and misses, but I now know that the very best thing I can do for me is stay healthy for life. And if I can make this happen for me—after my teary trauma of childhood and my careful evaluation of it all—you can most definitely make a more improved version of you. After decades of way too much doubt, I finally believe in me and I unequivocally believe in you, too. Besides learning to love yourself, which is key, grab a hold of some of the following things that have been important to me as I turn my transformation into a forever thing:

1. *Appreciate yourself now.* Don't wait to look a certain way or feel strong and powerful. Your body and brain do so much for you today, right this second. They deserve to be cherished, celebrated, and loved as soon as possible before any potential transformation.

2. *Do what you love.* Don't give up on the things you love. If you have a sweet tooth, don't skip sweets, just find more wholesome versions. If you drink wine judiciously, set up days when you get to have a glass or two.

3. *Be honest with yourself.* Don't ignore your successes or your setbacks. If you eat a bag of potato chips in between meetings, take note of it and accept it. Be truthful with yourself as it's the only way to reverse glitches and stick to a transformation long-term.

4. *Forgive any setbacks.* There will be complications and mishaps. There will be moments you may be tempted to let one of those setbacks impede all your progress. Please forgive yourself and move on swiftly. You're human and deserve heaps of compassion.

5. *Do not apologize for your process.* However you choose to transform, the process and all its steps are yours to own. Never apologize to anyone for what you need to do for you. For example, if you're avoiding dairy, do not let anyone (like a restaurant chef or a mother) put their disappointment or their preferences on you. Their issues or objections say a lot about them and nothing about you.

6. *Preserve important rituals.* It's true that life is short. If there are a handful of rituals that mean the moon to you, cultivate them in the healthiest way possible. If you gather with girlfriends to celebrate something regularly, figure out how to enjoy it in a way that makes it easy to forgive yourself the next day.

7. *Share your transformation.* At the right time, share your metamorphosis with your community. Once you share, it will feel very real and the support from people who love you will keep you motivated and enthusiastic.

8. *Keep transforming.* Don't stop growing, ever. Certainly, take a pause and relish recent accomplishments. When you're ready, get back into transformation mode and do something new like try a new food, learn meditation, or add movement to your life. The act of ongoing transformation provides incentive and inspiration to keep being the best version of you.

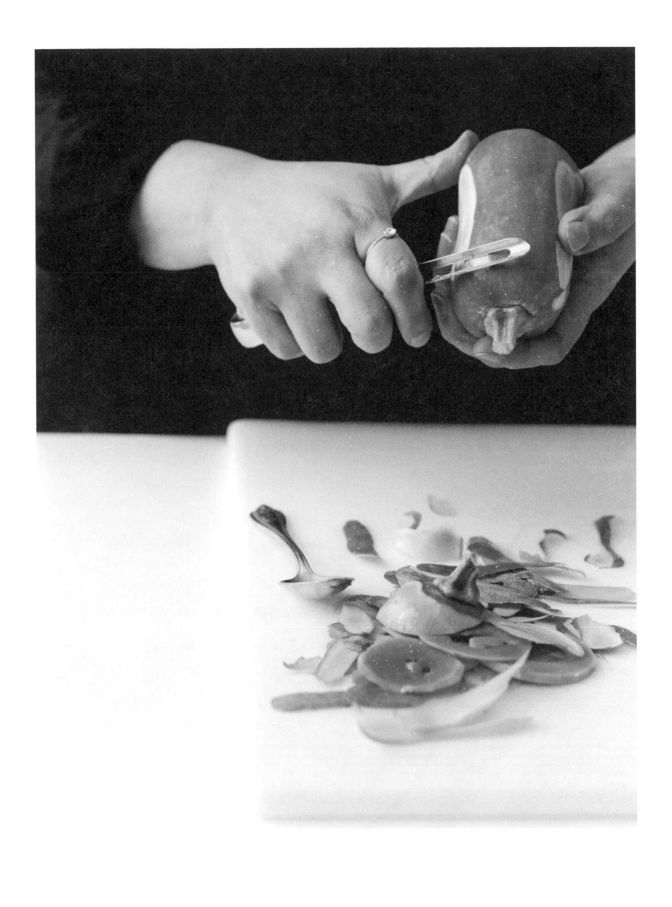

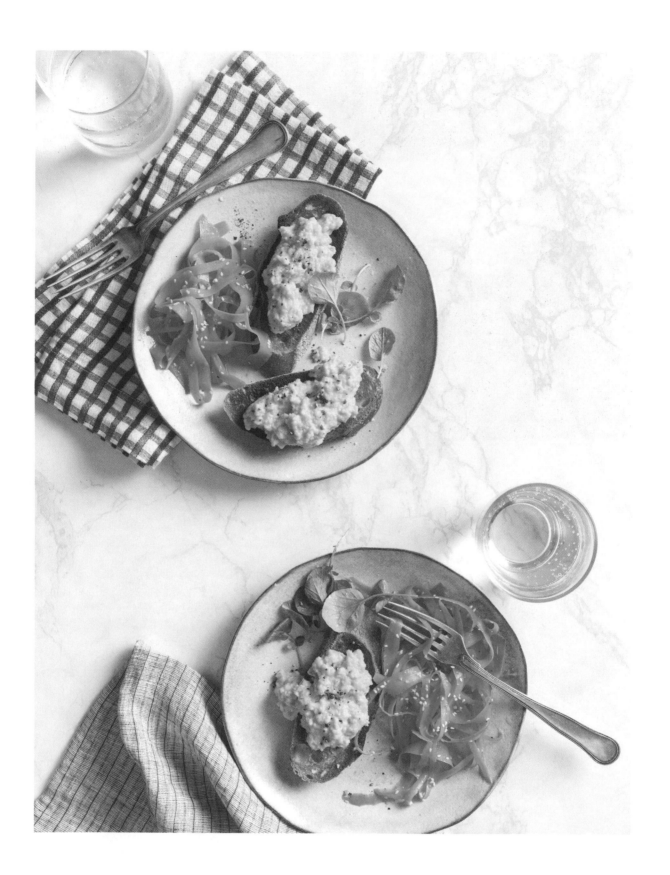

SCRAMBLED EGGS, CARROT SESAME SALAD, TOAST

There is nothing quite like a farm-fresh egg. The whites are heavy and solid, and the yolk is as bright as the center of an in-season orange. Since eggs are a significant enough part of my new way of eating, I source farm eggs from well-raised hens, the sort of chickens who roam freely, eat whole grain food, and spend no time in cages. These eggs, with their richer taste and improved nutrients, are worth the extra few dollars.

When I have more than a few moments for breakfast, I like to soft scramble my eggs. They get creamy and glossy and become a rich foil to a zippy carrot salad. I often make this dish in the fall, when carrots become an irresistible bulk buy at the farmers market and, as well, an omen to prepare for the long winter ahead by stocking up on root vegetables.

The carrot salad keeps in the fridge for a day so you're welcome to make two meals of it. Use two eggs and one table-spoon of almond milk for a single serving each day and, if you have it, a smaller pan in which to whisk the eggs.

Serves 2

FREQUENCY: *Once per week*

FOOD PREFERENCES: *DF, NF, GF, RSF, Veg*

HANDS-ON TIME: *15 minutes*

TOTAL TIME: *15 minutes*

. . . .

1 tablespoon coconut vinegar or white wine vinegar

1 tablespoon lime juice

2½ tablespoons extra-virgin olive oil, divided

½ teaspoon sea salt, divided, plus more for seasoning

6 twists freshly ground black pepper

3 or 4 small carrots, peeled and slivered lengthwise with a veg peeler or mandoline

1 teaspoon white sesame seeds

4 eggs

2 tablespoons unsweetened, plain plant milk

2 slices thick sourdough bread (or gluten-free type), toasted

1. Add the vinegar, lime juice, 1½ tablespoons of the oil, ¼ teaspoon of the salt, and the pepper to a jar. Shake until well combined.

2. Place the carrot slices in a medium bowl and pour over 2 tablespoons of the dressing. Toss them about a few times to ensure they're well coated. Sprinkle with the sesame seeds. Taste and add more dressing, if you'd like, or reserve the extra for tomorrow's salad.

3. Whisk together the eggs, milk, and remaining ¼ teaspoon salt in a small bowl.

4. Heat the remaining 1 tablespoon oil in a frying pan set over medium heat. Add the egg mixture and whisk continuously in the pan until fine curds are formed and the eggs become more solid and less wet, 3 to 4 minutes. Raise the heat slightly if it takes too long. Remove the pan from the heat when the eggs are cooked to your liking—I prefer mine to look a little wet and glossy.

5. Serve the eggs divided between the two toasted bread slices with a handful of the carrot salad on the side. Enjoy immediately.

Sweet Potato Cranberry SCONES

I am a scone fanatic: 30 minutes from bowl to my hot little hands can't be wrong. I've made the recipe a bit more wholesome and dairy-free, by swapping in maple sugar and coconut oil, respectively. They are, however, still filled with all-purpose flour, so as with any baked good, I like to enjoy one or two, and then share the rest with others, especially during the holiday season.

The long-lasting fuel in these scones comes from the sweet potato. Sweet potato is my kind of superfood. Filled with vitamins, beta-carotene, potassium, biotin, fiber, and niacin, sweet potatoes help to steady the pace of digestion and keep me full a bit longer. I also just like the taste so that makes me feel good, too.

Makes 8 large scones

FREQUENCY: *A couple times per month*

FOOD PREFERENCES: *DF, NF, RSF, Veg*

HANDS-ON TIME: *15 minutes*

TOTAL TIME: *35 minutes*

6 tablespoons coconut oil (in solid form),
    plus more for greasing the pan

3 cups (12¾ oz; 360 g) all-purpose flour

2 teaspoons baking powder

½ teaspoon sea salt

5 tablespoons maple sugar

2 eggs, separated

¾ cup dried cranberries

½ cup (120 ml) plus 2 tablespoons
    unsweetened, plain plant milk

1 large sweet potato, roasted and
    mashed, or one-half 15-ounce
    (425 g) can

½ teaspoon orange extract,
    or 1 tablespoon orange juice
    (from about ¼ orange)

1. Preheat the oven to 375°F (191°C). Line a baking sheet with parchment paper and grease it with a little coconut oil.

2. Combine the flour, baking powder, salt, and sugar in a large bowl.

3. Cut the coconut oil into small pieces and blend quickly and lightly into the flour mix, using your fingertips. Don't let it melt on your fingers.

4. Stir in the egg yolks lightly. The yolks will leave tiny yellow clumps throughout the bowl.

5. Stir in the cranberries.

6. Whisk the milk, sweet potato, and extract in a separate bowl until well combined. Lightly stir the wet ingredients into the dry ingredients, mixing just until the dough holds together without crumbling. Add additional milk, if needed.

7. Pour the dough onto the center of the parchment and—using the parchment paper or oiled hands—form it into a round, about 9 inches (23 cm) across and 1 inch (2.5 cm) deep. Slice the round into eight large uniform pie-shaped pieces, pulling them apart slightly as you cut. Brush the tops with the egg whites.

8. Bake the scones for 20 to 24 minutes, until lightly browned. Let cool before serving. Store in an airtight container at room temperature for up to 3 days.

MEGA KALE TARTINE *with Smoky Mayonnaise*

This dish is a gateway to kale. If you picked up this cookbook, you may not need a gateway dish to make you love the hearty green but maybe your partner or family does. The way I see it, everyone loves toasted bread and most everyone likes creamy mayonnaise. Top those two delights with salted, tangy kale and you've got a hefty, fiber-filled sandwich that will strengthen you for hours.

Makes 1 open-faced sandwich

FREQUENCY: *Once per week*

FOOD PREFERENCES: *DF, GF, NF, RSF, V, Veg*

HANDS-ON TIME: *15 minutes*

TOTAL TIME: *15 minutes*

⸱⸱⸱⸱⸱⸱⸱⸱⸱⸱⸱⸱⸱⸱⸱⸱⸱⸱⸱⸱⸱⸱

1 large bunch Lacinato kale
   (about 10 stalks), washed and dried

2 tablespoons extra-virgin olive oil

½ medium red onion, peeled
   and chopped

¼ teaspoon sea salt, plus more
   for seasoning

1 teaspoon red wine vinegar

2 slices sourdough bread
   (or gluten-free type), toasted

4 teaspoons Smoky Mayonnaise
   (page 55)

1. Slice the stems from each kale leaf, gathering the long leaves into a tall stack, one on top of the other. Slice across the width of the kale stack into 1-inch strips. Slice the stacks of strips into a ½-inch dice. You'll have a big pile of small rectangles of kale.

2. Warm the oil in a frying pan set over medium heat. Add the onion and sauté until wilted, 1 to 2 minutes. Add the kale and salt, and fry until the kale is soft and wilted, 2 to 3 minutes. Make sure to toss the kale frequently while cooking, ensuring that all pieces get cooked. Stir in the vinegar and turn the heat off.

3. Spread 2 teaspoons of Smoky Mayonnaise on each slice of bread. Pile half the kale on one slice and the rest on the other slice. Taste and add more salt, if you like. Serve immediately while it's still warm.

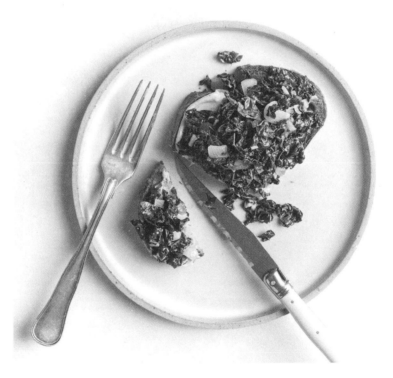

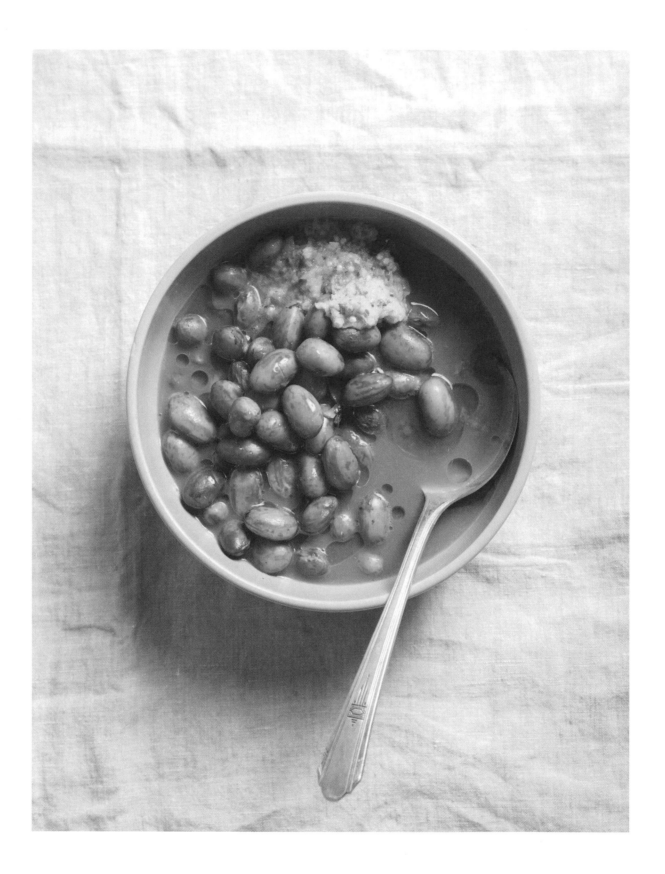

BEANS IN OLIVE OIL BROTH
with Tomatillo Salsa Verde

This is humble food, the sort my mother would make every day, almost like breathing, and eat while still piping hot over the kitchen sink, giving her a moment or two to ignore the rambunctious kiddos tumbling around her. It seemed to give her some sort of serenity, as it transported her back to her mountain village in Honduras.

Most mornings, she recalled, her grandmother and various cooks would place big pots of food—pinto beans, orange rice, pork or beef—over the fires, to get them ready for the farmers. As the cook's treat, they'd spoon the just-made beans into bowls and sip them like tea before the buzzing farmers descended on the kitchen. Any of the kids hanging nearby would get a small bowl too, and my mother was always there—she instinctively knew that a fresh bowl of beans, made from dried beans grown just feet away, salted and squeezed with juice from the lemons hanging outside the window, was sometimes more rewarding than any sweet treat.

I know, however, that this dish is not for everyone. In fact, some of you will whisper, "It's just a bowl of beans in their cooking liquid with salsa." You're so right. And, it's so much more. Come autumn, when dried beans go back into heavy rotation in my kitchen, I now drink this like tea, only it's far more nourishing. Like my mother back in 1940s Honduras, I use the best beans I can find (locally grown is wonderful) and an exceptional olive oil (something green and grassy). A scoop of any just-made salsa will do fine but I prefer my homemade Tomatillo Salsa Verde. If you'd like to replace the lemon juice in the salsa with lime juice, by all means, but the lemon makes it bright and subtle.

Makes 8 cups beans with broth

FREQUENCY: *Almost every day*

FOOD PREFERENCES: *DF, GF, NF, RSF, V*

HANDS-ON TIME: *25 minutes*

TOTAL TIME: *9 hours 10 minutes*

1 pound (454 g) dried navy, kidney, or calypso beans

1 bay leaf

5 medium garlic cloves, peeled

6 cups (1.4 L) vegetable stock or water, or combination of both

2 teaspoons sea salt, plus more for seasoning

Extra-virgin olive oil

Tomatillo Salsa Verde (page 56), to serve

1. Soak the beans in 10 cups of cold water in a very large bowl for at least 8 hours or overnight. Drain and rinse beans.

2. Add the beans, bay leaf, garlic, vegetable stock, and salt to a large pot with a lid. Bring to a boil and then lower the heat to let the beans simmer until tender, which should take 45 to 60 minutes. Put the lid on partially, so some steam stays in the pot and some is released. Stir once in a while, adding vegetable stock or water to keep the beans covered, as needed. Taste occasionally to determine when they're tender.

3. When they're as tender as you want them, turn off the heat, and remove the bay leaf and garlic cloves. Serve the beans by scooping 1 cup of warm beans plus the broth (at least ¼ cup liquid) into a soup bowl. Drizzle with oil—1 to 3 teaspoons—and more salt, to taste. Serve immediately with 1 or 2 spoonfuls of the salsa. Alternatively, you may cool the beans before storing in an airtight container in the fridge for up to 1 week, and reheat to serve when you'd like a warm bowl. You can also freeze the beans in 1-quart containers for up to 6 months.

INSTANT FAUX PHO *Jars*

This is lunch on-the-go in its saintly essence. Please don't allow the long list of ingredients to cause you stress, as the dish is really pure assembly and can work with whatever is surviving in the fridge, even a droopy chard leaf or a peeled limp beet. Just trim away the unrighteous parts and jam it into the jar.

The dried mushroom powder, however, is essential—it adds immense umami flavor—so grab some dried mushrooms stat and grind them up for your spice shelf. Except for that single ingredient, if you purchase everything else pre-cut or pre-cleaned, this jarred soup is a cinch. Of course, you may boil all the broth ingredients on a stove and pour it over everything else to make a straightforward sort of dinner but the eating-from-a-jar part is quite fun and, for me, a pleasurable part of the day.

Makes one 16-ounce (473 ml) jar

FREQUENCY: *Almost everyday*

FOOD PREFERENCES: *DF, GF, NF, RSF, V*

HANDS-ON TIME: *15 minutes*

TOTAL TIME: *22 minutes*

• •

1 tablespoon Mushroom Powder (page 54)

½ teaspoon minced fresh ginger

½ teaspoon minced fresh garlic

1 tablespoon soy sauce

1 teaspoon rice vinegar

1 teaspoon toasted sesame oil

¼ teaspoon chili paste

2 tablespoons lime juice (from about 1 lime)

Sea salt

ingredients continued

1. Gather a wide-mouth, 16-ounce jar that can fit the noodles and has a tight-fitting lid. Add the mushroom powder, ginger, garlic, soy sauce, vinegar, sesame oil, chili paste, lime juice, and salt and pepper to taste.

2. Add in the noodles. Then add the onion, cucumber, kale, mushrooms, cilantro, and scallion, tucking them in around the noodles.

3. When ready to eat, pour boiling water into the jar and seal. Let sit for 5 to 7 minutes, shaking a few times to disperse all the flavors. The pho is ready when the noodles are soft and the broth is flavorful.

4. If desired, garnish with sesame seeds, herbs, crispy shallots, or all three. Squeeze in extra lime juice to brighten it or drizzle in shallot oil to make it extra savory.

Freshly ground black pepper

1 block dried instant vermicelli-style noodles

½ medium white onion, peeled and thinly sliced

½ medium cucumber, thinly sliced

2 to 3 kale or chard leaves, stems removed, thinly sliced

3 large button mushrooms, thinly sliced

1 to 2 cilantro sprigs, stems cut and discarded

1 scallion, trimmed and thinly sliced

Sesame seeds, fresh herbs, or Crispy Shallots (page 49), for garnish (optional)

Extra lime wedges or Shallot Oil (page 49), for serving (optional)

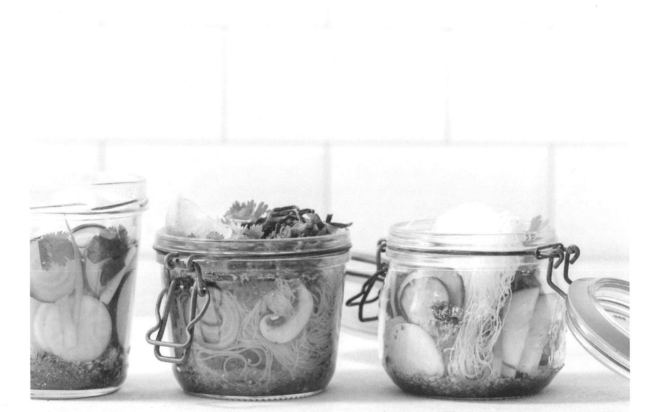

POTATO ZUCCHINI DUMPLINGS
with Green Sauce

Many satisfying restaurant-style dumplings are filled with a lot of sodium and a lot of pork, and I completely get that. Salt and fat are perhaps the champions of a gratifying meal; they offer true flavor and hearty mouthfeel. I can't live without my dumpling fix from time to time. To enjoy them most frequently, I make them from scratch.

I make dough by hand; it's an activity that, with the kneading, warms me up in cooler months. But if that seemingly large task threatens to halt your dumpling production, just purchase dumpling wrappers at your local grocery store. If you don't find a package explicitly labeled for dumplings, grab wonton, gyoza, or potsticker wrappers—any of them will work fine and make, more or less, the same style of dumpling, just likely a little larger than what I prescribe in this recipe.

Moving beyond the typical cabbage filling—you can find them at any Chinese restaurant—my first filling combination is potato mixed with green zucchini. If you'd rather not peel the potatoes, just proceed with them unpeeled. The green sauce is similar to a loose and briny pesto which you can most certainly use over and over again—on top of scrambled eggs, in tortilla-wrapped bundles, alongside fish, or over roasted sweet potatoes. A second dumpling recipe can be found on page 254.

Makes 36 to 40 dumplings

FREQUENCY: *Once per week*

FOOD PREFERENCES: *DF, NF, RSF, V*

HANDS-ON TIME: *1 hour 45 minutes*

TOTAL TIME: *2 hours*

· ·

FOR THE DUMPLING DOUGH

2½ cups (10⅔ oz; 300 g) all-purpose flour

¼ teaspoon sea salt

1 cup plus 2 tablespoons (280 ml) boiling water that's rested 10 minutes

MAKE THE DUMPLING DOUGH

1. Whisk together the flour and salt in a large bowl. Add the water and mix with a wooden spoon until a shaggy dough comes together. The dough will be warm and may seem dry, but trust me.

2. Dump the mixture onto a floured surface and knead until soft and smooth, up to 10 minutes, adding extra flour here or there to make a less sticky dough. Once it's smooth, cover with a damp towel and leave to rest on the counter for at least 10 minutes before you make your dumplings.

MAKE THE POTATO ZUCCHINI DUMPLINGS AND GREEN SAUCE

1. Add the potatoes with enough water to cover to a medium pot. Bring to a boil and simmer until cooked through or easily pierced with a fork, about 10 minutes. Drain the potatoes and return to the pot, off the heat, to dry out slightly. Mash well with a fork and let cool.

2. Toss the zucchini with ½ teaspoon of the salt. In a strainer, pile the shredded zucchini and let drain about 15 minutes. Squeeze any excess liquid from the zucchini before using.

continued

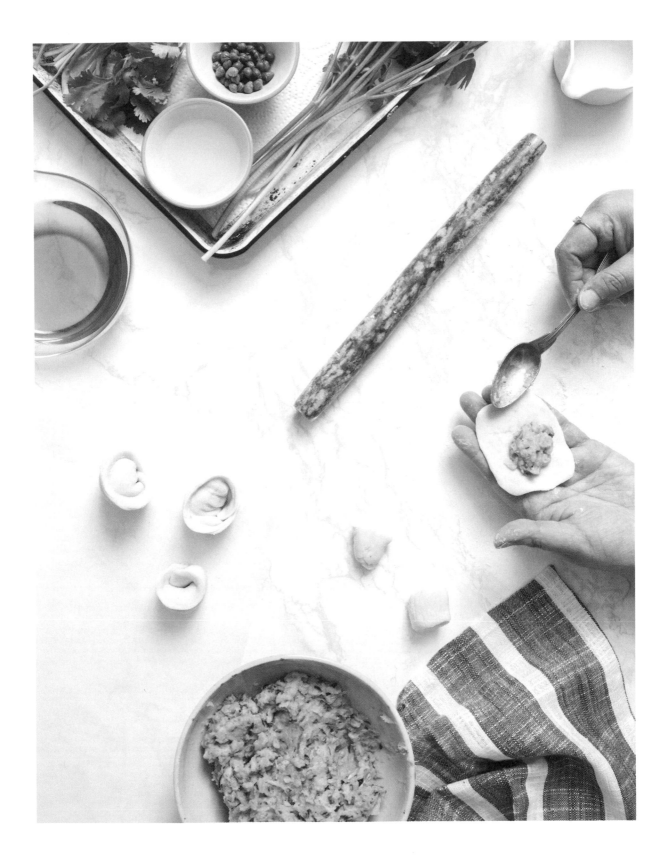

FOR THE POTATO ZUCCHINI DUMPLINGS

2 medium russet potatoes, scrubbed, peeled, and diced into 1-inch cubes

1 medium zucchini, shredded with box grater

¾ teaspoon sea salt

2 tablespoons all-purpose flour or buckwheat flour

2 tablespoons soy sauce

1 small bunch chives (about 20 stems), finely diced

Homemade Dumpling Dough (page 250) or store-bought dumpling wrappers

Safflower or grape seed oil

½ cup (120 ml) vegetable broth or water

Green Sauce, for serving (recipe follows)

FOR THE GREEN SAUCE

1 small bunch parsley (about 10 sprigs), finely diced

1 small bunch cilantro (about 10 sprigs), finely diced

1 small bunch chives (about 20 stems), finely diced

2 tablespoons lemon juice (from about 1 medium lemon)

1 tablespoon capers, drained

½ cup (120 ml) extra-virgin olive oil

3. Put the potatoes, zucchini, flour, soy sauce, and the remaining ¼ teaspoon salt in a medium bowl. Stir until the zucchini strands and soy sauce are evenly distributed and there are no flour streaks. Toss in the chives and do a final stir.

4. When you are ready to make dumplings, set aside a few tablespoons of cold water in a small bowl and place a piece of parchment paper on a baking sheet.

5. If using homemade dumpling dough, cut the dough into quarters and work with one quarter at a time; cover the remaining dough with a damp towel so it doesn't dry out. On a flourless surface, roll the quarter out into a long snake shape about 1-inch (2.5 cm) in diameter. Cut the dough into 1-inch pieces. Form one piece into a small round, generously dust it with flour, and flatten into little disks with the palm of your hand. Using a rolling pin, roll the round into a thin, ⅛-inch or so (0.3 cm), flat disk, flipping it as you go to ensure an even roll and that the dough doesn't stick to your work surface. Brush the excess flour from the dough by tossing it back and forth in your hands or wiping/patting it off.

6. Fill the center of each round of homemade dumpling dough (or store-bought dumpling wrapper) with 1 teaspoon of the filling mixture. Apply a light coat of water around the mixture with your finger. Fold the wrapper in half and seal the ends together with firm pressure. Take one half-moon end of the dumpling and fold it up and over the other end to form a rosebud shape. Add a drop of water to the dumpling dough ends to ensure both ends stick when you press them together.

7. Repeat until all the filling and dough or wrappers are filled. Place dumplings back on the parchment-lined sheet and cover with a damp cloth or freeze until ready to use.

8. To make the green sauce, add the parsley, cilantro, chives, lemon juice, capers, and oil to a blender. Whiz until well blended. Add a little cold water to loosen up the sauce, if needed.

9. To steam the dumplings: Set a steamer, the bottom filled with water, over medium-high heat. Line the top of the steamer with parchment paper. Once the water has come to a boil, place the dumplings in the top of the steamer, taking care to not let them touch. Cover and steam for 10 to 12 minutes, until cooked through.

10. To pan-fry the dumplings: Add a little oil to a frying pan with a tight-fitting lid over medium-high heat. Once warmed, swirl the oil around the pan and then place the dumplings upright in the pan, leaving just a little room between each. Fry the dumplings until they have a golden-brown color on the bottom. Add the broth to the pan carefully, as it will bubble up and create steam. Cover the dumplings and let cook about 5 minutes to cook the dough and filling. Remove the cover and let the remaining liquid in the pan evaporate. Transfer the dumplings to a serving platter, placing them upside down so the browned part is facing up and stays crispy.

11. Serve cooked dumplings with the green sauce.

PUMPKIN SCALLION DUMPLINGS
with Soy Chili Sauce

For my second dumpling offering, I use one of my favorite vegetables: pumpkin. I prefer to roast a pumpkin to make these dumplings. Canned pumpkin ends up tasting a little too bland and almost metallic. To roast your autumn gourd, just halve, seed, and roast it for 45 minutes in a 375°F (191°C) oven until it's tender when pierced with a fork. Let cool and spoon the flesh from the skin. For this recipe, whiz a one-pound portion of pumpkin flesh in a food processor or mash it by hand, and reserve the remaining pumpkin for another use.

Keep in mind that fresh pumpkin has more moisture than canned pumpkin so I let the filling mixture rest for 20 minutes and drain off any liquid that collects before making the dumplings. The accompanying soy chili sauce is salty and spicy—an appealing foil to the warm squash filling.

Makes 36 to 40 dumplings

FREQUENCY: *Once per week*

FOOD PREFERENCES: *DF, NF, RSF, V*

HANDS-ON TIME: *1 hour 45 minutes*

TOTAL TIME: *2 hours 15 minutes*

FOR THE PUMPKIN SCALLION
DUMPLINGS

4 cups roasted and mashed pumpkin
flesh (1 lb/454 g)

2 tablespoons all-purpose flour or
buckwheat flour

2 tablespoons soy sauce

½ teaspoon sea salt

8 to 10 scallions, trimmed and
finely diced

Homemade Dumpling Dough
(page 250) or store-bought
dumpling wrappers

Safflower or grape seed oil

½ cup (120 ml) vegetable broth or water

Soy Chili Sauce, for serving
(recipe follows)

1. Combine the pumpkin, flour, soy sauce, salt, and scallions in a medium bowl, stirring until the scallions are evenly distributed and there are no flour streaks.

2. When you are ready to make dumplings, set aside a few tablespoons of cold water in a small bowl and place a piece of parchment paper on a baking sheet.

3. If using homemade dumpling dough, cut the dough into quarters and work with one quarter at a time; cover the remaining dough with a damp towel so it doesn't dry out. On a flourless surface, roll the quarter out into a long snake shape about 1-inch (2.5 cm) in diameter. Cut the dough into 1-inch pieces. Form one piece into a small round, generously dust it with flour and flatten into little disks with the palm of your hand. Using a rolling pin, roll the round into a thin, ⅛-inch (0.3 cm) or so, flat disk, flipping it as you go to ensure an even roll and that the dough doesn't stick to your work surface. Brush the excess flour from the dough by tossing it back and forth in your hands or wiping/patting it off.

4. Fill the center of each round of homemade dumpling dough (or store-bought dumpling wrapper) with 1 teaspoon of filling mixture. Apply a light coat of water around half the wrapper with your finger. Fold wrapper in half and seal ends together with firm pressure. Take one half-moon end of the dumpling and fold it up and over the other end to form a rosebud shape. Add a drop of water to the dumpling dough ends to ensure both ends stick when you press them together.

continued

FOR THE SOY CHILI SAUCE

¼ cup (60 ml) soy sauce

2 tablespoons toasted sesame oil

½ teaspoon chili paste

1 teaspoon rice wine vinegar

1 teaspoon lime juice (from about
  ¼ medium lime)

1 to 2 scallions, trimmed and
  finely diced

5. Repeat until all the filling and dough or wrappers are filled. Place dumplings back on the parchment-lined sheet and cover with a damp cloth or freeze until ready to use.

6. To make the soy chili sauce, stir together the soy sauce, sesame oil, chili paste, vinegar, lime juice, and scallions in a small bowl. Taste and adjust the spice level by adding more chili paste, if desired.

7. To steam the dumplings: Set a steamer, the bottom filled with water, over medium-high heat. Line the top of the steamer with parchment paper. Once the water has come to a boil, place the dumplings in the top of the steamer, taking care to not let them touch. Cover and steam for 10 to 12 minutes, until cooked through.

8. To fry the dumplings, add enough oil to coat the bottom of a frying pan with a tight-fitting lid and place it over medium-high heat. Once warmed, swirl the oil around the pan and then place the dumplings upright in the pan, leaving just a little room between each. Fry the dumplings until they have a golden brown color on the bottom. Add the broth to the pan carefully, as it will bubble up and create steam. Cover the dumplings and let cook about 5 minutes to cook the dough and filling. Remove the cover and let the remaining liquid in the pan evaporate. Transfer dumplings to a serving platter, placing them upside down so the browned part is facing up and stays crispy.

9. Serve cooked dumplings with the soy chili sauce.

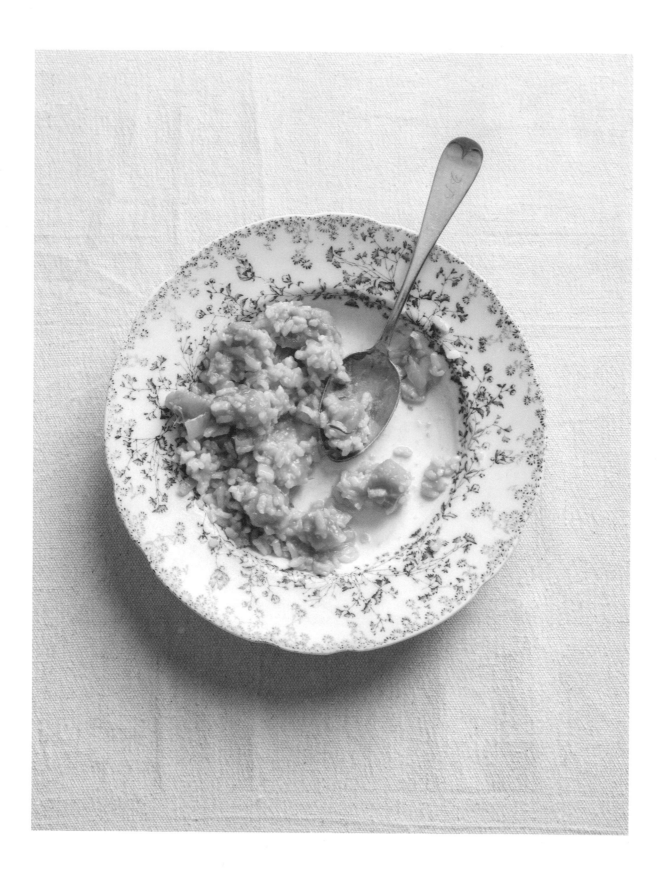

Roasted Pumpkin Saffron RISOTTO

Indisputably, this bowl of risotto is a hug in food form. The pumpkin, whether roasted or steamed, practically melts into the rice, creating a savory style of porridge that, quite frankly, I'll eat at any time of day, even breakfast. However, when I make such a large pot, I always prefer to spoon it up with friends.

Vegetable stock does the trick here but seafood stock ups the ante, making it taste like a light paella. I tend to have lobster stock around, not because we're rocking lobsters daily, but because one summer dinner of a few steamed lobsters will make eight to twelve quarts of stock for the freezer. It's a shame to let an animal carcass go to waste, especially nowadays when an electric pressure cooker makes easy work of all stocks.

Please don't use a canned pumpkin puree in this recipe. The savory porridge will turn more gloppy and taste a bit off. Real pumpkin will stay firm enough to chew with only its edges melting into the rice. Also, remember to taste the final dish and add extra salt to make the flavors come to life. This is a sizable dinner for four individuals but will go further if served with a salad or other sides.

Serves 4

FREQUENCY: *Once per week*

FOOD PREFERENCES: *DF, GF, NF, RSF, V*

HANDS-ON TIME: *15 minutes*

TOTAL TIME: *1 hour 30 minutes*

One 2-pound (904 g) sugar pumpkin

4 tablespoons extra-virgin olive oil, divided

1 tablespoon sea salt, plus more for seasoning

1 small white onion, peeled and chopped

2 large garlic cloves, peeled and finely diced

1 cup arborio rice

⅛ heaping teaspoon saffron

½ cup (120 ml) dry white wine

4½ cups (1 L) vegetable or seafood stock

Cilantro leaves, for garnish (optional)

1. Preheat the oven to 350°F (177°C). Line a rimmed baking sheet with parchment paper.

2. Slice the pumpkin into four or five big wedges and place them on the parchment. Divide 2 tablespoons of the oil and salt between the pumpkin wedges, drizzling it over each. Place the sheet in the oven. Roast for 45 to 50 minutes, until the pumpkin is tender when pierced with a fork. Remove from oven and let cool slightly.

3. When the pumpkin wedges are cool enough to handle, scoop out the seeds and reserve for another use (like snacking). Slice the pumpkin meat off each piece of skin, discard the skin, and slice the meat into ½-inch chunks. Set aside for the moment.

4. Warm the remaining 2 tablespoons oil in a large wide pan over medium heat. Add the onion and garlic, and sauté until wilted a bit and translucent. Add the rice and stir until well coated. Toast the rice until it appears to give a little and takes on a touch of golden color, 3 to 4 minutes . Stir in the saffron, wine, and 4 cups of the stock. Lower the heat to medium-low. Let the dish cook down on its own—the rice will plump up and soften, the stock will disappear into the rice, and the saffron will lend a faint red hue to the entire dish. After 25 minutes, stir and take a taste. It should be close to ready.

5. When it is close, place the pumpkin pieces into the rice so they have at least 5 minutes to warm up. At the 30-minute mark, taste and add the remaining ½ cup stock, if needed, to finish the cooking. It shouldn't need more than 35 minutes, tops. Taste and season with more salt, and if desired, garnish with cilantro before serving.

SWEET POTATO GNOCCHI
with Ghee and Pecans

In this dish, sweet potatoes are mashed and folded into a dough; the little nuggets are boiled and then pan-fried; and, ultimately, they're topped with lots of crispy, crunchy fixings. It's a recipe that's not without a little effort but it's also total comfort food that helps fall truly sink into place. When you take your first bite, you know summer is a world away and you don't care one bit because there's such a thing as homemade gnocchi.

The dough—and I use that term loosely—is made up mostly of bright orange potatoes and almond flour. The nuttiness from the flour is subtle but finds itself when topped with buttery ghee, which is indeed butter that's been simmered until all the milk solids are removed and lightly-viscous golden brown oil comes to life. Make your own ghee or pick up a jar at the grocery store. Hazelnuts are a wonderful stand-in for the pecans, too.

Serves 6

FREQUENCY: *Once per week*

FOOD PREFERENCES: *RSF*

HANDS-ON TIME: *30 minutes*

TOTAL TIME: *1 hour 45 minutes*

. . . .

6 medium orange sweet potatoes, cleaned

1 teaspoon sea salt, plus more for seasoning

1½ cups (2⅞ oz; 144 g) finely ground almond flour

½ cup (2⅛ oz; 60 g) all-purpose flour, a bit more or a bit less

2 tablespoons arrowroot powder or cornstarch

5 tablespoons Ghee, homemade (page 44) or store-bought

10 fresh sage leaves

1 tablespoon pecans, finely diced, per serving

Parsley, finely diced, for garnish (optional)

1. Preheat the oven to 350°F (177°C). Line a rimmed baking sheet with parchment paper. Place the whole sweet potatoes on the parchment and the sheet in the oven. Roast for 45 to 55 minutes, until the potatoes are tender when pierced with a fork. Remove from the oven and let cool. When the potatoes are cool enough to handle, peel them and discard the skin. Mash the potatoes well with a fork or masher until fluffy and smooth.

2. Sprinkle the salt on the potatoes and mash until combined. Add the almond flour, all-purpose flour, and arrowroot powder. Blend everything into the dough with a spatula (because it's very sticky) until all the white streaks disappear. Finally, flour your hands well and fold the dough over a few times (don't knead it) just to fully incorporate everything. Cover with a kitchen towel and rest for 5 to 10 minutes. Line another rimmed baking sheet with parchment paper.

3. With a well-floured knife or pastry cutter, cut a quarter of the dough off to work into gnocchi. Flour your surface and hands well, and roll the dough into a long snake ¾-inch (1.9 cm) in diameter. Cut 1-inch-wide (2.5 cm) pieces from the dough and flour each piece. Press each piece down the back of a fork to create a few ridges, if you like, or just place them directly onto the parchment-lined baking sheet. Place the sheet in the fridge for 10 minutes to let them get a little solid.

continued

4. Bring a large pot of water to boil and salt it well. Lightly oil a baking dish. The gnocchi cooks in just a few minutes. From the moment you pop them into the boiling water, you'll notice them buzz around and then float to the top. Stir once to make sure they don't stay on the bottom of the pot. Once they surface to the top of the water, they're done. Strain them out and place them in the baking dish while you cook the rest. I cook 8 to 10 gnocchi per person for an entree.

5. Melt the ghee in a wide pan set over medium heat. Add the sage leaves, and fry for 1 or 2 minutes. Push the sage leaves to the side of the pan. Add the cooked gnocchi and pan-fry for 1 to 2 minutes to impart the flavor from the ghee and get a golden color. Serve in a bowl with a sprinkle of pecans, parsley, if desired, and more salt to taste.

6. Freeze any uncooked gnocchi on the baking sheet and then store in an airtight bag or sealed container in the freezer for up to 3 months. Boil them by popping directly into boiling water from their frozen state.

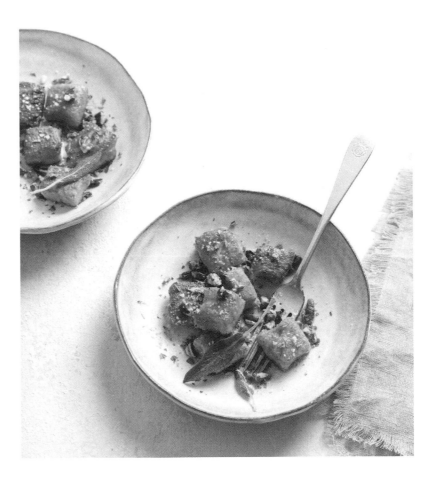

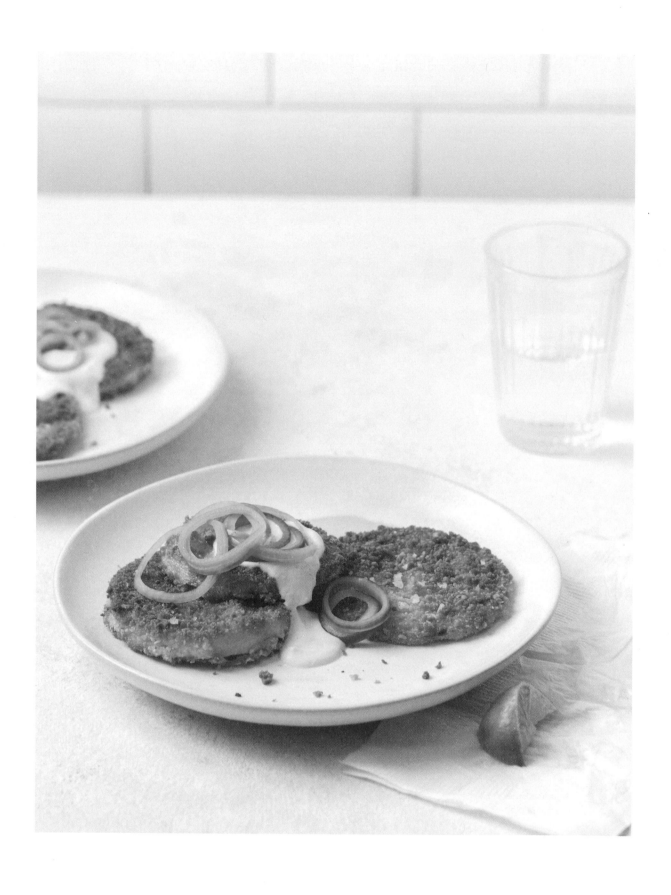

SQUASH SCHNITZEL *with Lime-Pickled Onions*

This surprising dish is inspired by all the sensational schnitzel I ate when I worked on and off in Berlin, Germany, several years ago. Schnitzel, which means cutlets, originated in Austria but it seems as if most countries have a version of thinly pounded and fried something or other. Through all my travels, I never saw a vegetable version so I took the matter into my own kitchen.

If you have a very large squash that produces lots of slices, just beat in another egg to the egg bowl, top off the flour and panko, and keep frying. This dish is most successful when using flat slices of squash. For that reason, I exclude the bulbous side of the squash because it's a little less predictable in its cooking time and you get enough slices from the other side of the squash anyway. However, if you'd like to use the entire squash, peel, halve, and clean the bulbous side. Slice, dip, and fry it as you would the round slices, understanding that it may take a minute or two less to cook through.

Makes 12 to 18 slices (3 to 4 servings)

FREQUENCY: *Once per week*

FOOD PREFERENCES: *DF, NF, RSF, V*

HANDS-ON TIME: *45 minutes*

TOTAL TIME: *45 minutes*

. . . .

¼ cup (1¹⁄₁₆ oz; 30 g) all-purpose flour

½ teaspoon sea salt, plus more
    for seasoning

12 twists freshly ground black pepper,
    plus more for seasoning

½ teaspoon smoked paprika powder

2 eggs

1 cup panko breadcrumbs
    (or a gluten-free style)

One 2-pound (904 g) butternut squash,
    peeled, cut into ¼-inch-thick
    slices (bulbous side reserved for
    another use)

Safflower oil, for frying

Lime-Pickled Onions (page 54),
    lime wedges, and unsweetened,
    plain plant-based yogurt, for serving

1. Set up three shallow bowls or plates. In one bowl, mix the flour, salt, black pepper, and smoked paprika. In another bowl, beat the eggs. In the third bowl, add the panko. Set aside a plate with a couple layers of paper towels.

2. Pour enough oil to go up about ⅛ inch in a shallow pan over medium heat. Coat a squash slice in the flour mixture. Transfer and dip into the egg mixture until coated. Let any extra egg drip off the slice and transfer into the panko—turn a few times until coated. Transfer the squash slice into the pan and cook until golden brown, 3 to 4 minutes per side. Repeat with remaining squash slices, taking care not to overcrowd the pan (which will bring the heat down and take longer to cook). You may need to add a little extra oil and discard any leftover panko crumbs that may get too dark between frying.

3. Blot cooked squash slices on the paper-towel-lined plate and season with extra salt and black pepper. Serve immediately with the pickled onions, a squeeze of lime juice, and a spoonful of yogurt.

SMOKY PAELLA *with Fennel*

This is my ideal meal for a celebration or just a Saturday night. While someone else may want to cook an entire fish or roast something meaty to recognize a certain moment, I want shellfish in rice. In fact, after decades of a love/hate relationship with rice, I've determined that this is one of the few ways in which rice can do no wrong: coated in a silky, smoky red stock and crammed in around mounds of shellfish and caramelized fennel.

This recipe feeds four without leftovers. And since you'll want leftovers for Paella Cakes (page 265), just make this for two and get those leftovers in your fridge. If you double the recipe to feed even more friends, make sure you have a very large paella pan. The rice swells up fast.

Serves 4

FREQUENCY: *Once per week*

FOOD PREFERENCES: *DF, GF, NF, RSF*

HANDS-ON TIME: *40 minutes*

TOTAL TIME: *40 minutes*

· ·

5 cups (1.2 L) seafood or veg stock

½ teaspoon smoked paprika

¼ teaspoon (pinch) saffron

6 tablespoons extra-virgin olive oil, divided

2 large fennel bulbs, trimmed, cored, and thinly sliced, and fennel fronds, finely diced

¾ teaspoon fine sea salt

3 medium tomatoes, diced and drained, or 1 cup canned whole peeled tomatoes, torn into small pieces, liquid reserved for another use

1 cup arborio rice

1 pound (454 g) mixed seafood (I use mussels, shrimp, ½-inch-thick white fish, and squid bodies)

1 small handful fresh herbs (like cilantro or parsley), finely chopped

Flaky sea salt, for seasoning

1. Pour the stock into a medium pot and bring to a low simmer on a back burner on your range. Add the smoked paprika and saffron to the stock. Once it simmers, turn the heat to low and keep warm.

2. Warm 2 tablespoons of the oil in a large paella pan over medium heat. Add the sliced fennel and ¼ teaspoon of the salt. Sauté until the fennel begins to wilt and take on a little golden color. Add the tomatoes and continue to sauté until any liquid that came out of the tomatoes has evaporated. Add the rice and toss with the veg. Sauté the rice until it's well coated and a little toasty.

3. Pour 4½ cups of warm seafood stock into the pan and make sure all the rice is covered with stock. Stir a few times to bring it together and then don't stir the rice again until the end of cooking. Let the rice slowly absorb the stock over the course of 25 minutes.

4. While the rice cooks, prepare the seafood.

Mussels: The mussels should be cleaned with beards removed. Steam the mussels in ½ inch of water until opened. If you're making a hands-free paella (meaning you won't need to use your hands to remove shells while eating), remove the mussels from the shells, set aside, and discard the shells. Otherwise, keep the mussels in the shells and set aside. Strain the leftover mussel liquid through cheesecloth and add to the stock pot.

Shrimp: The shrimp should be peeled (tails left intact) and deveined. Warm 2 tablespoons of the oil in a large paella pan or frying pan over medium heat. Add the shrimp to the pan, sprinkle with salt, and cook for 1 minute. Turn the shrimp, sprinkle with more salt, and cook just until the shrimp becomes mostly opaque, 30 to 60 seconds. Remove the shrimp to a plate and set aside.

White fish: The white fish should be skinless. Warm the remaining 2 tablespoons oil in a large paella pan or frying pan over medium heat. Add the fish to the pan, sprinkle with salt, and cook until the bottom half of the fish

continued

sizzles and becomes mostly opaque, 2 to 3 minutes. Turn the fish, sprinkle with more salt, and cook just until the fish becomes mostly opaque, 1 to 2 minutes longer. Remove the fish to a plate and set aside.

Squid bodies: This is the only seafood that I cook in the paella. Slice the bodies into ½-inch rings. During the last 3 minutes of cooking the paella, tuck the squid rings across the dish.

5. At the 25-minute mark, taste the rice to assess its tenderness. If it still has a bite, add the last ½ cup of stock and let it cook for 10 minutes longer. Add in the reserved cooked seafood during the last 5 minutes of cooking and sprinkle ½ teaspoon fine sea salt over the entire dish. Add the squid during the last 3 minutes of cooking. When the rice is plump and lovely, turn the heat off. Let cool for 5 minutes. Sprinkle the fennel fronds, soft herbs, and flaky sea salt over the entire pan before serving.

6. If you plan to make paella cakes for a follow-up meal, make sure to remove any shells (like tails from the shrimp, shells from the mussels) before you pack it away in the fridge. This will make assembly of the cakes far quicker.

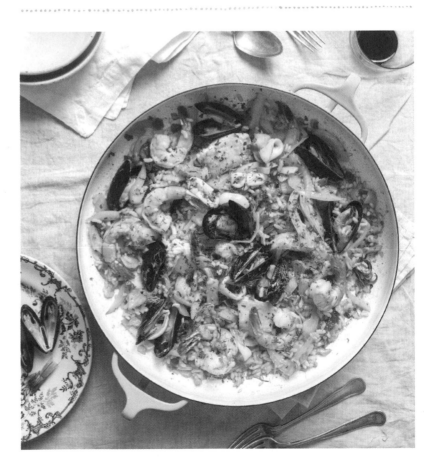

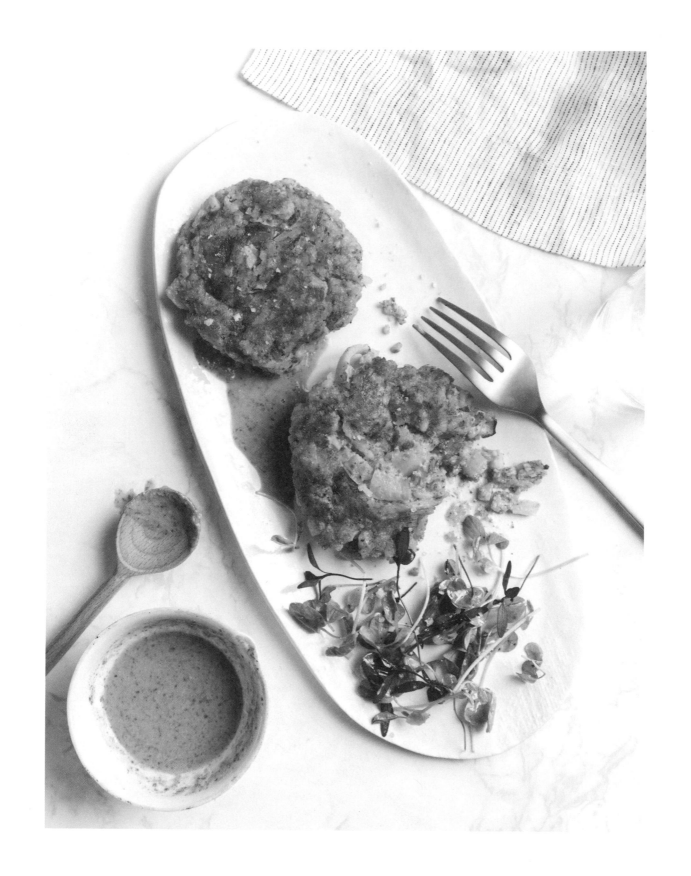

PAELLA CAKES *with Lemony Pesto Dressing*

For a weekend of really appreciable food, make the Smoky Paella with Fennel on Saturday night and these Paella Cakes on Sunday. You'll return to work mode on Monday feeling like you lived your best homespun food weekend ever.

The paella leftovers should be fairly moist, which is why it only needs a little almond flour. If your paella is very dry, add a beaten egg too. Since there's so much rice here, I eat them as they are with a fork and knife. However, if you decide to slide the cake and greens between two slices of toasted bread to become a makeshift burger, I won't judge you one bit.

Makes 4

FREQUENCY: *Once per week*

FOOD PREFERENCES: *DF, GF, RSF*

HANDS-ON TIME: *15 minutes*

TOTAL TIME: *45 minutes*

2 cups leftover Smoky Paella with
    Fennel (page 262) or any
    paella recipe

½ cup (1⅔ oz; 48 g) finely ground
    almond flour

½ teaspoon sea salt, plus more
    for seasoning

12 twists freshly ground black pepper,
    plus more for serving

2 teaspoons extra-virgin olive oil,
    more as needed

3 cups chopped fresh greens,
    such as spinach or arugula

1 tablespoon lemon juice (from about
    ½ medium lemon)

Lemony Pesto Dressing (page 53),
    for serving (optional)

1. Place a piece of parchment paper on a plate.

2. Turn your paella out onto a cutting board. Remove any shells. Dice it up with a large sharp knife until there are no pieces larger than ½ inch. Place the diced paella in a large bowl and add the almond flour, salt, and black pepper. Stir until everything is well incorporated and dispersed throughout the paella. Form the paella into four cakes, about 4 inches in diameter and 1 to 1½-inches tall. Place each on the parchment-lined plate and set the plate in the fridge for 30 minutes.

3. Heat the oil in a large non-stick frying pan over medium heat. Remove the cakes from the fridge and place two in the pan. Fry for 3 minutes on the first side, pressing down with a spatula to get a uniform fry. Flip the cakes and fry for 3 minutes on the other side. You want both sides to be golden brown and the cake to be warmed all the way through. Add another teaspoon of oil to the pan, as needed, and fry the remaining two cakes in the same way.

4. Toss the fresh greens with lemon juice, a sprinkle of salt, and pepper. Serve the cakes with the fresh greens and a spoonful of the dressing, if desired, or a little tartar sauce.

SIMPLE VEG BRAISE *with Polenta*

This is my satisfying stand-in for a cassoulet or any long-braised meat when I'm all vegetables, all the time. It's tasty, comforting, and has enough richness to satiate cooler weather cravings. The polenta makes it a complete, nourishing meal. If you'd rather bake than make a pot of polenta, this recipe goes brilliantly with the Shallot Thyme Soda Bread (page 193). It would also pair well with rice, or scoop it into a warm pita (just prepare to get a little messy).

I want to share a few side notes on this braise. Use vegetable stock (instead of water) if you want a richer dish. Any other stock will work fine, too, up to you. Increase the amount of chipotle in adobo sauce if you like your stew-like meals very spicy. While the mirepoix (onion, carrots, celery) should stay as is, feel free to swap in any veg you like for the potatoes, cabbage, and mushrooms. I quite like to use yams and any other sturdy wild mushrooms.

Serves 4

FREQUENCY: *Once per week*

FOOD PREFERENCES: *DF, GF, NF, RSF, V*

HANDS-ON TIME: *40 minutes*

TOTAL TIME: *1 hour 40 minutes*

· ·

FOR THE SIMPLE VEG BRAISE

5 tablespoons extra-virgin olive oil, divided

1 medium red onion, peeled and chopped

3 medium carrots, diced

2 large celery stalks, diced

4 garlic cloves, peeled and finely diced

2 bay leaves

1 tablespoon dried oregano

2 teaspoons sauce from a can of chipotle in adobo sauce

½ teaspoon smoked paprika

1½ cups (360 ml) dry red wine

One 15-ounce (425 g) can crushed tomatoes

2 cups (480 ml) vegetable stock or water

MAKE THE SIMPLE VEG BRAISE

1. Preheat the oven to 350°F (177°C).

2. Heat 3 tablespoons of the oil in a large heavy Dutch oven with a cover over medium-high heat. Add the onion, carrots, celery, and garlic, and sauté until all the veg are wilted a bit, about 5 minutes. Add the bay leaves, oregano, adobo sauce, smoked paprika, and wine, and cook until the wine is reduced by about half, 4 to 5 minutes.

3. Add the tomatoes and veg stock, and stir well to combine. Add the potatoes and cabbage as a sort of first layer in the pot. Add the beans and then top with the mushrooms, pressing some of them down into the water, leaving some above the water line. Sprinkle the salt on top and drizzle the remaining 2 tablespoons oil over the mushrooms. Cover and set the entire pot in the oven and braise for 50 minutes, until the veg become soft and the flavors mesh together. This is a good time to make the polenta (recipe follows).

4. After 50 minutes, remove the cover from the pot and cook uncovered for another 10 minutes. Remove from the oven and cool for 10 minutes— it will be very hot. Ladle some of the braise onto of a scoop of polenta, sprinkle with more salt, and serve.

continued

2 large white potatoes, thin skinned, diced into ½-inch cubes

½ large green cabbage, halved and sliced into 2-inch chunks

One 15-ounce (425 g) can cannellini beans, drained and rinsed

8 ounces (227 g) fresh shitake mushrooms, cleaned and sliced

1 tablespoon sea salt

Polenta (recipe follows), for serving

FOR THE POLENTA

5 cups (1.2 L) vegetable stock or water

1 teaspoon sea salt

1 cup medium coarse cornmeal

MAKE THE POLENTA

Set a medium heavy bottom pot with a lid on the stove. Add the veg stock to the pot. Whisk in the salt and cornmeal. Turn the heat to medium-high and bring the pot to a boil, stirring regularly with a rubber spatula or wooden spoon to prevent scorching on the bottom of the pan. Once it boils, lower the heat to low, partially cover the pot, and simmer for 1 hour, stirring frequently to prevent scorching. The cover should help prevent any bubbling from splattering out of the pot. Stir as frequently as you like, I tend to stir every 3 to 5 minutes, but bet on getting a little scorch on the bottom of the pot. The polenta is ready when it's creamy like a super thick soup and when a taste leaves no coarse grains in your mouth.

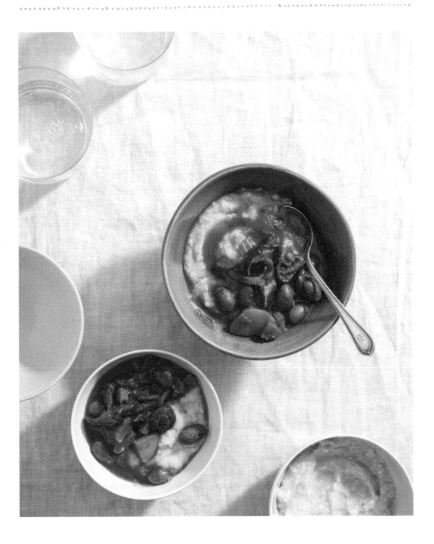

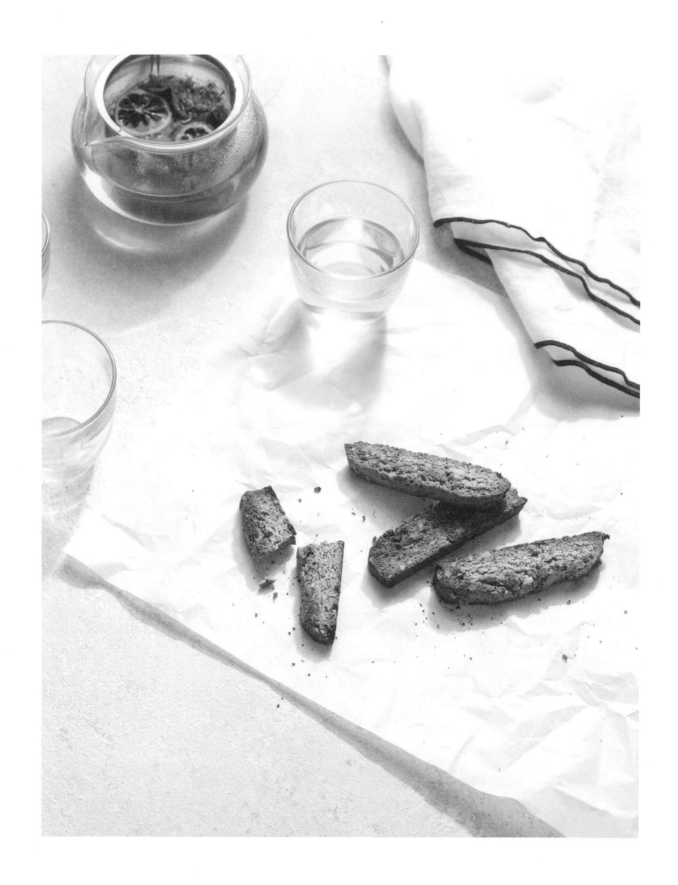

Pecan Poppy Seed BISCOTTI

I first made these biscotti with a dark hazelnut honey, a jar I picked up at a farmers market in northern Italy on a day trip across the border from France. The cookies were stunning. Lighter or colorless honeys just won't offer the desired depth of flavor, so choose the darkest honey you can find like hazelnut, buckwheat, tupelo, or honey from berry blossoms.

I am a purist and prefer simple biscotti. But a handful of dried sour cherries and orange zest would make these biscotti a lovely holiday treat.

Makes 24 cookies

FREQUENCY: *Once per week*

FOOD PREFERENCES: *DF, NF, RSF, Veg*

HANDS-ON TIME: *15 minutes*

TOTAL TIME: *1 hour*

. . . .

1½ cups (5¾ oz; 180 g) all-purpose flour

2 tablespoons poppy seeds

½ cup pecans, coarsely ground

½ teaspoon sea salt

1½ teaspoons baking powder

2 tablespoons coconut oil, melted and cooled

½ cup (2¾ oz; 80 g) lightly packed maple sugar

2 tablespoons dark honey

1 egg

1 teaspoon vanilla or hazelnut extract

1. Preheat the oven to 350° F (177°C). Line a baking sheet with parchment paper.

2. Whisk the flour, poppy seeds, pecans, salt, and baking powder together in a large bowl. Set aside.

3. Put the coconut oil, sugar, honey, egg, and vanilla together in a separate bowl and stir until creamy and well combined.

4. Pour the wet mixture into the dry ingredients. Mix with a wooden spoon or rubber spatula until just combined and no flour streaks remain. As the mixture gets more dough-like, you may need to use your hands to bring it together.

5. Shape the dough into a long, flat oval no more than 1-inch (2.5 cm) high on the lined baking sheet. Bake for 20 minutes, until golden brown.

6. Remove from the oven and let cool for 15 minutes. Slice the cookie loaf into ½-inch (1.25 cm) slices and return to the same baking sheet, placing each biscotti on its side. Bake, flipping once, for 10 to 12 minutes longer, or until each biscotti is golden. Remove from the oven to a cooling rack to cool before eating.

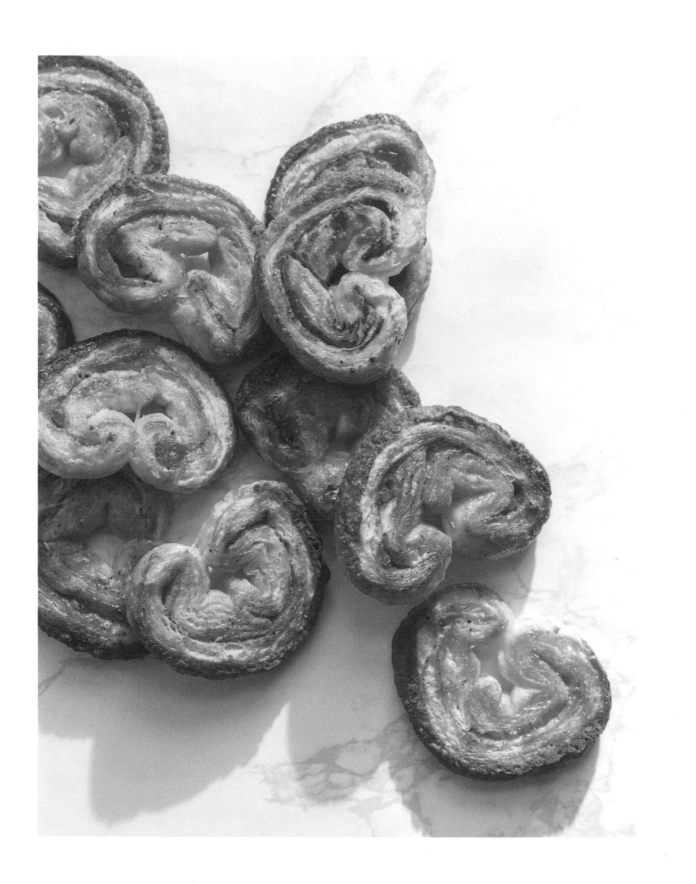

Masala-Spice PALMIERS

Place your puff pastry in the fridge to defrost overnight the moment the thought to make these cookies crosses your mind. Once it defrosts, you're so very close to Masala-spice bliss.

I often keep ground Masala spice mix—a blend of cinnamon, clove, cardamom, coriander, black pepper and fennel—on hand for these cookies or as a topping for a bowl of My Special Oatmeal (page 119). Add the sugar and salt to the spice mix for making these cookies. Roll out the dough and sprinkle, sprinkle, sprinkle. Don't forget the finely diced candied ginger—it's a nice surprise and bite in the final palmier.

After you've made all the correct folds, position your log in front of you and slice your cookies to life. Be careful to keep all the loose spices in between the thin layers. Bake them for a few minutes on one side and then flip—the flipping ensures that both sides caramelize nicely.

Makes 24 cookies

FREQUENCY: *Only on a special occasion*

FOOD PREFERENCES: *NF, Veg*

HANDS-ON TIME: *25 minutes*

TOTAL TIME: *40 minutes*

. . . .

1 teaspoon ground cinnamon

¼ teaspoon ground cloves

¼ teaspoon ground cardamom

¼ teaspoon ground coriander

¼ teaspoon freshly ground
    black pepper

¼ teaspoon ground fennel

½ cup (2¾ oz; 80 g) lightly packed
    maple sugar

½ teaspoon sea salt

One 14-ounce (397 g) puff pastry sheet,
    defrosted (I prefer Dufour)

2 tablespoons finely diced candied
    ginger

1 egg, beaten

1. Preheat the oven to 425°F (218°C) with the rack in the center position. Line two baking sheets with parchment paper.

2. Make the masala spice mix by whisking together the cinnamon, cloves, cardamom, coriander, black pepper, fennel, ¼ cup of the sugar, and the salt in a small bowl. Set aside.

3. On a clean work surface, sprinkle the remaining ¼ cup sugar and open your pastry out on top of the sugar. Sprinkle the masala mix all over the top of the pastry. Roll the dough out a little larger to be about 15 or 16 inches x 13 inches (41 x 33 cm). Sprinkle the candied ginger all over the top of the pastry.

4. Fold both long sides of the pastry into the middle of the dough, making sure the edges touch each other. Fold both long sides up and into the center again, getting the edges to touch each other. Brush off any excess sugar on the exposed side, the top side, of the pastry. (This will help the egg adhere to the dough.) Using a pastry brush, brush the egg on one of the long sides. Now, take the other long side and fold it up and over to cover the long side with the beaten egg. Tap the top of the dough lightly to nudge the dough and help it stick together.

5. Slice the dough into ⅜- or ½-inch (1 or 2.5 cm) slices and place them cut side up on the lined baking sheet 2 to 3 inches apart. Fit 12 cookies per baking sheet.

6. Place a single sheet in the oven (and the other sheet in the fridge for now) and bake the cookies for 6 to 7 minutes, until caramelized and cooked through. Carefully flip each cookie and bake again for 3 to 4 minutes, until caramelized on the other side. Repeat for the second baking sheet. Move to a cooling rack and cool completely before serving.

APPLE PEAR SAUCE *with Sweet Whipped Cream*

This is a nuanced take on classic applesauce, balanced with pears and made a touch more savory with rosemary. It's no-nonsense, in that you can keep it chunky or blend it until smooth. Make the sweet cream in advance, so the flavors and texture have some time to set up in the fridge.

Makes about 4 cups

FREQUENCY: *Once a season*

FOOD PREFERENCES: *DF, GF, RSF, V*

HANDS-ON TIME: *10 minutes*

TOTAL TIME: *40 minutes*

....

1 cup (240 ml) water

3 pounds (1.3 kg) apples, peeled, cored, and cut into large chunks

1 pound (454 g) pears, peeled, cored, and cut into large chunks

3 tablespoons lemon juice (from about 1½ medium lemons)

3 tablespoons maple sugar

One rosemary sprig

¼ teaspoon sea salt

Sweet Whipped Cream (page 62), to serve

1. Combine the water, apples, pears, lemon juice, sugar, rosemary, and salt in a large pot. Stir to coat the fruit with the ingredients and bring to a boil. Decrease the heat to low, cover the pot, and simmer until all the fruit is tender and falling apart, 30 minutes.

2. Remove the rosemary sprig and examine the mixture. Some fruit pieces will be totally mashed up and others may still be large but very soft. You may opt to cool the sauce and serve it just as it is, which is what I often do. Alternatively, you can pass it through a food mill or a powerful blender to get a fine and evenly smooth texture. Either way, make sure to cool the mixture before blending or serving.

3. Spoon ½ cup servings into bowls or dessert glasses and drizzle with whipped cream to serve.

Banoffee Pie PUDDING

Even before I visited Ireland, I knew about banoffee pie. It's a very sweet dessert served across the United Kingdom, though my husband's family will say it's Irish through and through. The original pie has only a few components: a graham cracker crust, a loose toffee filling, sliced bananas, and whipped cream. Some versions are garnished with light chocolate shavings. A slice is most definitely the stuff of sugary dreams and I typically make it once annually for my husband's birthday in the late spring.

Shifting toward a new way to food does not exclude enjoying your favorite treats. In fact, it's critical to make room for those dishes that cue certain food memories that make you feel all warm inside, that remind you that life is for living and not restriction. With that in mind, it was important to me to keep banoffee pie in my life; only I turned it into more of a small pudding that offers the same sweet kick without the dairy. It's still pretty high in sugar but it's also a once-a-year thing that makes me very happy and bonds me to my husband's history.

The work here is really in tending to a boiling pot of water for three hours; I do this while doing other kitchen projects. You can find cans of sweetened condensed coconut milk in the baking aisles of more progressive supermarkets or online. You can also find a few cans in my pantry for banoffee pie pudding emergencies—that's a thing.

Makes four 4-ounce (113 g) puddings

FREQUENCY: *Once per year, really*

FOOD PREFERENCES: *DF, V*

HANDS-ON TIME: *20 minutes*

TOTAL TIME: *11 hours 20 minutes*

One 11¼ ounce (320 g) can sweetened condensed coconut milk (dairy-free) or traditional condensed milk

1½ cups raw cashews

¾ cup (180 ml) filtered water

4 tablespoons coconut cream (or the solid part from a cold can of coconut milk)

2 tablespoons maple syrup

Pinch of sea salt

18 large whole grain graham crackers

2 medium ripe bananas

1. Fill a large handled pot with water and slide the can of sweetened condensed coconut milk (on its side) into the water until it's fully submerged. If your can of milk has a paper label on it, remove it first. Bring to a boil and boil for 3 hours over medium heat, always topping off the pot with additional water to make sure the can stays fully submerged at all times (under at least 1 inch of water). This process will turn the milk to something like toffee. Let the can cool completely, which could take as long as 4 hours, before opening.

2. To make the sweet cream, add the cashews, filtered water, coconut cream, maple syrup, and salt to a blender and whiz until thick and creamy. Chill for 1 to 2 hours. You can store the sweet cream in an airtight container in the fridge and use within 5 days.

3. Put the graham crackers in a sealable plastic bag and hit it with the back of a heavy spoon or rolling pin to turn the crackers to crumbs. Set aside.

4. When you're ready to make the puddings, pull out four glasses or small jars that hold at least 4 ounces each. Slice the bananas into thin coins.

continued

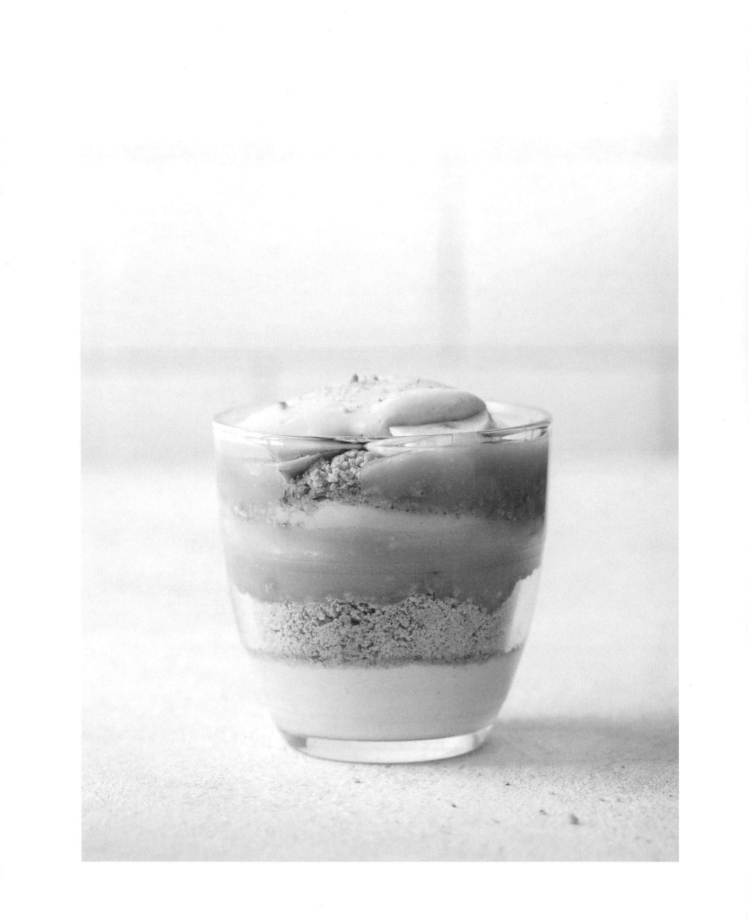

5. Form layers with all the ingredients: Place 2 tablespoons of sweet cream in the bottom of each glass. Add 3 tablespoons of graham cracker crumbs. Add 2 tablespoons of coconut toffee. Add four or five slices of banana. Repeat the layers until you reach the top of each glass, ending with extra sweet cream and a final sprinkle of graham cracker crumbs. Reserve any extra banana for a snack.

6. Seal the jars with plastic wrap or their lids and place in the fridge for at least 2 hours or up to overnight. Serve with a spoon for digging up every last bit.

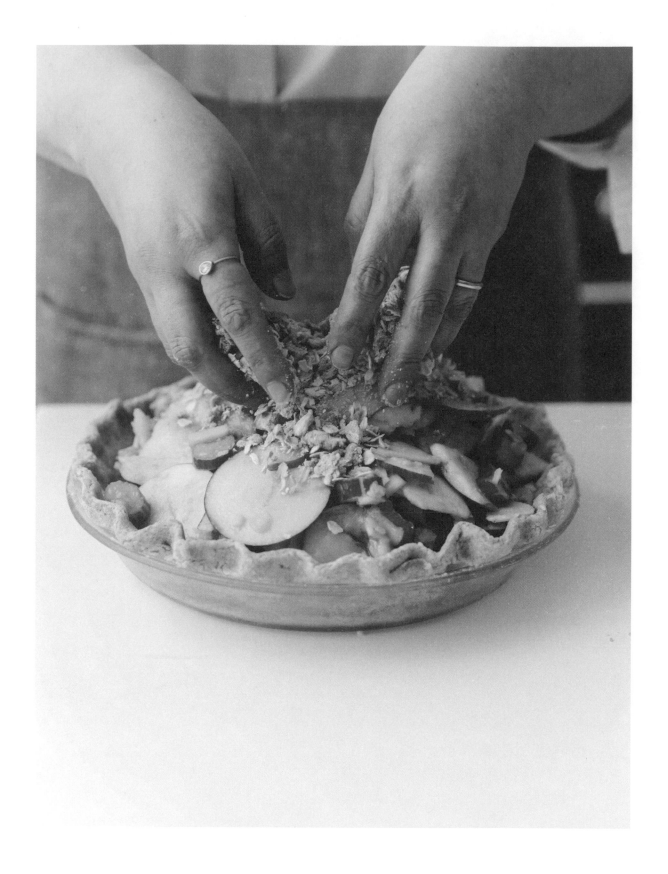

Rye Apple Rhubarb CRISP PIE

Apple pie is a wondrous thing; each bite ushers in fall. Instead of just apples, I like to add a bunch of rhubarb to the pie. Between the sweet apples and the rhubarb (probably coming from a frozen batch in your freezer during the fall), the pie enters an entirely new dimension and tastes heavenly.

To make a vegan rye pie dough, just replace the spelt flour in the Pie Dough recipe on page 58 with an equal amount of rye flour.

Makes one 9-inch (23 cm) pie

FREQUENCY: *Once a season*

FOOD PREFERENCES: *DF, RSF, V*

HANDS-ON TIME: *20 minutes*

TOTAL TIME: *1 hour 15 minutes*

. . . .

1 batch Pie Dough (page 58) or
 1 store-bought vegan pie crust
 in 9-inch (23 cm) foil shell
 (see headnote)

6 apples, peeled (if you prefer) and
 thinly sliced

2 long stalks rhubarb, fresh or frozen,
 thinly sliced

¼ cup plus 2 tablespoons (1⅜ oz; 40 g)
 lightly packed maple sugar, divided

¼ teaspoon sea salt, divided

2 tablespoons all-purpose flour

1 tablespoon lemon juice (from about
 ½ medium lemon)

1 cup old-fashioned oats

½ cup (1⅔ oz; 48 g) finely ground
 almond flour

⅛ teaspoon cinnamon

3 tablespoons coconut oil, solid form

1 tablespoon extra-virgin olive oil

1. Preheat the oven to 350°F (177°C).

2. Place the dough in a 9-inch pie plate or foil shell. Make sure that the dough fits snugly into all the corners of the plate. Trim off extra dough and crimp the edge as you prefer to create a design and hold the crisp topping in place. Set it in the fridge while you prepare the fruit and crisp. (If you are using a store-bought pie crust, set it in the fridge now.)

3. Add the apples, rhubarb, ¼ cup of the sugar, ⅛ teaspoon of the salt, the all-purpose flour, and lemon juice to a large bowl. Toss to coat evenly. Set aside.

4. Toss together the oats, almond flour, cinnamon, the remaining ⅛ teaspoon salt, and the remaining 2 tablespoons maple sugar in a medium bowl until well combined. Divide the coconut oil into teaspoon portions (9 total) and add it in 1 teaspoon at a time. With your clean hands, blend everything together until the mixture binds together a bit and looks like coarse breadcrumbs.

5. Remove your pie dough from the fridge. Pile in the fruit mixture, allowing any extra fruit to hump up in the center of the pie. Place your crisp mixture on top of the fruit, covering as much of it as you can, and allowing any extra crisp mixture to hump up in the center of the pie. Drizzle the olive oil across the top of the pie.

6. Place your pie on a rimmed baking sheet. Bake for 45 to 60 minutes, until the oats and pie crust are almost golden brown and any fruit that shows through is bubbling. Allow the pie to cool 20 minutes before serving or place in your fridge to cool completely.

Sweet Potato PIE

A favorite dessert, this Sweet Potato Pie is everything. My version is dairy-free and has a vegan pie crust. I like to make the pie filling well in advance. If you let it sit for an hour or even overnight in the fridge, the flavor deepens, becoming more like its sum and less like all the individual parts. If opening both a can and box of coconut milk is cumbersome, go with 100 percent canned coconut milk because it's a lot creamier. If you'd like to make the entire pie vegan, swap in three flaxseed eggs. As most people will tell you, canned sweet potato is just fine and works to make this recipe super fast but roasted or steamed sweet potato, mashed in your own kitchen, is way better.

Makes one 9-inch (23 cm) pie

FREQUENCY: *Once a season*

FOOD PREFERENCES: *DF, RSF, Veg*

HANDS-ON TIME: *20 minutes*

TOTAL TIME: *17 hours 5 minutes*

. . . .

1 batch Pie Dough, (page 58) or store-bought vegan pie crust in 9-inch (23 cm) foil shell

½ cup (2¾ oz; 80 g) lightly packed maple sugar

2 tablespoons all-purpose flour

½ teaspoon fine sea salt

1 teaspoon ground ginger

1 teaspoon ground cinnamon

3 eggs, beaten

2 medium sweet potatoes, cooked and mashed, or one 15-ounce (425 g) can sweet potato

½ cup (120 ml) unsweetened coconut milk from a can (stir the milk before measuring)

½ cup (120 ml) unsweetened coconut milk from a box (shake the box before measuring)

¼ cup (3 oz; 85 g) wildflower honey

1 teaspoon vanilla extract

1. Preheat the oven to 400°F (204°C).

2. Place the dough in a 9-inch pie plate or foil shell. Make sure that the dough fits snuggly into all the corners of the plate. Trim off extra dough and crimp the edge to your preferred design. Set it in the fridge while you prepare the pie filling. (If you are using a store-bought pie crust, set it in the fridge now.)

3. Whisk the maple sugar, flour, salt, ginger, and cinnamon together in a large bowl until everything is well dispersed. Break up any maple sugar clumps that appear. Set aside.

4. Whisk the eggs, sweet potato, canned milk, boxed milk, honey, and vanilla together in a medium bowl until well blended. Add the dry ingredients to the wet ingredients and whisk until well incorporated, a touch darker in color, and luscious. If you're not making your pie immediately, chill the filling for an hour or up to overnight to improve the flavor.

5. Remove your unbaked pie shell from the fridge. Place on a rimmed baking sheet. Pour the sweet potato filling into the unbaked pie shell. Bake for 45 minutes until the filling is set everywhere but the center 6 inches of the pie; that part should still be a bit wobbly. Allow the pie to cool, ideally on a rack, for at least 4 hours before serving—it will continue to cook outside the oven and that wobbly bit will get more solid. Serve or place in your fridge once cooled until ready to serve. The pie will still taste great up to 3 days if stored in the fridge covered with plastic wrap.

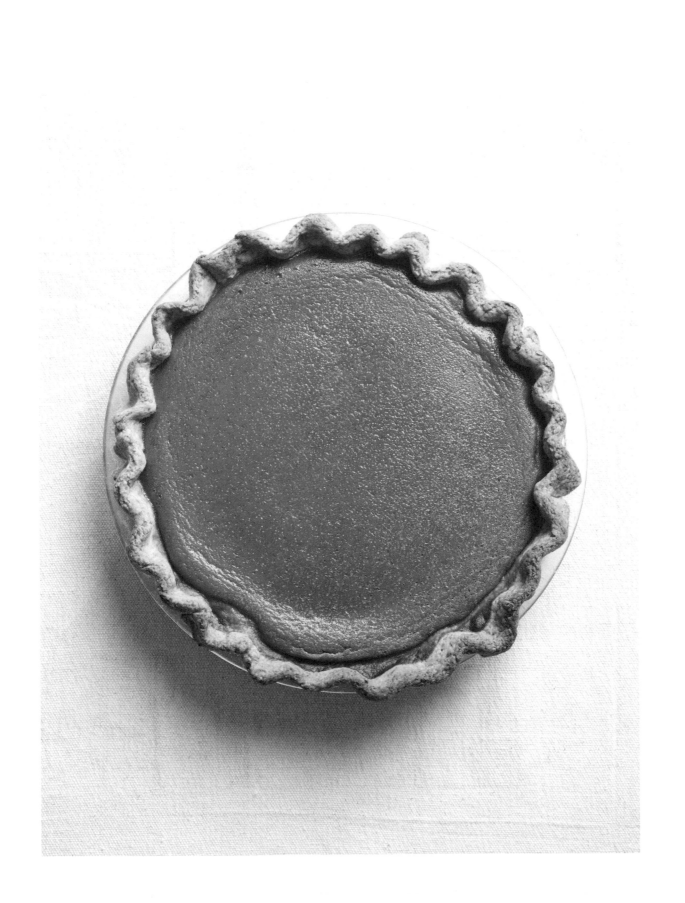

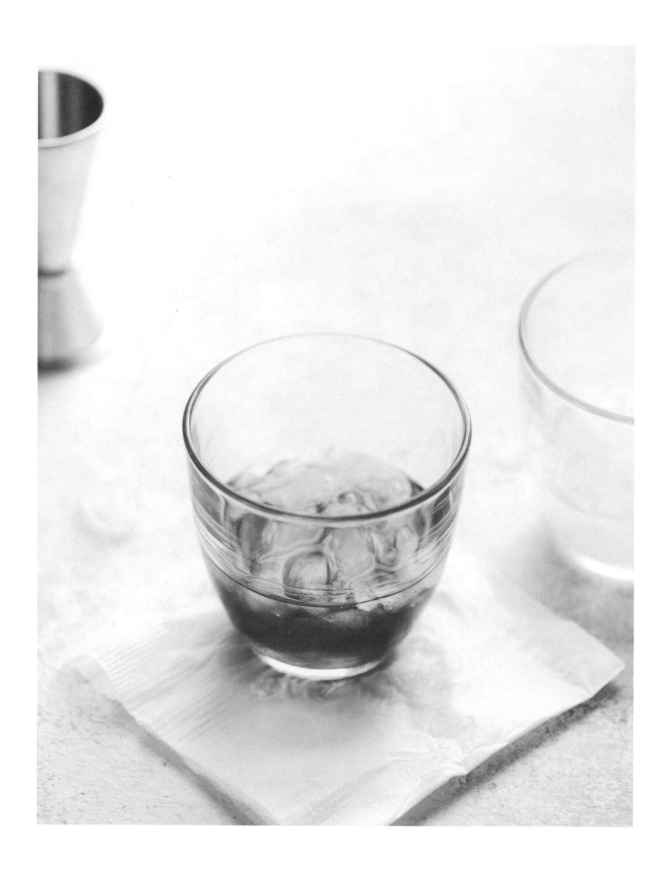

Acknowledgments

Thank you, Don. You're my top recipe taster and my heart.

Thank you and lots of hugs to Kate Knapp, for supporting me at every step in the process (in this book and in life), testing every recipe, and leading the best recipe testers: Cole Avenia-Fritzky, Catherine Braun, Connie Campbell, Shelby Dwyer, Leslie Goldenberg, Jessica Grosman, Catrine Kelty, Courtney Knapp, Mariah Lewis-Elliott, Rebecca Lord, Tracey Neret, Patricia Peck, Penelope Roberts, Lisa Smith, Deanna Welborn, Rachel Wilson, and Tiffany Zhou.

Big thanks to the village who made this cookbook: my editor, Jennifer Urban-Brown, who is patient and passionate; the entire team at Roost Books who brought this cookbook to life; my agent, Alison Fargis; ever-resourceful photographer Kristin Teig who makes a magical image (and her sweet dog, Olga); photographer and baker, Joseph Ferraro; stylist Heidi Robb who moved (and drove through) many mountains to make these images; Dana Sobota of Gris Studio for sharing so many gorgeous ceramics props; Billy Ritter for his lovely handmade ceramics; proposal designer Laura Palese; and all the friends who helped during the photo shoot, you know who you are.

Thank you, Sherrie, for being on my side and supporting me along this path. Never-ending appreciation to the yogis, therapist, acupuncturist, doctors, wellness experts, and dear friends who inspire me every single day.

Thank you, Universal Standard, for sharing some of the clothes I wear in these pages and in life.

Thank you to my cousin, Vanessa, whose wellness influence will stay with me long beyond her too-short life, and to her entire family—my family—for such fond memories of Chestnut Street.

Sending so much love and gratitude to my sister, Jennifer, who eats everything I make, takes all my veggie leftovers, and reminds me that our mother would celebrate every moment.

Thank you to my mother and my father. You're both gone now but I know you worked so hard to give me everything, including so many opportunities and a solid education. You both did your very best and I will always remember the good times, promise.

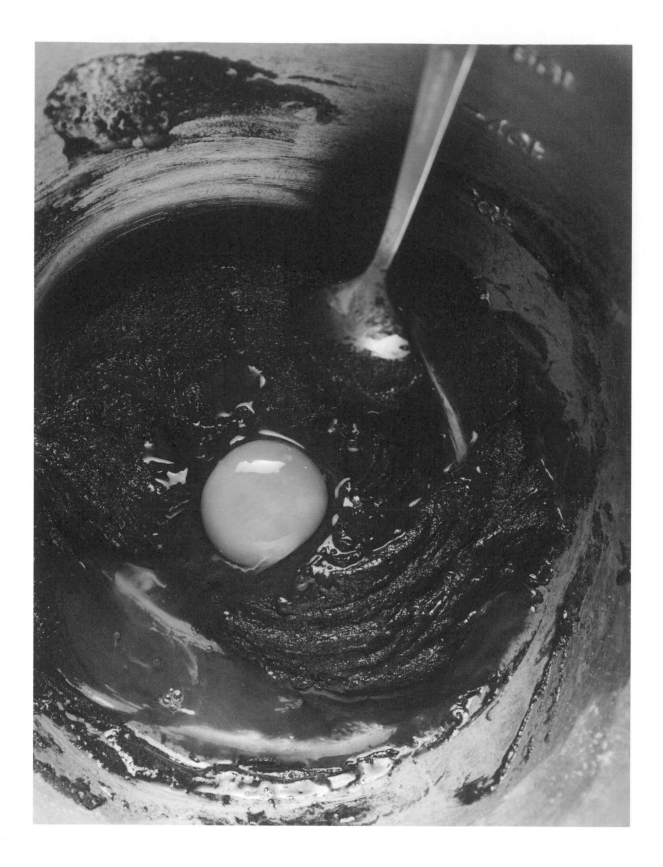

Resources

BOOKS

*10% Happier: How I Tamed the Voice in My Head,
Reduced Stress without Losing My Edge, and Found
Self-Help That Actually Works—A True Story*
by Dan Harris

*A Modern Way to Eat: Over 200 Satisfying, Everyday
Vegetarian Recipes (That Will Make You Feel Amazing)*
by Anna Jones

*Blood, Bones and Butter: The Inadvertent Education
of a Reluctant Chef*
by Gabrielle Hamilton

*Braving the Wilderness: The Quest for True Belonging
and the Courage to Stand Alone*
by Brené Brown

*Chickpea Flour Does It All: Gluten-Free, Dairy-Free,
Vegetarian Recipes for Every Taste and Season*
by Lindsey S. Love

Codependent No More
by Melody Beattie

*The Four Agreements: A Practical Guide to
Personal Freedom*
by Don Miguel Ruiz

Home Cooking: A Writer in the Kitchen
by Laurie Colwin

How to Cook Everything Vegetarian
by Mark Bittman

*How to Love; How to Eat; How to Walk; How to Sit;
How to Fight; How to Relax; No Mud, No Lotus;
The Art of Transforming Suffering*
—all by Thich Nhat Hanh

My Kitchen in Rome: Recipes and Notes on Italian Cooking
by Rachel Roddy

My New Roots: Inspired Plant-Based Recipes for Every Season
by Sarah Britton

*The Secret Life of Fat: The Science Behind the Body's Least
Understood Organ and What It Means for You*
by Sylvia Tara, PhD

*VB6: Eat Vegan Before 6:00 to Lose Weight and Restore
Your Health . . . for Good*
by Mark Bittman

The Vegan Pantry: The Art of Making Your Own Staples
by Miyoko Schinner

Whole Larder Love: Grow Gather Hunt Cook
by Rohan Anderson

WEBSITES

10% Happier (meditation)
10percenthappier.com
By Dan Harris

101 Cookbooks (recipe site)
101cookbooks.com
By Heidi Swanson

Call Your Girlfriend (podcast)
callyourgirlfriend.com
By Aminatou Sow and Ann Friedman

The First Mess (recipe site)
thefirstmess.com
By Laura Wright

The Goop Podcast (life inspiration)
goop.com/thepodcast
By Gwyneth Paltrow

Green Kitchen Stories (recipe site)
greenkitchenstories.com
By David Frenkiel and Luise Vindahl

Headspace (meditation)
headspace.com

Marie Forleo (business inspiration)
marieforleo.com
By Marie Forleo

Minimalist Baker (recipe site)
minimalistbaker.com
By Dana Shultz

Rich Roll (podcast)
richroll.com
By Rich Roll

Seeking Wisdom (business inspiration)
seekingwisdom.io
By David Cancel

She's All Fat (podcast)
shesallfat.com
By April K. Quioh and Sophia Carter-Kahn

Universal Standard (inclusive fashion)
universalstandard.com

With Food and Love (recipe site)
withfoodandlove.com
By Sherri Castellano

Yoga with Adriene (yoga videos)
yogawithadriene.com
By Adriene Mishler

INGREDIENTS

A&A Maple: maple sugar
aamaple.com

Abracadabra Coffee Co: coffee beans
abracadabracoffeeco.com

American Miso Company: organic American-made miso
great-eastern-sun.com

Apotheker's Bee Sweetened Goods: honey-sweetened
chocolate and confections
apothekerskitchen.com

Arrowhead Mills: organic and gluten-free flours
arrowheadmills.com

Beyond Meat: plant-based, soy-free protein crumbles
beyondmeat.com

Bob's Red Mill: oats, gluten-free grains, and whole grain flours
bobsredmill.com

Bragg: organic apple cider vinegar
bragg.com

Cento Tuna: wild caught, dolphin-safe tuna in olive oil
cento.com

Daiya Foods: dairy-free cheese shreds
daiyafoods.com

Garofalo: organic pasta
pastagarofalo.it

Jacobsen Salt Company: hand-harvested American sea salt
jacobsensalt.com

Jovial Foods: whole grain and gluten-free pasta
jovialfoods.com

King Arthur Flour: flours and baking supplies
kingarthurflour.com

Kite Hill: dairy-free cheese and yogurt
kite-hill.com

Lotus Foods: black and brown rice and rice noodles
lotusfoods.com

Maldon: flaky sea salt
maldonsalt.co.uk

Melt Organic: dairy-free, vegan butter spread
meltorganic.com

Miyoko's Kitchen: dairy-free smoked mozzarella and other dairy-free cheeses
miyokoskitchen.com

Mountain Rose Herbs: organic bulk herbs
mountainroseherbs.com

Mycoterra Farm: fresh mushrooms
mycoterrafarm.com

Nature's Bounty: probiotics and vitamins
naturesbounty.com

New England Tortilla: masa corn tortilla chips
mininatortilla.com

Nova Maple: maple sugar
novamaple.com

Nutiva: organic coconut oil
nutiva.com

Organic Valley: non-GMO ghee clarified butter
organicvalley.coop

Rancho Gordo: heirloom beans
ranchogordo.com

Ritual Chocolate: small-batch fine chocolate
ritualchocolate.com

Simply Organic: organic spices
simplyorganic.com

Smoke Show Sauce: maple-sweetened jalapeño hot sauce
smokeshowsauce.com

Terra Soul: organic pink sea salt, raw cacao powder, and other superfoods
terrasoul.com

Traditional Medicinals: organic herbal teas
traditionalmedicinals.com

Urban Moonshine: digestive bitters
urbanmoonshine.com

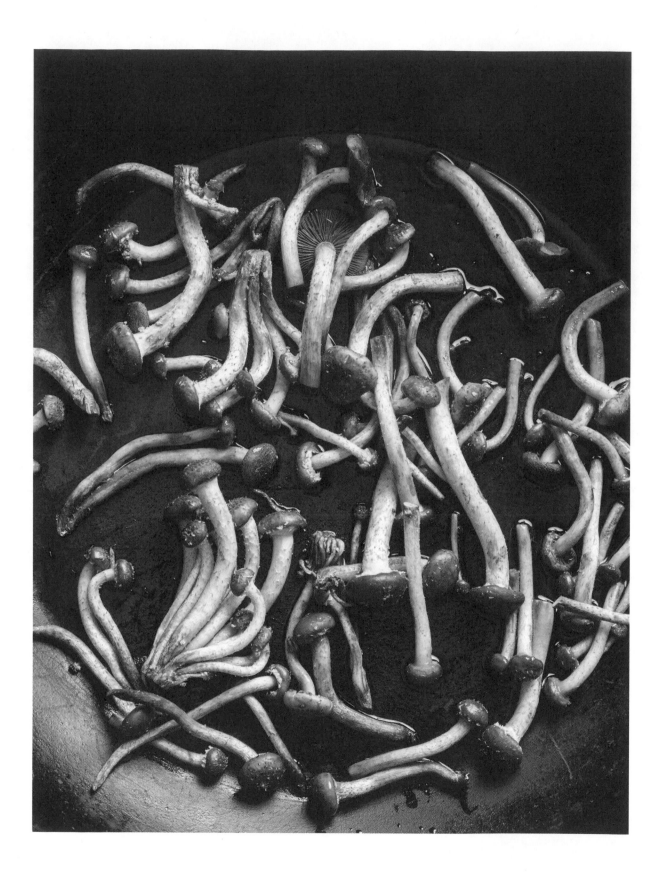

Valgosa: smoked Spanish paprika
valgosa.com

Vivido Natural: dried wild mushrooms
vividonatural.com

Wilderness Family Naturals: Wildly Organic
coconut vinegar
wildernessfamilynaturals.com

Oxo: cooking tools
oxo.com

Sarah Kersten: ceramics
sarahkersten.com

Vitamix: powerful blenders
vitamix.com

EQUIPMENT

Benriner: Japanese mandolines
benriner.com

Bialetti: Italian stovetop coffee maker
bialetti.com

Billy Ritter 77: ceramics
billyritter77.com

Cuisinart: food processors
cuisinart.com

Duralex: glassware
duralexusa.com

Hario: glass teapot
hario.jp

Kitchen Aid: mixers
kitchenaid.com

Le Parfait: French jars and terrines
leparfait.com

Luvhaus Ceramics: tumblers
luvhaus.com

Microplane: zesters
microplane.com

Recipes by Category

Index

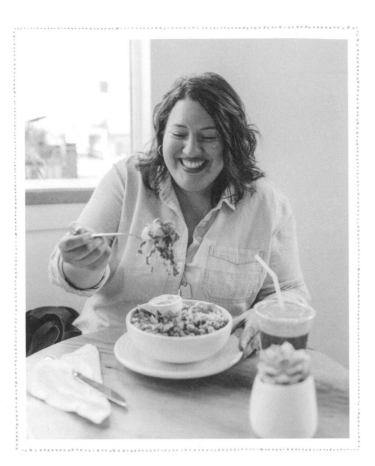

About the Author

Maggie Battista is a cookbook author, writer, creative business coach, and shop maker known for her wholehearted and empowering voice. In 2007, she founded Eat Boutique, an award-winning online food shop and story-driven recipe site. After hosting and creating pop-up food markets for 25,000 guests, she's currently working to open her first permanent Eat Boutique, a food retail concept space that provides a new way to shop for the very best food. She also shares her vast real life experience with other women in food by offering creative business coaching with heart.

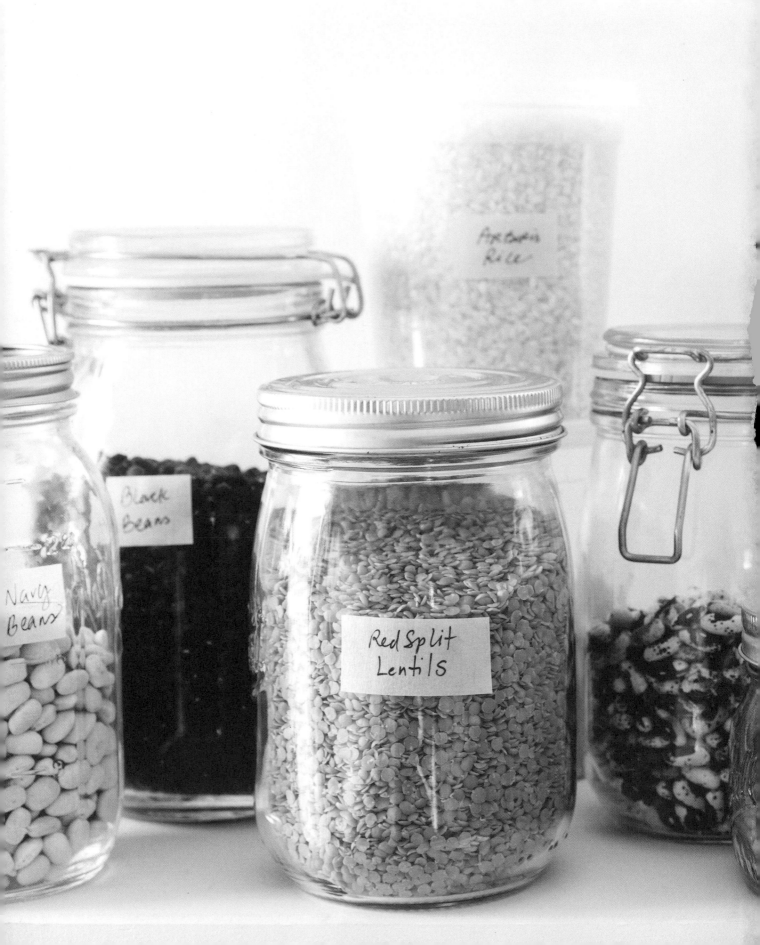